Dietary Supplements

Dietary Supplements

Fact versus Fiction

Myrna Chandler Goldstein and
Mark A. Goldstein, MD

BLOOMSBURY ACADEMIC
NEW YORK · LONDON · OXFORD · NEW DELHI · SYDNEY

BLOOMSBURY ACADEMIC
Bloomsbury Publishing Inc
1385 Broadway, New York, NY 10018, USA
50 Bedford Square, London, WC1B 3DP, UK
29 Earlsfort Terrace, Dublin 2, Ireland

BLOOMSBURY, BLOOMSBURY ACADEMIC and the Diana logo
are trademarks of Bloomsbury Publishing Plc

First published in the United States of America by ABC-CLIO 2020
Paperback edition published by Bloomsbury Academic 2024

Library of Congress Cataloging-in-Publication Data
Names: Goldstein, Myrna Chandler, 1948-author. | Goldstein, Mark A. (Mark Allan), 1947-author.
Title: Dietary supplements: fact versus fiction / Myrna Chandler Goldstein
and Mark A. Goldstein, MD.
Description: First edition. | Santa Barbara, California: Greenwood, an imprint
of ABC-CLIO, LLC [2020] | Includes bibliographical references and index.
Identifiers: LCCN 2019054808 (print) | LCCN 2019054809 (ebook) |
ISBN 9781440864223 (hardcover) | ISBN 9781440864230 (ebook)
Subjects: LCSH: Dietary supplements.
Classification: LCC RM258.5 G66 2020 (print) |
LCC RM258.5 (ebook) | DDC 613.2-dc23
LC record available at https://lccn.loc.gov/2019054808
LC ebook record available at https://lccn.loc.gov/2019054809

ISBN: HB: 978-1-4408-6422-3
PB: 979-8-7651-2688-2
ePDF: 978-1-4408-6423-0
eBook: 979-8-2160-7443-4

To find out more about our authors and books visit www.bloomsbury.com
and sign up for our newsletters.

This book discusses treatments (including types of medications and mental health therapies),
diagnostic tests for various symptoms and mental health disorders, and organizations. The authors have
made every effort to present accurate and up-to-date information. However, the information in this book
is not intended to recommend or endorse particular treatments or organizations, or substitute for the care
or medical advice of a qualified health professional, or used to alter any medical therapy without a medical
doctor's advice. Specific situations may require specific therapeutic approaches not included in this book.
For those reasons, we recommend that readers follow the advice of qualified healthcare professionals directly
involved in their care. Readers who suspect they may have specific medical problems should consult a
physician about any suggestions made in this book.

We dedicate this book with love to our five grandchildren:

Aidan Zev Goldstein, born February 8, 2008
Payton Maeve Goldstein, born December 4, 2009
Milo Adlai Kamras, born August 9, 2011
Erin Abigail Goldstein, born December 29, 2011
Zoe "Scout" Eames Kamras, born February 16, 2014

Contents

Introduction

According to the Dietary Supplement Health and Education Act (DSHEA) passed by Congress in 1994, a dietary supplement is a product that is intended to supplement the diet. Because they are not medications, they are not designed to treat, diagnose, mitigate, prevent, or cure illnesses. In the United States, the dietary supplement industry is a huge, multibillion-dollar, ever-growing market. According to estimates, at present, Americans spend more than $40 billion a year on supplements.

Dietary supplements contain one or more dietary ingredients including vitamins, minerals, herbs and other botanicals, amino acids, enzymes, and other substances. While they come in a variety of forms, such as pills, capsules, tablets, energy bars, and liquids, dietary supplements are generally taken by mouth. Somewhere on the front label should be the words "dietary supplement." The label should also contain a Supplement Facts panel listing the contents, amount of active ingredients per serving, and other added ingredients—fillers, binders, and flavorings—as well as the suggested serving size.

TYPES OF SUPPLEMENTS

In the United States, there are four main categories of supplements. People who use dietary supplements most often take vitamins and minerals, such as multivitamins, vitamin D, calcium, vitamin C, and vitamin B complex. (Vitamins and minerals are addressed in *Vitamins and Minerals: Fact versus Fiction* by the authors of this book.) Then there are the specialty supplements, such as omega-3 fatty acids, fiber products, probiotics, and glucosamine/chondroitin. Herbals and botanicals comprise a third category that includes green tea, garlic, cranberry, Echinacea, and ginseng. The fourth category includes sports nutrition and weight management. These include protein supplements, energy drinks and gels, garcinia cambogia, green coffee, and hydration drinks and gels.

Most people take vitamin supplements to support their health. In fact, many dietary supplements do just that. For example, calcium and vitamin D help keep bones strong. Because most people do not take in sufficient amounts of calcium and vitamin D from their diet, this supplementation is crucial for reducing bone loss. In addition, pregnant women take folic acid to prevent certain defects in babies.

It is important to underscore the fact that dietary supplements are not a substitute for a healthy diet. Eating a healthy diet is optimum. But, dietary supplements may help people obtain adequate amounts of essential nutrients. They may be particularly useful for people who have poor dietary habits, who take several prescription medications, who drink large amounts of alcohol, and who follow a restricted diet. Furthermore, dietary supplements may be useful for people suffering from certain medical conditions. (This book includes an appendix that lists supplements that may be useful for certain medical problems and conditions.) Dietary supplements do not replace medications prescribed by a healthcare provider.

SUPPLEMENT SAFETY

Some dietary supplements contain ingredients that may have a strong impact on the body and/or interfere with prescription medications. For example, fish oil is thought to increase the risk of bleeding. As a result, fish oil should not be taken before any type of surgical procedure. Similarly, Coumadin, a blood-thinning medication, should not be combined with vitamin E, which has blood-thinning properties. When someone takes Coumadin with vitamin E, they increase the risk for serious problems, such as internal bleeding and stroke. At the same time, vitamin K can reduce the ability of Coumadin to prevent blood from clotting. Further, St. John's wort may interfere with antidepressants and birth control bills and reduce their effectiveness. The herbs comfrey and kava may harm the liver. Antioxidant vitamins, such as vitamins C and E, may reduce the effectiveness of certain types of chemotherapy. Even dietary supplements marketed as "natural" may or may not be safe. A supplement's safety is a function of a variety of factors, such as chemical makeup, how it functions in the body, how it was made, and the dose. Plant-based supplements may be obtained from plants that were grown in soil with heavy metals or other contaminants. It is at least theoretically possible that the supplements contain these contaminants. Do you know if the manufacturer of your supplements has tested for these contaminants? Probably not. Additionally, researchers have found dietary supplements tainted with pharmaceutical medications. The vast majority of these were marketed for sexual enhancement or weight loss. A smaller percentage was for muscle building. Less than half of these were recalled.

The use of the terms standardized, verified, or certified on the label really has no meaning. Most dietary supplements have not been tested in pregnant women, nursing mothers, and children. Before beginning a supplement regime, it is a good idea to discuss the supplements with a healthcare provider. You should always tell your healthcare provider the dietary supplements you take. You might want to compile a list before an appointment; it may well be a good idea to list dosages. You may want to keep a copy of that list in your own files. And, if you suspect that you have had a serious reaction to a supplement, you should report your suspicions to your healthcare provider. Or, you can contact the FDA directly and complete a report at http://wwwsafetyreporting.hhs.gov. Supply as much information as possible as complete reports are the most helpful.

The FDA offers a long list of serious health-related reactions, also known as adverse effects, that may be associated with dietary supplements. These include

- itching, rash, hives, throat/lip/tongue welling, wheezing
- low blood pressure, fainting, chest pain, shortness of breath, palpitations, irregular heartbeat
- severe, persistent nausea, vomiting, diarrhea, or abdominal pain
- difficulty in urinating, decreased urination
- fatigue, appetite loss, yellowing skin/eyes, itching, dark urine
- severe joint/muscle pain
- slurred speech, one-sided weakness of face, arm, leg, vision
- abnormal bleeding from nose or gums
- blood in urine, stool, vomit, or sputum
- marked mood, cognitive, or behavioral changes, thoughts of suicide
- visit to emergency room or hospitalization

Always avoid dietary supplements that offer exaggerated and unrealistic results, such as weight loss supplements that will cause the pounds to melt away. Truly significant weight loss generally requires dietary modifications and increases in exercise. Do not expect any dietary supplement to trigger miraculous physical or psychological changes. While research has found that dietary supplements may improve a myriad of medical concerns, they are not panaceas. The federal government may take action against companies and websites that make false and deceptive claims about their products or sell products that are unsafe for human consumption. And, the growing popularity of dietary supplements has also seen increased numbers of misleading claims and potentially dangerous products.

Dietary supplements are sold without a prescription in many different retail outlets including grocery stores, warehouse stores, drugstores, many online stores, health food stores, and health and nutrition stores. How does one select a brand of supplements? The Office of Dietary Supplements of the National Institutes of Health does not test, analyze, or rate dietary supplements, and it does not recommend brands. However, it suggests asking healthcare providers for recommendations. If people have specific questions, they may contact the manufacturer. People may ask about any safety and efficacy testing the manufacturer may have completed, or they may want to know about any adverse effects that have been reported.

There are a few independent organizations that test various products. However, they can only assure consumers that the supplement was properly manufactured, that it contains the listed ingredients, and that it does not have harmful levels of contaminants. There is no guarantee of safety and efficacy.

Still, in the United States, dietary supplements are incredibly popular. Most adults take some form of dietary supplements; often they take them every day. A survey commissioned by the nonprofit Council for Responsible Nutrition found that the use of dietary supplements among adults in the United States increased by 10% from 2009 to 2018. In 2009, 65% of the adults took dietary supplements; by 2018, that figure was 75%. Seventy-eight percent of American adults aged 55 years or older take dietary supplements; 77% of those between the ages of 35 and 54 years take them, as do 69% between the ages of 18 and 34 years. Moreover, consumers appear to have confidence in the dietary supplement industry. Eighty-seven percent of adults have confidence in the "safety, quality, and effectiveness" of their dietary supplements, up from 84% in 2009. In addition, the 2018 survey found that 78% of Americans think the dietary supplement industry is "trustworthy." While the vitamins and minerals dietary supplement category remains the most popular, the use of herbals and botanicals is impressive. Forty-one percent of people who use supplements reported that they had taken herbals or botanicals during the previous 12 months. One such herb, turmeric, was not even on an earlier survey, and is now widely used.

Acknowledgments

Once again, we would like to thank our editor Maxine Taylor, who has edited several of our more recent books. Over the years that we have worked together, Maxine has repeatedly offered excellent suggestions and advice. She is one of the primary reasons that we continue to write books for ABC-CLIO.

REFERENCES AND FURTHER READING

Council for Responsible Nutrition. www.crnusa.org.
National Center for Complementary and Integrative Health. https://nccih.nih.gov.
Office of Dietary Supplements, National Institutes of Health. https://ods.od.nih.gov.

Regulation and Labeling of Dietary Supplements

It is commonly known that the U.S. Food & Drug Administration (FDA) must approve all prescription medications before they are sold to millions and millions of consumers. As a result, people taking prescription medications have a fairly good sense of how the medications work. In addition, they have an understanding of some of the side effects that they may experience.

However, because they are not classified as drugs, there is no such requirement for dietary supplements. Dietary supplements are essentially viewed as food products. Except in the case of the addition of a "new dietary ingredient," the FDA has no ability to evaluate dietary supplements before they are sold. So, manufacturers and distributors do not need any FDA approval to sell their supplements. The FDA does not keep any listing of the manufacturers and distributors and the products they sell.

While the FDA does not regulate supplements like drugs, since the Dietary Supplement Health and Education Act (DSHEA) of 1994, which was signed by President Bill Clinton, it does have some leverage over the dietary supplement industry. It is the responsibility of the manufacturers to ensure that the dietary supplements that they sell are safe. There are three types of claims that manufacturers may make about their dietary supplements—health claims, structure/function claims, and nutrient content claims. These may describe the benefits associated with using a specific supplement, the association between a supplement and a disease or medical problem, or the amount of a nutrient present in a supplement. If a dietary supplement label includes such claims, there must be a disclaimer noting that the FDA has not evaluated the claims(s). Furthermore, the disclaimer must state that this product is not intended to "diagnose, treat, cure, or prevent any disease." Only a drug evaluated by the FDA may make such a claim.

If the FDA learns that a product is unsafe or unfit for human consumption, it has the ability to take action. But, before it takes action, the FDA must prove that the product is unsafe. It may require that the product be removed from the marketplace, or it may force the manufacturer to recall the product. And, manufacturers and distributors are required to record, investigate, and forward to the FDA any reports they receive of serious adverse reactions associated with their dietary supplements.

Likewise, the FDA reviews labeling on dietary supplements, as well as the information on any package inserts. The Federal Trade Commission, which oversees advertising, also reviews this information. Of course, the overall goal of both agencies is to improve accuracy and eliminate inaccurate messaging. Still, the dietary supplement industry is literally growing exponentially, and it is impossible for the FDA to monitor all the products and their varying claims. Compared to the number of dietary supplements on the market, the resources available to the FDA are simply too small and inadequate to be a truly effective monitor.

LABELING OF DIETARY SUPPLEMENTS

The FDA requires that dietary supplement labels contain five key elements of information. These key elements must all be placed on the front label panel—known as the principal display panel—or on the information panel, which is usually the label panel immediately to the right of the principal display panel. The principal display panel is the part of the label that is most likely to be seen by consumers.

The first requirement is a statement of identity—the actual name of the dietary supplement. The statement of identity must be one of the most important features of the label. It should have bold type that must be more prominent than other elements on the front panel. The statement of identity must be located parallel to the base of the package.

The second requirement is the notation of the net quantity—the actual amount of the dietary supplement. The net quantity may be listed in weight, measure, numerical count, or a combination of these. When the net quantity is listed in weight or measure, the amount must be noted in metric and the U.S. Customary System terms (ounces, pounds, or fluid ounces). These figures must be placed parallel to the base of the container.

Except for some small-volume products or those produced by eligible small businesses, the third requirement is nutrition labeling. For a dietary supplement, this labeling is called a "Supplement Facts" panel. When they are present in measurable amounts, the Supplement Facts panel includes the following items: serving size, amount per serving, names and quantity of each ingredient, total calories, calories from fat, saturated fat, cholesterol, sodium, total carbohydrate, dietary fiber, sugars, protein, vitamin A, calcium, and iron. The dietary ingredients with no daily value must be listed by a common name, and the percent daily value must be declared on all dietary ingredients.

The fourth requirement is the ingredient list. The ingredient list includes all compounds used in the manufacturing of the dietary supplement, as well as the sources of the ingredients. However, this is not required if the ingredient are listed under the Supplements Facts panel. The ingredients must be listed in descending order of prominence by weight and should note any spices and natural or artificial flavors.

The fifth requirement is the name and place of business of the manufacturer, packer, or distributor. In addition, dietary supplements must have a warning statement. For example, they may say "Keep this products out of the reach of children." Print or type size must be "prominent, conspicuous and easy to read." Unless exempted, every supplement from a foreign country must note the English name of the country of origin. While no expiration date is required, many companies include a date somewhere on the package. It is not uncommon for consumers to check for an expiration date before purchasing a supplement. No one wants to purchase a product that will expire soon or has already expired.

Dietary supplement marketers are permitted to make certain health-related claims. Thus, it may note that a supplement addresses a specific nutrient deficiency or supports a certain aspect of health. But, as has previously been noted, such a claim must be followed by the words, "This statement has not been evaluated by the Food & Drug Administration. This product is not intended to diagnose, treat, cure, or prevent any disease."

U.S. PHARMACOPEIA (USP)

With offices and core laboratories in Maryland, China, Ghana, India, and Brazil, USP, which stands for the U.S. Pharmacopeia Convention, is a nonprofit committed to improving public health. One of the goals of the organization it to fill what it perceives is a gap in the Government's scrutiny of dietary supplements. That is why USP formed the Dietary Supplement Verification Program. With this program, USP serves as a objective independent party that evaluates the quality, purity, and potency of dietary supplements. According to USP, many companies have excellent quality assurance practices; but, regrettably, this is not true for all companies. According to USP, "a growing number of reports and recalls have raised concerns about inconsistent quality in the industry." According to its website, USP works with manufacturers to ensure that they are consistently using appropriate protocols; quality needs to be built into their everyday systems. It is important to underscore the fact that the USP evaluation is conducted as an impartial, independent, third-party oversight. USP is not associated in any way with the manufacturers.

During the evaluation process, USP meets with the owners of a company and inspects the manufacturing facilities. USP determines from where the company is sourcing dietary supplement ingredients and how it is testing the products. Are the tests the company is conducting appropriate and able to identify any harmful contaminants, such heavy metals, pesticides, and microbes? And, are these tests conducted at science-based quality standards? A supplement that successfully meets the USP "rigorous testing and auditing criteria" receives the USP Verified Mark. When the USP Verified Mark is on a dietary supplements it means that the supplements contains the ingredients listed on the label in the indicated strength and amounts, and that there are no harmful levels of contaminants. The supplement has been manufactured according to the FDA and USP Good Manufacturing Practices, sanitary and well-controlled, it will break down and dissolve in the body, and the active ingredients will be released and absorbed.

Why is quality so significant and worth all the effort? According to USP, there is an association between the quality of the products consumed and health.

Unfortunately, not all dietary supplements are of good quality. There are dietary supplements that do not contain the ingredients and/or the amounts listed on the label. How can ingredient and dosage recommendations be followed when the information is inaccurate? No one wants dietary supplements with contaminants, which may negatively impact health, and dietary supplements that do not dissolve cannot be absorbed by the body. They are more likely to pass unabsorbed through the gastrointestinal tract before being eliminated. Obviously, people do not obtain any benefits from them. "The USP Verified Mark makes quality visible so you can choose dietary supplements with confidence." To see a list of the products with this symbol, go to https://www.quality-supplements.org.

REFERENCES AND FURTHER READING

U.S. Food & Drug Administration. www.fda.gov.
U.S. Pharmacopeia (USP). www.usp.org.

Acai

Acai, also known as açai, pronounced AH-sigh-EE, is a berry fruit harvested from the tall, slender acai palm trees that are native to tropical regions of Central and South America. Not that long ago, acai was only available in areas where it was grown, being an important food source for the indigenous people of the region.

Acai berries look as if they are a cross between grapes and blueberries. However, they tend to be tender to travel longer distances. Most of the research on acai has been conducted in Brazil, and only a relatively small amount of this research has been conducted among humans.

HEALTH BENEFITS AND RISKS

Often called a superfood, acai berries have very high levels of antioxidants that protect the cells in the body against damage. While they are low in sugar, acai berries have high amounts of calcium, fiber, vitamin A, and anthocyanin compounds such as resveratrol. Acai berries are useful for a host of medical problems such as arthritis, inflammation, weight loss, high cholesterol, and general health and well-being. They are probably best known for supporting cardiovascular health.

People with certain health conditions should not take acai supplementation without discussing with a medical provider. For example, supplemental acai may interfere with treatment for high cholesterol and diabetes. In addition, acai has at least three compounds that promote blood thinning—flavonoids, salicylates, and oleic acid. People on blood thinning medications should probably avoid acai supplementation as they may increase the risk of internal bleeding.

HOW IT IS SOLD AND TAKEN

Acai is sold in juices and other beverages and in the freezer section of the supermarket or health food stores. Acai may be consumed as jellies, teas, freeze-dried powders, smoothie mixes, purees, capsule and softgel supplements, energy drinks, and ice creams.

There are no guidelines on recommended doses of acai. Recommendations seem to vary widely, fluctuating from product to product. Although dosage of 1000–2000 mg per day is often recommended, acai is sold in both lower and higher amounts. People who plan to supplement their diets with acai should discuss dosage with a medical provider.

RESEARCH FINDINGS

Acai May Be Useful for Atherosclerosis

In a study published in 2011 in the journal *Atherosclerosis*, researchers from Little Rock, Arkansas (USA), examined the association between consumption of an acai juice powder blend and atherosclerosis (the build-up of plaque in the arteries). The acai blend mostly contained freeze-dried and frozen acai pulp. For 20 weeks, the researchers fed mice that had a higher risk for atherosclerosis (ApoE) either with a regular mouse diet or with a mouse diet that included the acai blend. The researchers learned that the markers of oxidative stress were significantly lower in the serum and liver of the mice on the acai blend diet. In addition, the expression of two antioxidant enzyme genes, important to the vascular system, were higher in the aortas of the mice on the acai blend diet. From this research, it appears that the acai blend reduced plaque levels while increasing the activity of antioxidant enzymes.[1]

Acai May Have Neuroprotective Benefits against Alzheimer's Disease

In a study published in 2013 in the journal *Neuroscience Letters*, researchers from Australia investigated the ability of acai to prevent the build-up of plaque from beta-amyloid deposits. This build-up is associated with an increase in brain cell damage and death from oxidative stress, triggering a loss of cognitive functioning and a greater risk of Alzheimer's disease, the most common form of dementia. In this study, cells were pretreated with acai before being exposed to a specific form of beta-amyloid. The control cells were not treated before they were exposed to this same form of beta-amyloid. As the researchers had hypothesized, cells pretreated with acai were given a degree of protection from the beta-amyloid. The exposed cells experienced significantly less cell loss or improved cell viability. The researchers concluded that "inhibition of beta-amyloid aggregation may underlie a neuroprotective effect of açaí."[2]

Acai May Help Improve Memory

In a study published in 2017 in the journal *Nutritional Neuroscience*, researchers from Boston, Massachusetts (USA), wanted to determine if acai would improve the memory of aging rats. The cohort consisted of 60 19-month-old rats. For 8 weeks, the rats were divided into three groups. The rats in the first group were fed a diet supplemented with a type of acai known as *Euterpe oleracea* (EO); the rats in the second group were fed a diet supplemented with another type of acai known as *Euterpe precatoria* (EP); and the rats in the third group were fed a regular diet without any acai supplementation. During the seventh week of the dietary intervention, the rats were tested for spatial learning and memory. For four consecutive days, the testing was performed in the morning and afternoon. Compared to rats on the control diet, rats fed on acai had improvements in working memory when they were still learning a task. However, only rats fed on EO acai diet had improvements in reference memory. The researchers concluded that their findings "lend further evidence to support that the addition of açai pulp to the diet may improve brain health in aging, and may slow the aging process by reducing the incidence or delaying the onset of debilitating neurodegenerative disease."[3]

Acai Appears to Support Cardiovascular Health

In a study published in 2010 in the journal *Nutrition*, researchers from Brazil tested the ability of acai to lower levels of cholesterol in female rats. The cohort consisted of four groups of rats. Two groups ate a standard diet, and another two groups ate a high-fat diet containing 25% soy oil and 1% cholesterol. The rats in one of the standard groups and one of the high-fat groups also consumed 2% acai pulp. By the end of the trial, the rats in the high-fat group without acai had increase in total cholesterol, increase in non-high-density lipoprotein cholesterol, and decrease in high-density lipoprotein cholesterol ("good") cholesterol. These harmful changes were not seen in rats that ate the high-fat diet that included acai. The researchers commented that their findings "suggest that the consumption of acai improves antioxidant status and has a hypocholesterolemic effect on an animal model of dietary-induced hypercholesterolemia."[4]

In a study published in 2012 in the *Journal of Atherosclerosis and Thrombosis*, a different group of Brazilian researchers examined the association of acai and cholesterol in rabbits. The cohort consisted of 27 3-month-old adult male New Zealand white rabbits. For 12 weeks, they were fed a cholesterol-enriched diet. Then, for another 12 weeks, they were fed a cholesterol-enriched diet and randomized to receive acai extract (n = 15) or water (n = 12). At the end of the study, the researchers took blood samples and specimens from the aortas of the rabbits. Compared to the controls, those on acai extract had lower serum levels of total cholesterol, non-HDL-cholesterol, and triglycerides. Likewise, those on acai had smaller atherosclerotic plaque in their aortas. The researchers noted that their findings confirmed their belief that acai may attenuate atherosclerosis and "markedly improve the lipid profile."[5]

Acai May Be Useful for Helping Overweight Adults Lower Their Risk for Metabolic Disorders

In an open-label pilot study published in 2011 in the *Nutrition Journal*, researchers from California (USA) wanted to determine if acai would help healthy but overweight people lose weight and reduce their risk for metabolic disorders. The researchers recruited 10 overweight adults and provided them with a daily dose of 200 g of acai pulp for 1 month. At baseline and at the end of the trial, the researchers analyzed risk factors for metabolic disorders, including cholesterol levels, insulin and glucose levels, and blood levels of C-reactive protein, an inflammation marker. The researchers learned that acai pulp appeared to reduce levels of blood sugar, total cholesterol, and low-density lipoprotein ("bad" cholesterol). Acai consumption did not appear to have caused adverse events. The researchers suggested that there is a need for more trials including acai. According to the researchers, "conducting a larger placebo-controlled trial to determine the effects of acai on risk factors for chronic disease is warranted."[6]

Like Other Berries, Acai Is Useful in the Prevention of Esophageal Cancer in Rats

In a study published in 2010 in the journal *Pharmaceutical Research*, researchers from Columbus, Ohio (USA), compared the ability of different types of berries, including acai, to prevent chemically induced esophageal cancer. The cohort consisted of 10 groups of 15 rats. For 5 weeks, the rats were treated with a carcinogen that fosters the growth of esophageal cancer. Then, the rats were placed on diets containing 5% berries from seven different types of berries (acai, noni, goji, strawberry, blueberry, red raspberry, and black raspberry). Some rats were set aside as controls. The researchers learned that all berry types were equally effective in reducing the incidence of esophageal cancer; however, the berries had no significant effect on tumor size in any of the groups. The researchers noted that "seven berry types were about equally capable of inhibiting tumor progression in the rat esophagus in spite of known differences in levels of anthocyanins and ellagitannins."[7]

Acai Appears to Have Useful Properties against Bladder Cancer in Mice

In a study published in 2012 in the journal *Plant Foods for Human Nutrition*, researchers from Brazil tested the ability of acai to reduce the risk of bladder cancer. The cohort consisted of three groups of 20 male Swiss mice. They were chemically induced to develop urothelial bladder cancer for 10 weeks. Then, for another 10 weeks, the mice were fed a standard diet or a standard diet with 2.5% and 5% spray-dried acai pulp. There were also appropriate control groups. At week 20, the mice were evaluated for the incidence of bladder cancer. The researchers learned that the mice fed with 5% spray-dried acai pulp had significantly fewer lesions. This occurred without any notable negative impacts on the mice. The researchers concluded that acai "inhibited the tumor development in a suitable mouse urothelial bladder carcinogenesis model." To the researchers, the dietary intake of 5% spray-dried acai pulp may be "a potential food for cancer prevention."[8]

Acai Appears to Improve Overall Health

In a study published in 2016 in the journal *Nutrition*, researchers from Brazil examined the ability of acai supplements to improve the overall health of women. The researchers recruited 35 healthy women, between the ages of 18 and 35 years, and assigned all of them to take 200 g per day of acai pulp for 4 weeks. The study was conducted from April to December 2013, with each participant meeting the researchers once per week to receive enough pulp for the next week. Blood samples were collected at baseline and at the end of the trial. The samples showed significant increase in catalase activity, one of the main enzymes involved in the cellular antioxidative system. There were also significant increases in total anti-oxidant capacity. Apparently, consuming acai greatly increases the levels of antioxidants in the body. According to the researchers, "these results pave the way for better understanding the effects of the daily dietary intake of açai in humans."[9]

Daily Consumption of Acai May Reduce Pain and Improve Range of Motion

In an open-label, 12-week clinical pilot study published in the *Journal of Medicinal Food*, researchers from Oregon and Washington (USA) wanted to learn if the consumption of dietary acai would be useful for 14 people suffering from pain and range of motion problems. Some of the participants had age-related osteoarthritis. The participants consumed 120 mL per day of a juice that was "predominately" acai pulp, but contained other fruit concentrates too. They were monitored at baseline for 2, 4, 8, and 12 weeks. Blood sample was taken at each visit, and a nurse conducted structured interviews focusing primarily on assessing levels of pain and functionality. At the 2-week assessment, antioxidant levels had already improved and continued to improve throughout the study. By the end of the study, the participants experienced a decline in measures of pain and improvement in the range of motion in the spine and other extremities. According to the researchers, "the perceived pain changed significantly over the course of the study." Lumbar improvements were seen before improvements in the lower extremities. Still, no significant changes were observed in the levels of C-reactive protein, as a measure of inflammation. The researchers concluded that "the emerging recognition of the fact that intake of high-polyphenol foods, such as berries, fruits, and nuts, provides a broad-spectrum support of neurologic and vascular function may indeed change our management of many chronic health conditions."[10]

Acai May Be Somewhat Helpful to Teens Participating in Sports

In a pilot study published in 2015 in the journal *Biology of Sport*, researchers from Poland hoped to learn if acai would improve the sprint performance, antioxidant status, and lipid profile in junior athletes. The cohort consisted of seven "elite" junior hurdlers who participated in a preseason conditioning camp. For 6 weeks, every day the athletes consumed 100 mL of a juice blend containing acai. At the start and the end of the camp, the athletes performed a 300-m sprint running test on an outdoor track. Blood samples were taken before and immediately after the test and after 1 hour of recovery. While the researchers learned that consuming juice had no impact on the athletic performance of the teens, it did lead to increased levels of serum antioxidants and significant improvements in lipid profile. In addition, there was a moderate attenuation of exercise-induced muscle damage. The researchers concluded that their "findings strongly support the view of the health benefits of supplementation with acai berry-based juice blend, mainly attributed to its high total polyphenol content and the related high in vivo antioxidant and hypocholesterolemic activities of this supplement."[11]

NOTES

1. Xie, C., J. Kang, R. Burris, et al. "Açai Juice Attenuates Atherosclerosis in ApoE Deficient Mice through Antioxidant and Anti-Inflammatory Activities." *Atherosclerosis* 16, no. 2 (June 2011): 327–333.

2. Wong, D. Y., I. F. Musgrave, B. S. Harvey, and S. D. Smid. "Açai (*Euterpe oleraceae Mart.*) Berry Extract Exerts Neuroprotective Effects against β-Amyloid Exposure in Vitro." *Neuroscience Letters* 556 (November 27, 2013): 221–226.

3. Carey, A. N., M. G. Miller, D. R. Fisher, et al. "Dietary Supplementation with the Polyphenol-Rich Açai Pulps (*Euterpe oleracea* Mart. and *Euterpe precatoria* Mart.) Improves Cognition in Aged Rats and Attenuates Inflammatory Signaling in BV-s Microglial Cells." *Nutritional Neuroscience* 20, no. 4 (May 2017): 238–245.

4. de Souza, M. O., M. Silva, M. E. Silva, et al. "Diet Supplementation with Acai (*Euterpe oleracea* Mart.) Pulp Improves Biomarkers of Oxidative Stress and the Serum Lipid Profiles in Rats." *Nutrition* 26, no. 7–8 (July–August 2010): 804–910.

5. Feio, Claudine A., Maria C. Izar, Silvia S. Ihara, et al. "*Euterpe Oleracea* (Açai) Modifies Sterol Metabolism and Attenuates Experimentally-Induced Atherosclerosis." *Journal of Atherosclerosis and Thrombosis* 19, no. 3 (2012): 237–245.

6. Udani, Jay K., Betsy B. Singh, Vijay J. Singh, and Marilyn L. Barrett. "Effects of Açai (*Euterpe oleracea* Mart.) Berry Preparation on Metabolic Parameters in a Healthy Overweight Population: A Pilot Study." *Nutrition Journal* 10 (December 2011): 45–51.

7. Stoner, Gary D., Li-Shu Wang, Claire Seguin, et al. "Multiple Berry Types Prevent N-nitrosomethylbenzylamine-Induced Esophageal Cancer in Rats." *Pharmaceutical Research* 27 (2010): 1138–1145.

8. Fragoso, Marianna F., Monize G. Prado, Luciano Barbosa, et al. "Inhibition of Mouse Urinary Bladder Carcinogenesis by Açai Fruit (*Euterpe oleraceae* Martius) Intake." *Plant Foods for Human Nutrition* 67 (2012): 235–241.

9. Barbosa, P. O., D. Pala, C. T. Silva, et al. "Açai (*Euterpe oleracea* Mart.) Pulp Dietary Intake Improves Cellular Antioxidant Enzymes and Biomarkers of Serum in Healthy Women." *Nutrition* 32, no. 6 (June 2016): 674–680.

10. Jensen, Gitte S., David M. Ager, Kimberlee A. Redman, et al. "Pain Reduction and Improvement in Range of Motion After Daily Consumption of an Açai (*Euterpe oleracea* Mart.) Pulp-Fortified Polyphenolic-Rich Fruit and Berry Juice Blend." *Journal of Medicinal Food* 14, no. 7–8 (2011): 702–711.

11. Sadowska-Krępa, E., B. Kłapcińska, T. Podgórski, et al. "Effects of Supplementation with Acai (*Euterpe oleracea* Mart.) Berry-Based Juice Blend on the Blood Antioxidant Defence Capacity and Lipid Profile in Junior Handlers: A Pilot Study." *Biology of Sport* 32, no. 2 (June 2015): 161–168.

REFERENCES AND FURTHER READING

Barbosa, P. O., D. Pala, C. T. Silva, et al. "Açai (*Euterpe oleracea* Mart.) Pulp Dietary Intake Improves Cellular Antioxidant Enzymes and Biomarkers of Serum in Healthy Women." *Nutrition* 32, no. 6 (June 2016): 674–680.

Carey, A. N., M. G. Miller, D. R. Fisher, et al. "Dietary Supplementation with the Polyphenol-Rich Açai Pulps (*Euterpe oleracea* Mart. and *Euterpe precatoria* Mart.) Improves Cognition in Aged Rats and Attenuates Inflammatory Signaling in BV-2 Microglial Cells." *Nutritional Neuroscience* 20, no. 4 (May 2017): 238–245.

de Souza, M. O., M. Silva, M. E. Silva, and M. L. Pedrosa. "Diet Supplementation with Acai (*Euterpe oleracea* Mart.) Pulp Improves Biomarkers of Oxidative Stress and the Serum Lipid Profile in Rats." *Nutrition* 26, no. 7–8 (July–August 2010): 804–810.

Feio, Claudine A., Maria C. Izar, Silvia S. Ihara, et al. "*Euterpe Oleracea* (Açai) Modifies Sterol Metabolism and Attenuates Experimentally-Induced Atherosclerosis." *Journal of Atherosclerosis and Thrombosis* 19, no. 3 (2012): 237–245.

Fragoso, Marianna F., Monize G. Prado, Luciano Barbosa, et al. "Inhibition of Mouse Urinary Bladder Carcinogenesis by Açai Fruit (*Euterpe oleraceae* Martius) Intake." *Plant Foods for Human Nutrition* 67 (2012): 235–241.

Jensen, Gitte S., David M. Ager, Kimberlee A. Redman, et al. "Pain Reduction and Improvement in Range of Motion After Daily Consumption of an Açai (*Euterpe oleracea* Mart.) Pulp-Fortified Polyphenolic-Rich Fruit and Berry Juice." *Journal of Medicinal Food* 14, no. 7–8 (2011): 702–711.

Sadowsk-Krępa, E., B. Kłapcińska, T. Podgórski, et al. "Effects of Supplementation with Acai (*Euterpe oleracea* Mart.) Berry-Based Juice Blend on the Blood Antioxidant Defence Capacity and Lipid Profile in Junior Hurdlers. A Pilot Study." *Biology of Sport* 32, no. 2 (June 2015): 161–168.

Stoner, Gary D., Li-Shu Wang, Claire Seguin, et al. "Multiple Berry Types Prevent N-nitrosomethylbenzylamine-Induced Esophageal Cancer in Rats." *Pharmaceutical Research* 27 (2010): 1138–1145.

Udani, Jay K., Betsy B. Singh, Vijay J. Singh, and Marilyn L. Barrett. "Effects of Açai (*Euterpe oleracea* Mart.) Berry Preparation on Metabolic Parameters in a Healthy Overweight Population: A Pilot Study." *Nutrition Journal* 10 (December 2011): 45–51.

Wong, D. Y., I. F. Musgrave, B. S. Harvey, and S. D. Smid. "Açai (*Euterpe oleraceae* Mart.) Berry Extract Exerts Neuroprotective Effects against β-Amyloid Exposure in Vitro." *Neuroscience Letters* 556 (November 27, 2013): 221–226.

Xie, C., J. Kang, R. Burris, et al. "Açai Juice Attenuates Atherosclerosis in ApoE Deficient Mice Through Antioxidant and Anti-Inflammatory Activities." *Atherosclerosis* 16, no. 2 (June 2011): 327–333.

Aloe Vera

Although often used interchangeably, aloe and aloe vera have slight differences. Aloe vera is a plant belonging to a cacti family known as Aloe. While there are hundreds of species of the genus Aloe, aloe vera (*Aloe barbadensis*) is popular and is recognized throughout the world.

Traced back 6,000 years to ancient Egypt, where the plant was depicted on stone carvings, aloe vera was historically considered useful for a wide variety of medical problems, including wounds, hair loss, constipation, and hemorrhoids.

HEALTH BENEFITS AND RISKS

Today, aloe vera gel is primarily used topically as a remedy for skin conditions such as burns, frostbite, psoriasis, acne, radiation-induced skin damage, genital herpes in men, diaper rash, minor burns, and cold sores. It is generally considered safe for these problems. When taken orally in a juice, which is also called aloe latex, it may have some benefits for osteoarthritis, weight loss, itching, high cholesterol, gastrointestinal problems such as constipation, seborrhea, immune system deficiencies, and fever. However, there have been reports of side effects such as abdominal cramps and diarrhea. People with diabetes who take glucose lowering medication should not consume aloe vera without consulting their healthcare provider. It may also lower glucose levels. Pregnant women should never consume aloe vera orally as it may trigger uterine contractions and miscarriage. Because how aloe vera may impact a child is unknown, nursing moms should avoid oral aloe vera. In addition, because oral aloe vera lowers potassium levels in the body, the product should not be taken by people on diuretics or digoxin, which lower potassium levels. This combination may make the potassium levels reduce significantly.

HOW IT IS SOLD AND TAKEN

Aloe vera may be obtained simply by breaking off leaves of the plant. Aloe vera is a perennial plant, with the leaves holding large quantities of water. The plant may grow up to 4 feet, and the tough, spear-shaped leaves can grow up to 36 inches. The thick, clear gel inside the leaves is usually used for treating cuts and burns.

Aloe vera is sold as a cream, gel, juice, softgel, lotion, and in capsules. The creams and gels containing aloe vera vary widely in dosage ranging from approximately 0.5% to 70%. There are no set dosages for oral aloe vera. When used for constipation, some recommend 100–200 mg of juice per day for a limited period of time, such as a week. High doses should be avoided as they may cause kidney damage.

RESEARCH FINDINGS

Aloe Vera May Be Useful against Susceptible and Resistant *Helicobacter pylori*

In a study published in 2014 in the journal *Letters in Applied Microbiology*, researchers from Italy wanted to learn more about the antibacterial properties of aloe vera against *Helicobacter pylori*, which is associated with peptic ulcer disease. Therefore, they tested the inner gel of leaves from a 5-year-old aloe vera plant against 14 clinical strains and one reference strain of *H. pylori*. The researchers learned that the antibacterial properties of aloe vera were similar to other bactericidal agents. In addition, they suggested that combining aloe vera with a traditional *H. pylori* antibacterial treatment may improve outcomes. The researchers concluded that "in combination with antibiotics, [aloe vera] could represent a novel strategy for the treatment of the infection of *H. pylori*, especially in cases of multiresistance."[1]

Obese People, with or without Diabetes, May Benefit from Aloe Vera

In a double-blind, placebo-controlled, randomized trial published in 2013 in the journal *Nutrition*, researchers from South Korea noted that very little is known about how aloe vera could affect obese people who do not have type 2 diabetes or are in the early stages of type 2 diabetes and not yet on diabetes medication. Would supplemental aloe vera have any impact on the biomarkers of obesity such as body weight, body fat mass, serum insulin levels, and fasting blood sugar? The initial cohort consisted of 136 participants who were randomly assigned to an aloe vera intervention or a control group. Participants in the control group took placebos. Evaluations were conducted at baseline, at 4 weeks and at 8 weeks. The study lost eight participants in the intervention group and six in the control group; the final analysis included 60 participants in the intervention group and 62 in the control group. The researchers learned that at 8 weeks, the body weight and body fat mass were significantly lower in the intervention group. At 4 weeks, serum insulin levels were lower in the intervention group; they were also lower at 8 weeks, "with borderline significance." At 8 weeks, the fasting blood glucose "tended to decrease in the intervention group," however, the difference was not significant. The researchers stressed the need for more studies on the effects of the long-term use of aloe vera supplementation in people with diabetes.[2]

Aloe Vera Appears to Be Useful for Healing Wounds

In a study published in 2013 in the *Journal of the Pakistan Medical Association*, researchers from Pakistan compared the wound healing efficacy of aloe vera gel with 1% silver sulfadiazine cream, a common topical antimicrobial agent. From July 2008 to December 2010, 50 patients with second-degree burns were divided into two groups. The patients in one group had their burns treated with aloe vera gel, whereas the patients in the other group had their burns treated with 1% silver sulfadiazine cream. The wounds were dressed twice each day until healing was complete. The researchers learned that the patients in the aloe vera group achieved pain relief faster than those in the sulfadiazine cream group. Among the 25 patients in the aloe group, 24 experienced complete recovery. Of the 25 patients in the cream group, 19 experienced complete recovery. These differences were statistically significant. Even the cost of using aloe was significantly less than the cream. According to the researchers, the healing properties of aloe vera "may be explained by its cell proliferation and anti-inflammatory effects."[3]

In another study published in 2012 in the journal *Anatomy & Cell Biology*, researchers from Iran compared the use of aloe vera gel, thyroid hormone cream, and 1% silver sulfadiazine cream on incisions in 36 Wistar rats. The rats were equally divided into experimental and control groups. Each rat in the experimental group received four incisions, and the control rats received one incision. The wounds in the experimental rats were treated with the above-mentioned agents; the wounds of the control rats were not treated. The researchers learned that the wounds healed best when they were treated with aloe vera gel. The researchers concluded that "therefore, AV is recommended as the treatment of choice for surgically induced incisions."[4]

Aloe Vera Appears Useful for Peritonitis in Rats

In a study published in 2014 in the *Indian Journal of Pharmacology*, researchers from Turkey tested the use of aloe vera leaf gel for peritonitis in rats. (Peritonitis is an inflammation of the peritoneum, the tissue that lines the inner wall of the abdomen and covers and supports most of the abdominal organs.) The cohort consisted of 38 rats. A control group had six rats; the remaining groups, with eight rats in each, were an aloe vera treatment group, a peritonitis group, a peritonitis plus aloe vera group, and a peritonitis and antibiotic therapy group. The researchers learned that aloe vera appeared to have antioxidant and anti-inflammatory properties in rats with peritonitis. Moreover, there were no toxic side effects. The researchers concluded that "results were suggestive for the use of AV in peritonitis."[5]

Aloe Vera Cream Appears to Be a Useful Treatment for Chronic Anal Fissures

In a study published in 2014 in the journal *European Review for Medical and Pharmacological Sciences*, researchers from Iran investigated the ability of aloe vera cream containing 0.5% aloe vera juice powder to help reduce pain associated with chronic anal fissures. The initial cohort consisted of 60 patients with a confirmed diagnosis of chronic anal fissures. Thirty patients used the aloe vera cream, whereas 30 patients in the control group used a placebo cream. The researchers found that there were statistically significant differences in pain levels among the patients using the aloe cream and those who did not. The patients using aloe cream had statistically significant less pain and bleeding and more wound healing without any side effects or allergic reactions. The researchers concluded that "topical aloe vera cream is an effective and safe form of treatment and represents a new therapeutic avenue toward treating chronic anal fissures."[6]

Aloe Vera May Be Useful for Mild-to-Moderate Plaque Psoriasis

In a randomized, double-blind, 8-week study published in 2010 in the *Journal of the European Academy of Dermatology and Venereology*, researchers from Thailand compared the efficacy of topical aloe vera to 0.1% triamcinolone acetonide, a synthetic corticosteroid, in treating mild-to-moderate plaque psoriasis. Forty participants were randomly assigned to the aloe vera group and 40 to the triamcinolone acetonide group. Each participant was examined at baseline and again after 2, 4, and 8 weeks of treatment. Thirty-seven people completed the aloe vera treatment, and 38 completed the triamcinolone acetonide treatment. Interestingly, after 8 weeks, no one had complete clearance from psoriasis. However, there were definite clinical improvements in symptoms, especially in the aloe vera group. The researchers concluded that "however, both treatments have similar efficacy in improving the quality of life of patients with mild to moderate psoriasis."[7]

Oral Aloe Vera May Be Beneficial to the Skin

In a study published in 2015 in the journal *Clinical, Cosmetic and Investigational Dermatology*, researchers from Japan wanted to determine if oral intake of aloe vera would have any impact on human skin. They first investigated the capability of aloe sterols to stimulate human dermal fibroblasts in the laboratory; subsequently, they examined whether the intake of aloe vera gel powder would improve the skin of Japanese women. In the laboratory tests, aloe increased the production of collagen and hyaluronic acid. The double-blind, placebo-controlled trial among Japanese women initially included a cohort of 56 women with dry skin. The women were randomly assigned to the aloe vera or placebo groups. For 8 weeks, all the participants ingested five tablets per day. After the baseline testing, one participant in each group withdrew from the study. Therefore, data were analyzed from 54 participants. By the end of the trial, both groups had significant increase in facial skin hydration, and the aloe vera group had an increase in arm skin hydration. Meanwhile, the percentage change in the mean wrinkle depth was significantly lower in the aloe vera group than the control group. To conclude, daily intake of aloe vera "significantly reduced facial wrinkles in women" who were 40 years old and older.[8]

Aloe Vera May Be Useful for Acne

In an 8-week, randomized, double-blind trial published in 2014 in the *Journal of Dermatological Treatment*, researchers from Iran wanted to learn if the combination of aloe vera gel and tretinoin, a retinoid used to treat acne, would be useful for mild and moderate acne. The cohort consisted of 60 participants with mild-to-moderate acne. Half of the participants were treated with 0.05% tretinoin cream combined with 50% aloe vera topical gel; the other half were treated with tretinoin cream and moisturizer. The researchers determined that the combination therapy "showed superior efficacy" to the use of tretinoin with moisturizer. Moreover, the combination therapy was significantly more effective in reducing noninflammatory, inflammatory, and total lesion scores. The members of the combination group also had significantly less skin redness. While a large number of participants in both groups had some type of adverse reaction to the products, the number of severe reactions was relatively small. The researchers concluded that "this combination therapy effectively treated both inflammatory and non-inflammatory lesions, and showed less AEs [adverse reactions], especially in skin erythema [redness]."[9]

Aloe Vera Gel Extract May Be Useful in the Prevention of Intestinal Polyps

In a study published in 2013 in the *Asian Pacific Journal of Cancer Prevention*, researchers from Japan tested the ability of aloe vera gel extract to impact intestinal polyp formation in male mice at higher risk for colorectal cancer that are fed a high-fat diet. The mice were divided into four groups—normal diet, high-fat diet, low-dose aloe vera gel and high-fat diet, and high-dose aloe vera gel and high-fat diet. At the end of 7 weeks, the mice were sacrificed and their small and large intestines were searched for polyps. While no significant differences were observed in either the incidence or multiplicity of polyps, when the polyps were characterized by size, the incidence and multiplicity of large polyps in the intestines in the high-fat diet with high amounts of aloe vera were significantly lower than those in the high-fat diet group.[10]

Aloe Vera May Help with Weight Loss

In a study published in 2012 in the *Journal of Nutritional Science and Vitaminology*, researchers from Japan wanted to learn more about the antiobesity properties of aloe vera gel in male Sprague–Dawley rats with diet-induced obesity. The researchers divided the rats into four groups—standard diet group, high-fat diet control group, high-fat diet with low-dose aloe vera, and high-fat diet with high-dose aloe vera. The rats were sacrificed when they were 24 weeks old. The researchers found that the subcutaneous and visceral fat weight and body fat were reduced significantly in the rats treated with aloe vera. The researchers commented that their findings indicated that aloe vera gel "may prevent and improve obesity caused by a high-fat diet, and its health-promoting effect could be beneficial to reduce the risk of obesity-associated disease, that is, metabolic syndrome."[11]

Aloe Vera May Benefit People with Type 2 Diabetes

In a randomized, double-blind, placebo-controlled clinical trial published in 2012 in the journal *Planta Medica*, researchers from Iran wanted to learn if aloe vera would benefit people with type 2 diabetes with high lipid levels and/or high glucose levels. The initial cohort consisted of 67 men and women with type 2 diabetes between the ages of 40 and 60 years. The intervention group took aloe capsules at a dose of one 300 mg capsule every 12 hours for 2 months; the other group took a placebo tablet every 12 hours for the same period. Compared to the members of the placebo group, the researchers determined that aloe vera significantly lowered the levels of glucose, total cholesterol, and low-density lipoprotein in the members of the intervention group. The researchers concluded that "the results suggest that aloe gel may be a safe anti-hyperglycemic and anti-hypercholesterolemic agent for hyperlipidemic type 2 diabetes patients."[12]

Oral Aloe Vera Has the Potential to Trigger Hepatitis

In an anecdotal report published in 2007 in the journal *Annals of Pharmacotherapy*, researchers from Des Moines, Iowa (USA), described a 73-year-old female who was admitted to the hospital with hepatitis. She reported feeling general malaise, poor appetite, nausea, right shoulder pain, and weight loss. After she developed jaundice, she sought medical care. Extensive laboratory testing was unable to reveal the cause of the woman's illness. It was only after repeated questioning that she mentioned taking oral aloe vera for constipation. In fact, she had been taking aloe vera for 5 years. After the oral aloe vera was discontinued, the liver markers of hepatotoxicity returned to normal levels. The researchers commented that clinicians are now dealing with the widespread use of many types of herbal products. Clinicians faced with acute hepatitis that is not readily diagnosed need to "question patients specifically about herbal product use and should consider aloe vera as a possible cause."[13]

NOTES

1. Cellini, L., S. Di Bartolomeo, E. Di Campli, et al. "In Vitro Activity of Aloe Vera Inner Gel against *Helicobacter pylori* Strains." *Letters in Applied Microbiology* 59, no. 1 (July 2014): 43–48.

2. Choi, Ho-Chun, Seok-Joong Kim, Ki-Young Son, et al. "Metabolic Effects of Vera Gel Complex in Obese Prediabetes and Early Non-Treated Diabetic Patients: Randomized Controlled Trial." *Nutrition* 29 (2013): 1110–1114.

3. Shahzad, Muhammad Naveed, and Naheed Ahmed. "Effectiveness of Aloe Vera Gel Compared with 1% Silver Sulphadiazine Cream." *Journal of the Pakistan Medical Association* 63 (2013): 225–230.

4. Tarmeshloo, Mahsa, Mohsen Norouzian, Saeed Zarein-Dolab, et al. "Aloe Vera Gel and Thyroid Hormone Cream May Improve Wound Healing in Wistar Rats." *Anatomy & Cell Biology* 45 (2012): 170–177.

5. Altincik, A., F. Sönmez, C. Yenisey, et al. "Effects of Aloe Vera Leaf Gel Extract on Rat Peritonitis Model." *Indian Journal of Pharmacology* 46, no. 3 (May–June 2014): 322–327.

6. Rahmani, N., M. Khademloo, K. Vosoughi, and S. Assadpour. "Effects of Aloe Vera Cream on Chronic Anal Fissure Pain, Wound Healing and Hemorrhaging upon Defection: A Prospective Double Blind Clinical Trial." *European Review for Medical and Pharmaceutical Sciences* 18, no. 7 (2014): 1078–1084.

7. Choonhakarn, C., P. Busaracome, B. Sripanidkulchai, and P. Sarakarn. "A Prospective, Randomized Clinical Trial Comparing Topical Aloe Vera with 0.1% Triamcinolone Acetonide in Mild to Moderate Plaque Psoriasis." *Journal of the European Academy of Dermatology and Venereology* 24, no. 2 (February 2010): 168–172.

8. Tanaka, M., E. Misawa, K. Yamauchi, et al. "Effects of Plant Sterols Derived from Aloe Vera Gel on Human Dermal Fibroblasts in Vitro and on Skin Condition in Japanese Women." *Clinical, Cosmetic and Investigational Dermatology* 8 (February 20, 2015): 95–104.

9. Hajheydari, Zohreh, Majid Saeedi, Katayoun Morteza-Semnani, and Aida Soltani. "Effect of *Aloe vera* Topical Gel Combined with Tretinoin in Treatment of Mild and Moderate Acne Vulgaris: A Randomized, Double-Blind, Prospective Trial." *Journal of Dermatological Treatment* 25, no. 2 (April 2014): 123–129.

10. Chihara, Takeshi, Kan Shimpo, Hidehiko Beppu, et al. "Reduction of Intestinal Polyp Formation in Min Mice Fed a High-Fat Diet with *Aloe Vera* Gel Extract." *American Pacific Journal of Cancer Prevention* 14, no. 7 (2013): 4435–4440.

11. Misawa, E., M. Tanaka, K. Nabeshima, et al. "Administration of Dried *Aloe vera* Gel Powder Reduced Body Fat Mass in Diet-Induced Obesity (DIO) Rats." *Journal of Nutritional Science and Vitaminology* 58, no. 3 (2012): 195–201.

12. Huseini, H. F., S. Kianbakht, R. Hajiaghaee, and F. H. Dabaghian. "Anti-Hyperglycemic and Anti-Hypercholesterolemic Effects of *Aloe vera* Leaf Gel in Hyperlipidemic Type 2 Diabetic Patients: A Randomized Double-Blind Placebo-Controlled Clinical Trial." *Planta Medica* 78, no. 4 (March 2012): 311–316.

13. Bottenberg, M. M., G. C. Wall, R. L. Harvey, and S. Habib. "Oral Aloe Vera-Induced Hepatitis." *Annals of Pharmacotherapy* 41, no. 10 (October 2007): 1740–1743.

REFERENCES AND FURTHER READING

Altincik, A., F. Sönmez, C. Yenisey, et al. "Effects of Aloe Vera Leaf Gel on Rat Peritonitis Model." *Indian Journal of Pharmacology* 46, no. 3 (May–June 2014): 322–327.

Bottenberg, M. M., G. C. Wall, R. L. Harvey, and S. Habib. "Oral Aloe Vera-Induced Hepatitis." *Annals of Pharmacology* 41, no. 10 (October 2007): 1740–1743.

Cellini, L., S. Di Bartolomeo, E. Di Campli, et al. "In Vitro Activity of Aloe Vera Inner Gel against *Helicobacter pylori* Strains." *Letters in Applied Microbiology* 59, no. 1 (July 2014): 43–48.

Chihara, Takeshi, Kan Shimpo, Hidehiko Beppu, et al. "Reduction of Intestinal Polyp Formation in Min Mice Fed a High-Fat Diet with *Aloe Vera* Gel Abstract." *Asian Pacific Journal of Cancer Prevention* 14, no. 7 (2013): 4435–4440.

Choi, Ho-Chun, Seok-Joong Kim, Ki-Young Son, et al. "Metabolic Effects of Aloe Vera Gel Complex in Obese Prediabetes and Early-Non-Treated Diabetic Patients: Randomized Controlled Trial." *Nutrition* 29 (2013): 1110–1114.

Choonhakarn, C., P. Busaracome, B. Sripanidkulchai, and P. Sarakarn. "A Prospective, Randomized Clinical Trial Comparing Topical Aloe Vera with 0.1% Triamcinolone Acetonide in Mild to Moderate Plaque Psoriasis." *Journal of the European Academy of Dermatology and Venereology* 24, no. 2 (February 2010): 168–172.

Hajheydari, Zohreh, Majid Saeedi, Katayoun Morteza-Semnani, and Aida Soltani. "Effect of *Aloe vera* Topical Gel Combined with Tretinoin in Treatment of Mild and Moderate Acne Vulgaris: A Randomized, Double-Blind, Prospective Trial." *Journal of Dermatological Treatment* 25, no. 2 (April 2014): 123–129.

Huseini, H. E., S. Kianbakht, R. Hajiaghaee, and F. H. Dabaghian. "Anti-Hyperglycemic and Anti-Hypercholesterolemic Effects of *Aloe vera* Leaf Gel in Hyperlipidemic Type 2 Diabetic Patients: A Randomized Double-Blind Placebo-Controlled Clinical Trial." *Planta Medica* 78, no. 4 (March 2012): 311–316.

Misawa, E., M. Tanaka, K. Nabeshima, et al. "Administration of Dried *Aloe vera* Gel Powder Reduced Body Fat Mass in Diet-Induced Obesity (DIO) Rats." *Journal of Nutritional Science and Vitaminology* 58, no. 3 (2012): 195–201.

Rahmani, N., M. Khademloo, K. Vosoughi, and S. Assadpour. "Effects of Aloe Vera Cream on Chronic Anal Fissure Pain, Wound Healing and Hemorrhaging upon Defection: A Prospective Double Blind Clinical Trial." *European Review for Medical and Pharmacological Sciences* 18, no. 7 (2014): 1078–1084.

Shadzad, Muhammad Naveed, and Naheed Ahmed. "Effectiveness of Aloe Vera Gel Compared with 1% Silver Sulphadiazine Cream as Burn Wound Dressing in Second Degree Burns." *Journal of the Pakistan Medical Association* 63 (2013): 225–230.

Tanaka, M., E. Misawa, K. Yamauchi, et al. "Effects of Plant Sterols Derived from Aloe Vera Gel on Human Fibroblasts in Vitro and on Skin Condition in Japanese Women." *Clinical, Cosmetic and Investigational Dermatology* 8 (February 20, 2015): 95–104.

Tarameshloo, Mahsa, Mohsen Norouzian, Saeed Zarein-Dolab, et al. "Aloe Vera Gel and Thyroid Hormone Cream May Improve Wound Healing in Wistar Rats." *Anatomy & Cell Biology* 45 (2012): 170–177.

Alpha Lipoic Acid

Alpha lipoic acid, also known as lipoic acid, is an organic compound that acts as a powerful antioxidant in the body. While the human body naturally produces alpha lipoic acid in the mitochondria of the cells, it is found in small amounts in all human cells, and it is both water and fat soluble.

Red and organ meats are great sources of alpha lipoic acid. However, it is also found in plant-based foods such as broccoli, tomatoes, spinach, and Brussels sprouts.

HEALTH BENEFITS AND RISKS

Alpha lipoic acid is believed to have a wide variety of health benefits, including reducing inflammation, insulin resistance, and fasting glucose levels; slowing skin aging; and improving nerve functioning. It may lower the risk of metabolic syndrome and reduce the incidence of complications associated with diabetes, such as diabetic retinopathy and nerve damage. There is some evidence that alpha lipoic acid may slow the progression of disorders characterized by memory loss, such as Alzheimer's disease, and may support cardiovascular health by reducing levels of triglycerides and low-density lipoprotein or "bad" cholesterol. In addition, alpha lipoic acid may slow the progression of carpal tunnel syndrome and numbness or tingling in hands. Further, taking this supplement after surgery for carpal tunnel may improve recovery outcomes.

Side effects of alpha lipoic acid supplementation include nausea, rashes, and itching. These supplements may react with medications for diabetes and further lower blood sugar levels. In addition, because of a lack of sufficient studies, they may or may not be safe in pregnant women. Although there is little research on the association, according to some researchers, people who have thyroid disease should probably avoid this supplement, contending that it may have thyroid hormone lowering properties.

HOW IT IS SOLD AND TAKEN

While it may be present in topical products, alpha lipoic acid is generally sold in capsules, caplets, softgels, and tablets. There are no recommended dosages for this supplement. Evidence suggests that people should take between 300 and 600 mg per day. However, people have taken up to 2400 mg per day without experiencing any side effects. It is probably best to follow the instructions on the label. These supplements should be taken on an empty stomach.

RESEARCH FINDINGS

Alpha Lipoic Acid Appears to Have Benefits for People with Diabetic Polyneuropathy and Neuropathy

In a systematic review published in 2018 in the *Journal of Pharmacy & Pharmaceutical Sciences*, researchers from Tyler, Texas (USA), evaluated the use of alpha lipoic acid for diabetic polyneuropathy. Their analysis included 25 articles, five randomized controlled trials and three open-label studies. All but one of the studies used oral forms of alpha lipoic acid, and the duration of treatments ranged from 3 to 20 weeks. The researchers learned that alpha lipoic acid, at a dose of 600 mg per day for at least 3 weeks, benefited people with diabetes who had polyneuropathy. People on alpha lipoic acid supplements had improved nerve function and neuropathic pain. Doses above 600 mg per day did not show any statistical or clinical difference. Common side effects of the supplements were rash and nausea. The researchers concluded that it is now "appropriate" to consider alpha lipoic acid as a treatment for diabetic polyneuropathy.[1]

In a 40-day clinical trial published in 2018 in the *Journal of International Medical Research*, researchers from Greece tested the ability of alpha lipoic acid to provide relief to diabetic neuropathy patients. The cohort consisted of 72 patients who have diabetic neuropathy. All patients were treated with 600 mg per day of oral alpha lipoic acid. Assessments were conducted at baseline and at the end of the trial. All patients completed the trial. The researchers learned that the alpha lipoic acid supplement was associated with a clinically significant and prompt reduction in neuropathy and an overall improvement in quality of life parameters. The researchers commented that "it remains to be determined if the improvement in neuropathy symptoms could be further enhanced by treatment prolongation beyond 40 days and more importantly if this will have an impact on the long-term course of diabetic neuropathy."[2]

In a meta-analysis and systematic review published in 2018 in the journal *Drug, Design, Development and Therapy*, researchers from China compared the use of the medication epalrestat alone or in combination with alpha lipoic acid to treat diabetic peripheral neuropathy. Their analysis included 12 clinical trials. The researchers noted that the quality of the trials were high in terms of "randomization, completeness of outcome data, selective reporting, and other potential biases." However, most of the trials had a poor methodology. The researchers found that the combination therapy was "superior" to monotherapy with epalrestat. According to the researchers, their findings provide a promising option for people with diabetes who have peripheral neuropathy, a common disorder. In particular, it may offer relief to those who have had poor clinical outcomes to treatment only with epalrestat. The researchers commented that their findings need to be verified by larger randomized controlled trials.[3]

In a systematic literature review published in 2010 in *The Netherlands Journal of Medicine*, researchers from the Netherlands evaluated the use of alpha lipoic acid for neuropathic pain in people with diabetes. They found five randomized controlled trials, with participants ranging from 18 to 74 years, and one meta-analysis that met their criteria. Three of the studies examined the effects of oral alpha lipoic acid, two were about the intravenous (IV) administration of alpha lipoic acid, and one study had both oral and IV administration. The dosages ranged from 100 to 1800 mg per day. The oral administration studies ranged from 3 weeks to 6 months; the IV administration study was 3 weeks in duration. The final analysis did not include one of the randomized controlled trials as many participants had dropped out. The researchers concluded that the short-term IV administration of alpha lipoic acid resulted in "a significant and clinically relevant" reduction in neuropathic pain when used for 3 weeks at a dose of 600 mg per day. However, they were unable to conclude that the oral administration was clinically relevant. Moreover, there were additional problems. All studies were sponsored by a pharmaceutical company that manufactures alpha lipoic acid, and several of the authors received salaries from the company. In addition, the company had representatives serving as advisors for some studies.[4]

Switching from Alpha Lipoic Acid to Other Analgesics to Treat Diabetic Neuropathy May Not Be Advised

In a retrospective, "real-world" study published in 2009 in the *Journal of Diabetes and Its Complications*, a researcher from Germany, assisted by other researchers, examined what happened when patients with painful diabetic neuropathy were switched from alpha lipoic acid treatment to another analgesic, such as gabapentin. Specifically, the researcher reviewed the efficacy, safety, and cost-effectiveness of the change in treatment. The researcher assembled a cohort of 443 patients (mean age 65 years) with chronic painful neuropathy who were treated with 600 mg per day of alpha lipoic acid for a mean period of 5 years. After stopping the treatment, 293 patients were switched from 600 to 2400 mg per day of gabapentin, while 150 patients were not treated with pain medication. Among the group on gabapentin, 132 were responders on an average dose of 1200 mg per day and 161 were nonresponders on an average dose of 2400 mg per day. The nonresponders were placed on an alternative analgesics medication or a combination of medications. One hundred and thirty-one patients on gabapentin stopped taking the medication because of "intolerable side effects," such as dizziness, somnolence, vertigo, and a tendency to fall. One hundred and ten patients in the untreated group developed neuropathic symptoms as soon as 2 weeks after their alpha lipoic acid treatment ended. In addition, the researcher found that the cost of using alpha lipoic acid was considerably less than the other treatments, and when the participants stopped using alpha lipoic acid, they had about twice the number of visits to medical providers. The researchers concluded that "switching from long-term treatment with α-lipoic acid to gabapentin or other central analgesic drugs in patients with painful diabetic neuropathy is not warranted."[5]

Alpha Lipoic Acid Supplementation May Help Obese People Lose Weight

In a randomized, double-blind, placebo-controlled, 20-week trial published in 2011 in the *American Journal of Medicine*, researchers from Korea wanted to learn if alpha lipoic acid would help obese people lose weight. The initial cohort consisted of 360 obese participants between the ages of 18 and 65 years; some participants had related medical problems, such as hypertension, diabetes, or elevated cholesterol levels. During the course of the trial, the participants took either 1200 or 1800 mg per day of alpha lipoic acid supplementation or a placebo. They were also advised how to restrict their caloric intake. Two hundred and twenty-eight participants completed the trial. The withdrawal rates did not differ among the three groups. The most common adverse effect was an itching sensation. The researchers learned that the participants in both the supplement groups had significant reductions in body weight, starting as early as 4 weeks. At 20 weeks, the mean body weight reduction was significantly greater in the 1800-mg group than the placebo group. Further, they had modest but significant reductions in body weight and body mass index (BMI). While the researchers acknowledged that there is a need for similar studies in other non-Korean populations, there is also a need for research comparing the effectiveness of alpha lipoic acid to other anti-obesity products.[6]

In a randomized, double-blind, placebo-controlled trial published in 2015 in the journal *Obesity*, researchers from Spain divided 97 overweight and obese women into four similar groups. For 10 weeks, one group took 0.3 g per day of alpha lipoic acid, one group took 1.3 g per day of eicosapentaenoic acid (an omega-3 fatty acid), one group took the same dose of alpha lipoic acid and the same dose of eicosapentaenoic acid, and one group served as the control. Everyone was advised to follow an energy-restricted diet. Seventy-seven women completed the trial. The researchers found that weight loss was significantly higher among women who took alpha lipoic acid supplementation. In addition, these women had significant reductions in hip circumference and fat mass. The researchers concluded that "this pattern was observed in the α-lipoic [alpha lipoic] acid-supplemented groups from the first weeks of treatment and became more prominent during the trial."[7]

In a meta-analysis published in 2017 in the journal *Obesity Reviews*, researchers from New Haven, Connecticut (USA), identified 11 randomized, double-blind, placebo-controlled studies that addressed alpha lipoic supplementation and weight loss in overweight and obese people. All studies were between 8 and 52 weeks long and reported weight and/or BMI before and after intervention. In total, there were 534 participants in the alpha lipoic acid supplement groups and 413 patients in the placebo groups. Supplement doses ranged from 300 to 1800 mg per day. The researchers learned that, compared to participants taking placebos, those treated with alpha lipoic acid had significant reductions in body weight and BMI. Upon further analysis, the researchers found that shorter duration of supplementation achieved more reduction of BMI than the longer interventions. Both the supplement and placebo groups had similar rates of side effects and discontinuations. The researchers concluded that alpha lipoic acid may "be considered in clinical practice due to its benign side-effect profile … and low cost comparing to the available weight loss medications."[8]

When Combined with Superoxide Dismutase, Alpha Lipoic Acid Supplementation May Be Useful for Chronic Low Back Pain

In a prospective, nonrandomized, open-label trial published in 2013 in the *European Journal of Physical and Rehabilitation Medicine*, researchers from Italy investigated the use of alpha lipoic acid and superoxide dismutase, an enzyme that speeds up certain chemical reactions in the body, for chronic low back pain. The researchers recruited 98 adult participants who had chronic low back pain for at least 12 weeks. The mean age at baseline was 72 years. For 60 days, the participants were treated with 600 mg alpha lipoic acid supplementation per day and superoxide dismutase. Assessments were conducted at baseline, 20 days, 40 days, and when the trial ended. At baseline, 72 participants regularly took analgesics. By the end of the trial, only 8 participants needed treatment with analgesics. There were statistically significant reductions in perceived pain and reported disabilities. The researchers concluded that the combination therapy "may be a powerful adjuvant in multimodal therapy of chronic LBP [low back pain] patients."[9]

A Topical Gel Containing Alpha Lipoic Acid May Be Useful for Aging Skin

In a single-blind, placebo-controlled, right-left comparative clinical trial, researchers from Egypt evaluated the efficacy of 5% cubosomal alpha lipoic acid. For 6 months, 20 women, who complained of facial aging, applied the gel formulation over the right half of their faces and a placebo gel over the left half of their faces twice daily. The researchers used the Global Aesthetic Improvement Scale to assess the faces, and evaluated the thickness of the epidermis and dermis on each side of the face before treatment and at the end of the trial. All the participants, whose ages ranged from 38 to 64 years, completed the trial. The researchers found variable degrees of improvement in 90% of the actively treated sides; this was in contrast to 60% in the placebo sides. There was a significant increase in the epidermal skin and a nonsignificant increase in the dermal skin thickness. Regarding side effects, three participants reported mild skin tightness on the treated side. The researchers concluded that the topical gel containing alpha lipoic acid "seems to be an effective and safe modality for improving the appearance of the aging face with a rather rapid onset of action."[10]

Alpha Lipoic Acid Appears to Reduce Levels of C-Reactive Protein

In a systematic review and meta-analysis published in 2018 in the journal *Nutrition, Metabolism & Cardiovascular Diseases*, researchers from Iran investigated the association between alpha lipoic acid supplementation and levels of C-reactive protein, a marker of cardiovascular inflammation. Their analysis included 11 randomized, placebo-controlled trials with 264 participants in the supplement groups and 287 in the control groups. The trials were carried out in Korea, United States, Italy, Iran, China, and Spain between 2007 and 2017; the duration of the trials ranged from 2 to 51.4 weeks, with a median range of 8 weeks. Supplement dosages ranged from 300 to 1200 mg per day, with a median dose of 600 mg per day. The researchers learned that alpha lipoic acid significantly lowered the levels of C-reactive protein. In addition, neither the supplement dose nor duration of intervention appeared to have an effect on the final levels of C-reactive protein. The researchers concluded that their findings demonstrated that alpha lipoic acid supplementation "could significantly decrease CRP [C-reactive protein] level in patients with elevated levels of this inflammatory marker."[11]

In This Study, Alpha Lipoic Acid Was Found to Be Safe during Pregnancy

In an observational retrospective study published in 2017 in the journal *European Review for Medical and Pharmacological Sciences*, researchers from Italy collected data on 610 expectant mothers who had been treated with alpha lipoic acid during pregnancy. The supplements were prescribed at a dose of 600 mg per day by physicians for a variety of medical concerns, such as treatment for uterine contractions and threatened miscarriage. Four hundred and twenty participants took the supplement for at least 20 weeks. Data on both the mothers and the fetuses/newborn infants were collected and reviewed. The researchers determined that alpha lipoic acid supplementation during pregnancy was "completely safe." The supplementation did not result in adverse effects in the mothers or the infants. All the monitored parameters were not significantly different in the treated or control groups. The researchers concluded that "in some cases, [the results] were better in the treated group."[12]

NOTES

1. Nguven, N., and J. K. Takemoto. "A Case for Alpha-Lipoic Acid as an Alternative Treatment for Diabetic Polyneuropathy." *Journal of Pharmacy & Pharmaceutical Sciences* 21, no. 1s (2018): 177s–191s.

2. Agathos, Evangelos, Anastasios Tentolouris, Ioanna Eleftheriadou, et al. "Effect of α-Lipoic Acid on Symptoms and Quality of Life in Patients with Painful Diabetic Neuropathy." *Journal of International Medical Research* 46, no. 5 (2018): 1779–1790.

3. Wang, Xiaotong, Haixiong Lin, Shuai Xu, et al. "Alpha Lipoic Acid Combined with Epalrestat: A Therapeutic Option for Patients with Diabetic Peripheral Neuropathy." *Drug Design, Development and Therapy* 12 (2018): 2827–2840.

4. Mijnhout, G. S., A. Alkhalaf, N. Kleefstra, and H. J. G. Bilo. "Alpha Lipoic Acid: A New Treatment for Neuropathic Pain in Patients with Diabetes?" *The Netherland Journal of Medicine* 68, no. 4 (April 2010): 158–162.

5. Ruessmann, H. J. "Switching from Pathogenetic Treatment with Alpha-Lipoic Acid to Gabapentin and Other Analgesics in Painful Diabetic Neuropathy: A Real-World Study in Outpatients." *Journal of Diabetes and Its Complications* 23, no. 3 (May–June 2009): 174–177.

6. Koh, Eun Hee, Woo Je Lee, Sang Ah Lee, et al. "Effects of Alpha-Lipoic Acid on Body Weight in Obese Subjects." *The American Journal of Medicine* 124, no. 1 (January 2011): 85.e1–85.e8.

7. Huerta, A. E., S. Navas-Carretero, P. L. Prieto-Hontoria, et al. "Effects of α-Lipoic Acid and Eicosapentaenoic Acid in Overweight and Obese Women During Weight Loss." *Obesity* 23, no. 2 (February 2015): 313–321.

8. Kucukgoncu, Suat, Elton Zhou, Katherine B. Lucas, and Cenk Tek. "Alpha-Lipoic Acid (ALA) as a Supplementation for Weight Loss: Results from a Meta-Analysis of Randomized Controlled Trials." *Obesity Reviews* 18, no. 5 (May 2017): 594–601.

9. Basttisti, E., A. Albanese, L. Guerra, et al. "Alpha Lipoic Acid and Superoxide Dismutase in the Treatment of Chronic Low Back Pain." *European Journal of Physical and Rehabilitation Medicine* 49, no. 5 (October 2013): 659–664.

10. El-Komy, M., S. Shalaby, R. Hegazy, et al. "Assessment of Cubosomal Alpha Lipoic Acid Gel Efficacy for the Aging Face: A Single-Blinded, Placebo-Controlled, Right-Left Comparative Clinical Study." *Journal of Cosmetic Dermatology* 16, no. 3 (September 2017): 358–363.

11. Saboori, S., E. Falahi, E. Eslampour, et al. "Effects of Alpha-Lipoic Acid Supplementation on C-Reactive Protein Levels: A Systematic Review and Meta-Analysis of Randomized Controlled Clinical Trials." *Nutrition, Metabolism & Cardiovascular Diseases* 28, no. 8 (August 2018): 779–786.

12. Parente, E., G. Colannino, O. Picconi, and G. Monastra. "Safety of Oral Alpha-Lipoic Acid Treatment in Pregnant Women: A Retrospective Observational Study." *European Review for Medical and Pharmacological Sciences* 21 (2017): 4219–4227.

REFERENCES AND FURTHER READING

Agathos, Evangelos, Anastasios Tentolouris, Ioanna Eleftheriadou, et al. "Effect of α-Lipoic Acid on Symptoms and Quality of Life in Patients with Painful Diabetic Neuropathy." *Journal of International Medical Research* 46, no. 5 (2018): 1779–1790.

Battisti, E., A. Albanese, L. Guerra, et al. "Alpha Lipoic Acid and Superoxide Dismutase in the Treatment of Chronic Back Pain." *European Journal of Physical and Rehabilitation Medicine* 49, no. 5 (October 2013): 659–664.

El-Komy, Mohamed, Suzan Shalaby, Rehab Hegazy, et al. "Assessment of Cubosomal Alpha Lipoic Acid Gel Efficacy for the Aging Face: A Single-Blinded, Placebo-Controlled, Right-Left Comparative Clinical Study." *Journal of Cosmetic Dermatology* 16, no. 3 (September 2017): 358–363.

Huerta, A. E., S. Navas-Carretero, P. L. Prieto-Hontoria, et al. "Effects of α-Lipoic Acid and Eicosapentaenoic Acid in Overweight and Obese Women During Weight Loss." *Obesity* 23, no. 2 (February 2015): 313–321.

Koh, Eun Hee, Woo Je Lee, Sang Ah Lee, et al. "Effects of Alpha-Lipoic Acid on Body Weight in Obese Subjects." *The American Journal of Medicine* 124, no. 1 (January 2011): 85.e1–85.e8.

Kucukgoncu, Suat, Elton Zhou, Katherine B. Lucas, and Cenk Tek. "Alpha-Lipoic Acid (ALA) as a Supplementation for Weight Loss: Results from a Meta-Analysis of Randomized Controlled Trials." *Obesity Reviews* 18, no. 5 (May 2017): 594–601.

Mijnhout, G. S., A. Alkhalaf, N. Kleefstra, H. J. G Bilo. "Alpha Lipoic Acid: A New Treatment for Neuropathic Pain in Patients with Diabetes?" *The Netherlands Journal of Medicine* 68, no. 4 (April 2010): 158–162.

Nguyen, N., and J. K. Takemoto. "A Case for Alpha-Lipoic Acid as an Alternative Treatment for Diabetic Polyneuropathy." *Journal of Pharmacy & Pharmaceutical Sciences* 21, no. 1s (2018): 177s–191s.

Parente, E., G. Colannino, O. Picconi, and G. Monastra. "Safety of Oral Alpha-Lipoic Acid Treatment in Pregnant Women: A Retrospective Observational Study." *European Review of Medical and Pharmacological Sciences* 21 (2017): 4219–4227.

Ruessmann, H. J. "Switching from Pathogenetic Treatment with Alpha-Lipoic Acid to Gabapentin and Other Analgesics in Painful Diabetic Neuropathy: A Real-World Study in Outpatients." *Journal of Diabetes and Its Complications* 23, no. 3 (May–June 2009): 174–177.

Saboori, S., E. Falahi, E. Eslampour, et al. "Effects of Alpha-Lipoic Acid Supplementation on C-Reactive Protein Level: A Systematic Review and Meta-Analysis of Randomized Controlled Clinical Trials." *Nutrition, Metabolism & Cardiovascular Diseases* 28, no. 8 (August 2018): 779–786.

Wang, Xiaotong, Haixiong Lin, Shuai Xu, et al. "Alpha Lipoic Acid Combined with Epalrestat: A Therapeutic Option for Patients with Diabetic Peripheral Neuropathy." *Drug Design, Development and Therapy* 12 (2018): 2827–2840.

Ashwagandha

Also known as *Withania somnifera*, Indian ginseng, winter cherry, and somnifera root, ashwagandha is an ancient medicinal herb derived from a plant in the nightshade (*Solanaceae*) family. It is an important herb in Ayurveda, a form of alternative medicine based on the Indian principles of natural healing that has been used for over 3000 years.

The name ashwagandha is derived from the Sanskrit language and is a combination of the word ashua, horse, and the word gandha, smell. The root has a strong "horse-like" aroma. In India, ashwagandha has traditionally been used to strengthen the immune system after illnesses; supposedly, people will develop the strength and vitality of a horse.

HEALTH BENEFITS AND RISKS

Ashwagandha is believed to be useful for a wide variety of medical concerns. Because ashwagandha is an adaptogen, it helps the body deal with stress and reduces cortisol levels, the stress hormone. It has anticancer and anti-inflammation properties and lowers anxiety and depression. In addition, ashwagandha decreases levels of blood sugar and cholesterol and possibly increases muscle mass and strength. Many of these health benefits are attributed to high concentrations of withanolides, naturally occurring steroids.

Ashwagandha is thought to be safe for most people. However, its safety is yet to be determined for pregnant and breastfeeding women. Moreover, because it may speed up the immune system, people with autoimmune disorders may be advised to avoid this supplement. People with diabetes should discuss the use of ashwagandha with a medical provider as it may interfere with diabetes medications. Moreover, it may increase the response of sleeping medications, making people overly sleepy. Ashwagandha supplementation should be discontinued 2 weeks before any surgical procedure.

HOW IT IS SOLD AND TAKEN

Ashwagandha is sold as capsules, tablets, powder, and liquid extract. It is usually prepared from the roots and leaves of the plant. Although there are no overall dosage recommendations, some suggest starting with 300 to 500 mg per day. It is not uncommon to recommend between 1000 and 1500 mg per day. It is best to follow the package directions.

RESEARCH FINDINGS

Ashwagandha Seems to Support Health in Healthy People

In a prospective open-label trial published in 2012 in the *Journal of Ayurveda & Integrative Medicine*, researchers in India evaluated the tolerability, safety, and activity of ashwagandha. The researchers enrolled 18 "apparently healthy" volunteers between the ages of 18 and 30 years, with a mean age of 24.33 years. After conducting several different baseline assessments, all the participants took ashwagandha capsules daily in two divided doses with increase in daily doses every 10 days for 30 days. (750 mg per day for 10 days, 1000 mg per day for 10 days, and 1250 mg per day for 10 days.) During the trial, there were a number of additional assessments. The researchers determined that ashwagandha was safe even in the higher doses used in the study. No intolerances or adverse effects were observed in vital functions, such as body temperature, pulse rate, respiratory rate, and systolic and diastolic blood pressure. While sleep duration did not exhibit significant change, the quality of sleep improved in six participants. The supplementation also appeared to improve muscle strength, and had lipid-lowering properties.[1]

Ashwagandha May Have Antianxiety and Antistress Properties

In a systematic review published in 2014 in the *Journal of Alternative and Complementary Medicine*, researchers from Syracuse, New York, and New Haven, Connecticut (USA), assessed the ability of ashwagandha to help people with anxiety and stress. Five human trials met their inclusion criteria; sample sizes varied as did the doses of ashwagandha and the methodologies. Still, the researchers found that, compared to placebos, ashwagandha generally produced favorable results. In fact, four of the five trials found significant differences between ashwagandha and placebos. In the fifth study, which had the shortest trial duration and the smallest sample size, there was a difference between ashwagandha and the placebo, but it failed to achieve significance. Yet, according to the researchers, all the studies probably had a moderate-to-high risk of bias. At the same time, no study reported any significant adverse effects of the supplement. The researchers concluded that, although ashwagandha appears to alleviate symptoms of anxiety and stress, "additional research in larger samples and in more clinical contexts is essential to validate its therapeutic capabilities for widespread use."[2]

In a prospective, randomized, double-blind, placebo-controlled trial published in 2012 in the *Indian Journal of Psychological Medicine*, researchers from India examined the safety and efficacy of high-concentration full-spectrum ashwagandha root for reducing stress and anxiety. The initial cohort consisted of 64 patients with a history of chronic stress; there were 41 males and 23 females. For 60 days, the participants took either one capsule twice daily of 300 mg of high-concentration full-spectrum extract from the root of the ashwagandha plant or a placebo. Sixty-one participants completed the trial. The researchers determined that the participants taking ashwagandha had "substantial reduction" in several measures of stress. For example, their levels of serum cortisol, which tends to increase in stressful situations, decreased. The researchers found evidence that ashwagandha mitigated "not only the focal aspects of stress but also some of the precursors, consequences and associated symptoms of stress," which was accomplished both "directly and indirectly."[3]

Ashwagandha Appears to Be Useful for Knee Joint Pain

In a prospective, randomized, double-blind, placebo-controlled trial published in 2016 in the *Journal of Ayurveda and Integrative Medicine*, researchers from India investigated the ability of ashwagandha to relieve knee joint pain. The cohort consisted of 60 participants (43 males and 17 females) with a mean age of 57.78 years. For 12 weeks, the participants with knee pain took 250 mg per day of ashwagandha, 500 mg per day of ashwagandha, or a placebo. The participants were evaluated at baseline, 4 weeks, 8 weeks, and at the end of the trial. The researchers conducted symptom and tolerability assessments. All the participants completed the trial. By the end of the trial, participants taking supplements had significant symptom reduction, with a greater reduction among those on higher doses. Participants taking the high-dose supplement were the least likely to use the rescue medication, Paracetamol (acetaminophen). Participants in the placebo group were most likely to use the rescue medication. Participants on the higher dose had earlier and better symptoms relief, "thus increasing patient compliance and satisfaction." In addition, the researchers concluded that "the therapeutic response appears to be dose-dependent and free of any significant GI disturbances."[4]

Ashwagandha Seems to Support Muscle Strength and Recovery

In an 8-week, randomized, prospective, double-blind, placebo-controlled clinical trial published in 2015 in the *Journal of the International Society of Sports Nutrition*, researchers from India investigated the ability of ashwagandha supplementation to support muscle strength and recovery. The cohort consisted of 57 males between the ages of 18 and 50 years who had little experience with resistance training. Twenty-nine participants were placed in a treatment group, who took 300 mg of ashwagandha root extract supplementation twice daily. Twenty-eight participants in the control group took placebos. Three times each week, the participants in both groups participated in an upper and lower body resistance training program. The researchers learned that the participants in both groups experienced "a substantial degree of improvement in muscle-related parameters." Still, the participants taking the supplement had better gains in muscle strength, body composition, and testosterone. The researchers commented that their findings "confirmed previous data regarding the adaptogenic properties of ashwagandha and suggests it might be a useful adjunct to strength training."[5]

Ashwagandha May Help People with Subclinical Levels of Hypothyroidism (Low Levels of Thyroid Hormones)

In a prospective, randomized, double-blind, placebo-controlled pilot trial published in 2018 in the *Journal of Alternative and Complementary Medicine*, researchers from India evaluated the efficacy and safety of ashwagandha supplementation for people with subclinical hypothyroid disease. For 8 weeks, 50 participants between the ages of 18 and 50 years with subclinical hypothyroidism were placed on 600 mg per day of ashwagandha root extract (n = 25) or a placebo (n = 25). During the trial, two participants from each group withdrew from the study. Assessments were conducted at baseline and during the trial. The researchers learned that the ashwagandha supplement "effectively normalized" the thyroid indices, and it was "safe and tolerable, with few mild and temporary adverse effects." The researchers underscored the need for future studies with larger sample sizes for longer periods of time.[6]

Ashwagandha Supplementation May Support Cognition and Psychomotor Performance

In a prospective, double-blind, multidose, placebo-controlled, crossover trial published in 2014 in the journal *Pharmacognosy Research*, researchers from India examined the cognitive and psychomotor effects of ashwagandha supplementation in healthy humans. The initial cohort consisted of 26 healthy males between the ages of 20 and 35 years. For 14 days, they took 500 mg twice each day of an aqueous extract of ashwagandha roots and leaves or a matching placebo. Periodic assessments were conducted on cognitive and psychomotor performance. After a washout period of 14 days, the participants were placed on alternative treatment, and the same assessments were completed. Six participants did not complete all the requirements of the trial. Therefore, the final analyses included findings from 20 participants. The researchers determined that the supplementation improved the cognitive and psychomotor performance in all but one of the various tests. Still, the researchers cautioned that "multicentric long-term clinical studies in patients are required to confirm its therapeutic efficacy in disease states associated with impaired cognition and psychomotor function."[7]

Ashwagandha Supplementation May Support Cardiovascular Health, at Least in People with Schizophrenia

In a randomized, double-blind, placebo-controlled clinical trial published in 2013 in the *Indian Journal of Pharmacology*, researchers from India wanted to learn if ashwagandha supplement would support cardiac health in people with schizophrenia. Why is this important? People taking second-generation antipsychotic medications have an increased risk of metabolic syndrome, which in turn is associated with cardiovascular problems, such as elevated serum triglyceride and fasting blood glucose levels. The cohort consisted of 30 schizophrenia patients; at baseline, the patients had similar demographic characteristics. For 1 month, half of the patients took three 400 mg capsules per day of the ashwagandha supplement, and the other half took a placebo. Tests were conducted at baseline and at the end of the trial. Five patients were lost to follow-up. While no changes were observed in the placebo group, after 1 month, the patients in the treatment group had a statistically significant reduction in serum triglycerides and fasting blood glucose levels. The researchers emphasized the need for more research, concluding that "the results of this trial, if confirmed through large clinical trials, will certainly aid the therapeutics not only for patients having drug-induced MS [metabolic syndrome] but also for those having MS due to other causes."[8]

Ashwagandha Supplementation May Help Some People Lose Weight

In an 8-week, prospective, double-blind, randomized, placebo-controlled trial published in 2017 in the *Journal of Evidence-Based Complementary & Alternative Medicine*, researchers from India evaluated the ability of ashwagandha supplement to help chronically stressed people deal with stress and their weight. According to the researchers, it is well-known that stress has been linked to weight gain, obesity, and metabolic syndrome. The cohort consisted of 52 participants who were overweight and under chronic stress; there were 38 males and 14 females between the ages of 18 and 60 years. Symptoms of stress included difficulty in concentration, insomnia, anxiety, and restlessness. During the trial, participants took either 600 mg per day of ashwagandha supplement or a placebo. Both the supplement and placebo were identical in appearance. The final analyses were conducted on 50 participants, who were assessed at baseline and at 4 and 8 weeks. The researchers learned that the participants taking the supplementation had significantly greater reduction in stress than those in the placebo group. In addition, by the end of the trial, the participants taking the supplement had significant lower levels of food cravings than those in the placebo group, with a statistically significant reduction in body weight and body mass index. Almost all the participants in both groups reported "excellent" tolerability of their supplements. The researchers concluded that ashwagandha root extract may "be useful for body-weight management in patients experiencing chronic stress."[9]

Ashwagandha Supplement Appears to Have a Limited Ability to Support Cognition in People with Bipolar Disorder

In an 8-week, randomized, double-blind, placebo-controlled trial published in 2013 in the *Journal of Clinical Psychiatry*, researchers from Pittsburgh, Pennsylvania (USA), and Ontario, Canada noted that there are few data on treatment options for cognitive impairment in people with bipolar disorder. As a result, they decided to test the ability of ashwagandha supplement to assist people with this serious psychiatric problem. The initial cohort consisted of 60 euthymic patients with bipolar disorder, who were assigned to take a dose that led up to 500 mg per day of ashwagandha supplement or a placebo. Almost all the patients were maintained on a dose of 500 mg per day. Three patients were titrated back to 250 mg per day because of "vivid dreams" and "sleepiness." Approximately 60 min of cognitive testing was conducted at baseline and at the end of the trial. One time-point at 4 weeks was added to assess a secondary outcome. Fifty-three patients completed the trial (24 in the supplement group and 29 in the placebo group). There were only minor reports of adverse events. The researchers learned that the patients taking ashwagandha supplement had significantly greater improvement compared to those on placebo in three cognitive tests—mean digital span backward, neutral mean response time, and mean social cognition response rating. However, none of the other cognitive tests they conducted found significant differences between the two groups. The researchers commented that they had expected that the supplement would have "a broader profile of cognitive benefits." In addition, they underscored the need for more research, "given the paucity of data for improving cognitive capacity in bipolar disorder."[10]

Ashwagandha Supplementation May Help People with Mild Cognitive Impairment

In a pilot, prospective, randomized, double-blind, placebo-controlled trial published in 2017 in the *Journal of Dietary Supplements*, researchers from India wanted to learn if ashwagandha supplementation would improve memory in people with mild cognitive impairment. The cohort consisted of 50 adults who were at least 35 years old; all the participants had mild cognitive impairment: "a transitional state between normal cognitive aging and dementia." At baseline, the demographic characteristics and degree of cognitive impairment in both groups were similar. For 8 weeks, the participants were treated with 300 mg ashwagandha root extract twice each day, or a placebo. All the participants were assessed at baseline, after 4 weeks, and at the end of the trial. The researchers commented that they conducted "a battery of cognitive tests." By the end of the trial, compared to those taking the placebo, the participants taking ashwagandha demonstrated significant cognitive improvement. The treatment group also had improvement in executive function, sustained attention, and information processing speed. The results of the testing for working memory and visuospatial processing were inconclusive. The researchers concluded that ashwagandha supplementation appears to be useful for mild cognitive impairment.[11]

Ashwagandha Supplementation May Benefit People with Obsessive-Compulsive Disorder

In a randomized, double-blind, placebo-controlled trial published in 2016 in the journal *Complementary Therapies in Medicine*, researchers from Iran and Australia wanted to learn if ashwagandha supplement would help people suffering from obsessive-compulsive disorder. The cohort consisted of 30 patients with obsessive-compulsive disorder who were being treated with selective serotonin reuptake inhibitor medication. For 6 weeks, the participants took either 120 mg per day of ashwagandha supplementation or a lactose placebo; there were 15 participants in each group. Participants were monitored for side effects such as diarrhea; however, there were no reports of adverse side effects. The researchers learned that ashwagandha was an effective adjunct therapy for people dealing with obsessive-compulsive disorder. Participants in the treatment group had significant improvement in their obsessive-compulsive symptoms. The researchers concluded that ashwagandha extract "may be beneficial as an adjunct therapy to regular treatments of OCD."[12]

NOTES

1. Raut, Ashwinikumar A., Nirmala N. Rege, Firoz M. Tadvi, et al. "Exploratory Study to Evaluate Tolerability, Safety, and Activity of Ashwagandha (*Withania somnifera*) in Healthy Volunteers." *Journal of Ayurveda & Integrative Medicine* 3, no. 3 (July–September 2012): 111–114.

2. Pratte, Morgan A., Kaushal B. Nanavati, Virginia Young, and Christopher P. Morley. "An Alternative Treatment for Anxiety: A Systematic Review of Human Trial Results Reported for the Ayurvedic Herb Ashwagandha (*Withania somnifera*)." *Journal of Alternative and Complementary Medicine* 20, no 12 (December 1, 2014): 901–908.

3. Chandrasekhar, K., Jyoti Kapoor, and Sridhar Anishetty. "A Prospective, Randomized Double-Blind, Placebo-Controlled Study of Safety and efficacy of a High-Concentration Full-Spectrum Extract of *Ashwagandha* Root in Reducing Stress and Anxiety in Adults." *Indian Journal of Psychological Medicine* 34, no. 3 (July–September 2012): 255–262.

4. Ramakanth, G. S. H., C. Uday Kumar, P. V. Kishan, and P. Usharani. "A Randomized, Double-Blind Placebo-Controlled Study of Efficacy and Tolerability of *Withania somnifera* Extracts in Knee Joint Pain." *Journal of Ayurveda and Integrative Medicine* 7 (2016): 151–157.

5. Wankhede, Sachin, Deepak Langade, Kedar Joshi, et al. "Examining the Effect of *Withania somnifera* Supplementation on Muscle Strength and Recovery: A Randomized Controlled Trial." *Journal of the International Society of Sports Nutrition* 12 (2015): 43–53.

6. Sharma, A. K., I. Basu, and S. Singh. "Efficacy and Safety of Ashwagandha Root Extract in Subclinical Hypothyroid Patients: A Double-Blind, Randomized Placebo-Controlled Trial." *Journal of Alternative and Complementary Medicine* 24, no. 3 (2018): 243–248.

7. Pingali, Usharani, Raveendranadh Pilli, and Nishat Fatima. "Effect of Standardized Aqueous Extract of *Withania somnifera* on Tests of Cognitive and Psychomotor Performance in Healthy Human Participants." *Pharmacognosy Research* 6, no. 1 (January–March 2014): 12–18.

8. Agnihotri, Akshay P., Smita D. Sontakke, Vijay R. Thawani, et al. "Effects of *Withania somnifera* in Patients of Schizophrenia: A Randomized, Double Blind, Placebo Controlled Pilot Trial Study." *Indian Journal of Pharmacology* 45, no. 4 (July–August 2013): 417–418.

9. Choudhary, Dnyanraj, Sauvik Bhattacharyya, and Kedar Joshi. "Body Weight Management in Adults under Chronic Stress through Treatment with Ashwagandha Root Extract: A Double-Blind, Randomized, Placebo-Controlled Trial." *Journal of Evidence-Based Complementary & Alternative Medicine* 22, no. 1 (2017): 96–106.

10. Chengappa, K. N. Roy, Christopher R. Bowie, Patricia J. Schlicht, et al. "Randomized Placebo-Controlled Adjunctive Study of the Extract of *Withania somnifera* for

Cognitive Dysfunction in Bipolar Disorder." *Journal of Clinical Psychiatry* 74, no. 11 (2013): 1076–1083.

11. Choudhary, Dnyanraj, Sauvik Bhattacharyya, and Sekhar Bose. "Efficacy and Safety of Ashwagandha (*Withania somnifera* (L.) *Dunal*) Root Extract in Improving Memory and Cognitive Functions." *Journal of Dietary Supplements* 14, no. 6 (2017): 599–612.

12. Jahanbakhsh, S. P., A. A. Manteghi, S. A. Emammi, et al. "Evaluation of the Efficacy of *Withania somnifera* (Ashwagandha) Root Extract in Patients with Obsessive-Compulsive Disorder: A Randomized Double-Blind Placebo-Controlled Trial." *Complementary Therapies in Medicine* 27 (August 2016): 25–29.

REFERENCES AND FURTHER READING

Agnihotri, Akshay P., Smita D. Sontakke, Vijay R. Thawani, et al. "Effects of *Withania somnifera* in Patients of Schizophrenia: A Randomized, Double Blind, Placebo Controlled Pilot Trial Study." *Indian Journal of Pharmacology* 45, no. 4 (July–August 2013): 417–418.

Chandrsaekhar, K., Jyoti Kapoor, and Sridhar Anishetty. "A Prospective, Randomized Double-Blind, Placebo-Controlled Study of Safety and Efficacy of a High-Concentration Full-Spectrum Extract of *Ashwagandha* Root in Reducing Stress and Anxiety in Adults." *Indian Journal of Psychological Medicine* 34, no. 3 (July–September 2012): 355–262.

Chengappa, K. N. Roy, Christopher R. Bowie, Patricia J. Schlicht, et al. "Randomized Placebo-Controlled Adjunctive Study of an Extract of *Withania somnifera* for Cognitive Dysfunction in Bipolar Disorder." *Journal of Clinical Psychiatry* 74, no. 11 (2013): 1076–1083.

Choudhary, Dnyanraj, Sauvik Bhattacharyya, and Sekhar Bose. "Efficacy and Safety of Ashwagandha (*Withania somnifera* (L.) *Dunal*) Root Extract in Improving Memory and Cognitive Functions." *Journal of Dietary Supplements* 14, no. 6 (2017): 599–612.

Choudhary, Dnyanraj, Sauvik Bhattacharyya, and Kedar Joshi. "Body Weight Management in Adults under Chronic Stress, through Treatment with Ashwagandha Root Extract: A Double-Blind, Randomized, Placebo-Controlled Trial." *Journal of Evidence-Based Complementary & Alternative Medicine* 22, no. 1 (January 2017): 96–106.

Jahanbakhsh, S. P., A. A. Manteghi, S. A. Emami, et al. "Evaluation of the Efficacy of *Withania somnifera* (Ashwagandha) Root Extract in Patients with Obsessive-Compulsive Disorder: A Randomized Double-Blind Placebo-Controlled Trial." *Complementary Therapies in Medicine* 27 (August 2016): 25–29.

Pingali, Usharani, Raveendranadh Pilli, and Nishat Fatima. "Effect of Standardized Aqueous Extract of *Withania somnifera* on Tests of Cognitive and Psychomotor Performance in Healthy Human Participants." *Pharmacognosy Research* 6, no. 1 (January–March 2014): 12–18.

Pratte, Morgan A., Kaushal B. Nanavati, Virginia Young, and Christopher P. Morley. "An Alternative Treatment for Anxiety: A Systematic review of Human Trial Results Reported for the Ayurvedic Herb Ashwagandha (*Withania somnifera*)." *Journal of Alternative and Complementary Medicine* 20, no. 12 (December 1, 2014): 901–908.

Ramakanth, G. S. H., C. Uday Kumar, P. V. Kishan, and P. Usharani. "A Randomized, Double-Blind Placebo-Controlled Study of Efficacy and Tolerability of *Withania somnifera* Extracts in Knee Joint Pain." *Journal of Ayurveda and Integrative Medicine* 7 (2016): 151–157.

Raut, Ashwinikumar A., Nirmala N. Rege, Firoz M. Tadvi, et al. "Exploratory Study to Evaluate tolerability, Safety, and Activity of Ashwagandha (*Withania somnifera*) in Healthy Volunteers." *Journal of Ayurveda & Integrative Medicine* 3, no. 3 (July–September 2012): 111–114.

Sharma, A. K., I. Basu, and S. Singh. "Efficacy and Safety of Ashwagandha Root Extract in Subclinical Hypothyroid Patients: A Double-Blind, Randomized Placebo-Controlled Trial." *Journal of Alternative and Complementary Medicine* 24, no. 3 (2018): 243–248.

Wankhede, Sachin, Deepak Langade, Kedar Joshi, et al. "Examining the Effect of *Withania somnifera* Supplementation on Muscle Strength and Recover: A Randomized Controlled Trial." *Journal of the International Society of Sports Nutrition* 12 (2015): 43–53.

Black Cohosh

Native to North America, black cohosh is a member of the buttercup family. For more than two centuries, it has been used for menstrual cramps and menopausal problems, such as hot flashes. Because of these alleged properties, it has become one of the most popular supplements, especially among menopausal women concerned with the risks associated with hormone therapy. Still, the benefits may not be as notable as some believe. Black cohosh should not be confused with blue cohosh, which is a different herb.

HEALTH BENEFITS AND RISKS

Black cohosh is thought to be useful for numerous medical problems, such as premenstrual syndrome, anxiety, and vaginal dryness. In some instances, black cohosh has been used to induce labor. Yet, the research on using black cohosh for these medical problems is mixed and often inconclusive.

Black cohosh may interact negatively with other herbs or traditional remedies. Some commercial black cohosh products contain the wrong herb or mixture of black cohosh and other ingredients that are not listed on the label. For example, black cohosh mixed with salicylic acid, the active component in aspirin. This supplement can be very harmful, even dangerous, to people who are intolerant or allergic to aspirin. In some people, especially those who have a liver disorder, black cohosh may trigger liver problems, which may include symptoms such as abdominal pain, dark urine, and jaundice.

High doses of black cohosh may result in a number of side effects including abdominal pain, shortness of breath, diarrhea, dizziness, headaches, joint pains, nausea, slow heart rate, tremors, visual dimness, vomiting, and weight gain.

Because the pediatric use of black cohosh has not been studied, children should not ingest black cohosh in any form. To be safe, pregnant and breastfeeding women should also avoid black cohosh. Because the long-term effects of black cohosh are unknown, its long-term use is not recommended. In general, black cohosh should not be used for more than a year.

HOW IT IS SOLD AND TAKEN

Black cohosh is sold as a dried root tea, an extract, liquid tincture, and in tablets and capsules. The recommended dose of black cohosh ranges from 20 to 80 mg per day. Black cohosh tincture of 2 to 4 mg can be consumed one to three times per day in water or tea. However, some sources recommend higher doses. It is not known whether black cohosh should be taken with or without food.

RESEARCH FINDINGS

Black Cohosh May Be Useful for Postmenopausal Women with Sleep Disturbances

In a randomized, double-blind, placebo-controlled trial published in 2015 in the journal *Climacteric*, researchers from China and the United Kingdom wanted to determine if black cohosh supplementation would be useful for early postmenopausal women experiencing sleep disturbances. The initial cohort consisted of 48 women between the ages of 45 and 60 years who had sleep disturbances. They were placed on daily black cohosh supplementation or a placebo for 6 months. Forty-two women completed the entire trial. Sleep was both objectively and subjectively assessed. Compared to the placebo group, the women on black cohosh had increased sleep efficiency and were less likely to awaken after falling asleep. In addition, black cohosh "had the potential to ameliorate perceived sleep quality." The researchers concluded that their findings "open the possibility that black cohosh might be useful in menopause-related sleep disturbance."[1]

It Is Not Clear If Women Who Have Already Been Diagnosed with Breast Cancer or Are at Increased Risk from Breast Cancer Benefit from Black Cohosh

In a systematic review published in 2014 in the journal *Integrative Cancer Therapies*, researchers from Canada examined the use of black cohosh in women who were diagnosed with breast cancer or who were at an increased risk for breast cancer. The researchers included 26 articles—14 randomized controlled trials, seven uncontrolled trials, and five observational studies. Although the results were mixed, the overall impression was that there is no current evidence to support an association between the use of black cohosh and an increased risk for breast cancer. In four studies that investigated the impact of black cohosh on breast cancer risk, two studies found no significant association and two reported an inverse relationship—black cohosh supplementation was associated with a significantly reduced risk of primary breast cancer risk incidence or breast cancer recurrence. Black cohosh appeared to have "limited estrogen activity." The researchers commented that "more evidence is required to confirm these early findings before the question of black cohosh's safety and efficacy in this population can be conclusively answered."[2]

Postmenopausal Women Might Benefit from Black Cohosh Supplementation

In a study published in 2016 in the journal *Rejuvenation Research*, researchers from Beijing (China) examined the long-term effect of black cohosh on glucose and lipid metabolism in a postmenopausal rat model. The researchers divided 40 female Sprague–Dawley rats into four groups of 10 rats. While one group served as control, other rats were ovariectomized. One group of the ovariectomized rats was not treated. Two groups of ovariectomized rats were treated with estradiol valerate, a hormone, and black cohosh. The researchers monitored body weight, body composition, and blood glucose levels. Before the treatments began, the rats in all groups had similar body weights. After 3 months, the rats in the two treatments groups had lower body weight, lower glucose levels, lower low-density lipoprotein levels, and lower serum triglyceride levels than those in the ovariectomized group that received no treatment. The researchers concluded that "black cohosh at a proper dose is promising for the treatment of metabolic derangements in women around or after menopause."[3]

Preparations Containing Black Cohosh Appear to Improve Menopausal Symptoms

In a meta-analysis published in 2010 in the journal *Alternative Therapies in Health and Medicine*, researchers from Canada wanted to learn if black cohosh supplementation would help menopausal symptoms, such as hot flashes. Their review included nine randomized placebo-controlled trials, with more than 1,400 participants. Five trials had black cohosh combined with another product, and the average age of the women ranged from 50.5 to 59 years. Six of the studies demonstrated a significant improvement in the black cohosh group compared to the placebo group. The researchers concluded that black cohosh appeared to be effective in treating menopausal symptoms. Interestingly, the trial with the longest follow-up (12 months) and the highest dose of black cohosh (160 mg) did not demonstrate significant improvement in the black cohosh group compared to the placebo group. Still, when black cohosh was combined with other products, such as St. John's wort, it was even more efficacious in treating symptoms. The researchers found no differences in side effects in both black cohosh and placebo groups. Further, they underscored the need for more research on black cohosh, concluding that "given that black cohosh is one of the most frequently used herbal medications for vasomotor symptoms in North America and Europe, more research about its effectiveness and safety is warranted."[4]

In Another Study, Black Cohosh Did Not Relieve Hot Flashes

In a 12-month trial published in 2009 in the journal *Menopause*, researchers from Chicago, Illinois (USA), compared the ability of black cohosh, red clover, conjugated equine estrogens, and a placebo to help manage the vasomotor symptoms of menopause, specifically hot flashes. The initial cohort included 89 women; 80 women completed the trial. The average age of the participants was 53 years, with the last menstrual period averaging 4.3 years earlier. The researchers found that the average number of hot flashes experienced by women decreased in all four groups. Compared to the placebo group, the women in the estrogen group had a significant reduction in vasomotor symptoms. While black cohosh and red clover appeared to be safe during daily administration, neither of the supplement significantly reduced the women's vasomotor symptoms. The researchers concluded that "positive safety outcomes are important because women may be expected to continue to use black cohosh and red clover, regardless of scientific clinical findings."[5]

Black Cohosh Supplementation May Be a Good Choice for Women Who Have Fibroids and Menopausal Symptoms

In a study published in 2014 in the journal *Holistic Nursing Practice*, a researcher from Philadelphia, Pennsylvania (USA), investigated the use of black cohosh in women with menopausal symptoms who also have fibroids. She described a randomized, double-blind, parallel-group study that compared the use of black cohosh to tibolone on Chinese women with menopausal symptoms. (Tibolone is a hormone replacement therapy medication.) This 3-month trial included 244 women between the ages of 40 and 60 years and took place at three medical centers located at three cities in China. After a baseline appointment and examination, the women were assigned to consume black cohosh or tibolone. They were evaluated again at 4 weeks and 12 weeks. The researchers learned that the two treatments were statistically equivalent in efficacy, "including [in women with] moderate to severe symptoms."

It was later determined that 34 women consuming black cohosh and 28 consuming tibolone had uterine fibroids. Did consumption of black cohosh or tibolone alter the size of the fibroids? The researchers found that the women consuming black cohosh experienced decreases in the size of their fibroids. Although some women had decreases in fibroid size, on average, the women consuming tibolone tended to have small increases in the size of their fibroids. Thus, while both therapies were efficacious for relieving menopausal symptoms, black cohosh appeared to be a better choice for women with fibroids. The researchers concluded that black cohosh "seems to be a valid treatment option in patients with uterine fibroids, as it provides adequate relief from menopausal symptoms and avoids increase in uterine fibroid size, which is usually a cause of concern for the patient."[6]

Black Cohosh May Improve Oral/Mouth Dryness

In a study published in 2018 in the journal *Biomedicine & Pharmacotherapy*, researchers from China explained that a common feature of menopause is oral dryness or dry mouth. Estrogen is known to be useful for this medical problem. The researchers wanted to determine if black cohosh could alleviate this problem. The researchers purchased 44 female Sprague–Dawley rats and divided then into four groups—control rats, ovariectomized rats, ovariectomized rats on estradiol, and ovariectomized rats on black cohosh. The treatments continued for 4 weeks. All rats and water bottles were weighed. The researchers determined that the non-treated ovariectomized rats drank far more water than those treated with estradiol or black cohosh. Similar to estradiol, black cohosh "exerted a protective effect on salivary gland function." The researchers concluded that "black cohosh may be considered as an alternative therapy for relieving oral dryness" in women with menopausal symptoms.[7] While such a conclusion may or may not be warranted, women experiencing oral dryness may wish to try black cohosh supplementation.

Use of Black Cohosh during Labor and Delivery May Be Associated with Undesirable Outcomes

In an article published in 2016 in the *American Journal of Perinatology Reports*, physicians from Manhasset, New York (USA), described the case of a 39-year-old woman in labor who presented to their emergency department. For more than 2 days, she had been in labor at her home under the guidance of a midwife. During that time, in an effort to facilitate labor, she had consumed several doses of black cohosh, following which she had become disoriented and lethargic. When she arrived at the hospital, the woman was awake but very tired, nonverbal, and unable to follow commands. She had dangerously low levels of sodium in her blood, a condition known as hyponatremia. (Symptoms of hyponatremia include confusion, seizures, and coma.) After less than an hour, she became "uncooperative and combative," and the decision was made to proceed with a cesarean delivery. After the child was delivered, the woman was transferred to the intensive care unit, where her sodium levels were monitored and gradually corrected. Her mental status also improved, and she was transferred to a postpartum floor and subsequently discharged. The physicians noted that it is not uncommon for midwives to use herbal preparations to stimulate labor. In fact, it has been reported that 45% use black cohosh. The physicians underscored the need for more information on the use of black cohosh and other herbal supplements during pregnancy and labor. They concluded that "given the paucity of literature on black cohosh and other herbal supplements commonly used during pregnancy and labor, further investigation is warranted to evaluate their safety and efficacy."[8]

In Some People, Black Cohosh May Be Toxic to the Liver

In an article published in 2014 in the journal *Case Reports in Gastrointestinal Medicine*, researchers from Oklahoma City, Oklahoma (USA), Chicago, Illinois (USA), Phoenix, Arizona (USA), and Pakistan described the case of a 44-year-old woman who had painless jaundice for a month. Her primary care physician determined that she had elevated liver function. She did not improve on steroid medications. After she was admitted to the hospital, physicians conducted a number of tests including an ultrasound of the abdomen, which showed "nodular contour of the liver consistent with cirrhosis," caused by her intake of black cohosh. When she stopped consuming black cohosh, her symptoms and laboratory results improved. The researchers concluded that "remarkable improvement in the liver function after stopping the drug clearly demonstrates that there is a causal relationship."[9]

In a report published in 2009 in the journal *Alternative Therapies in Health and Medicine*, researchers from Italy summarized the case of a 37-year-old woman who was admitted to the infectious disease department of a hospital in Grosseto, Italy. The patient suffered from a variety of medical problems including nausea, widespread and unbearable itching, cough, and jaundice. She also had very high levels of a liver enzyme (alanine transaminase), as well as high levels of bile salts. At discharge, and thereafter, the patient continued to have high levels of the liver enzyme. After 10 months, a liver biopsy was performed, and she was found to have a mild form of hepatitis. At that point, the patient commented that she thought she had been taking a supplement that contained black cohosh. When the supplement was discontinued, she experienced complete recovery. The researchers noted that upon admission and during her hospitalization no medical provider asked her about the use of botanical medicines. The researchers concluded that their findings highlight "the importance of conducting a thorough medical investigation of complementary and alternative use."[10]

Black Cohosh Does Not Appear to Be Toxic in Other People

In a study published in 2011 in the journal *Evidence-Based Complementary and Alternative Medicine*, researchers from Italy noted that they frequently recommend black cohosh supplementation for women experiencing menopausal symptoms. In general, they recommend a dose of 500 or 1000 mg per day as a dry extract. To their knowledge, they have had no reports of adverse reactions. However, they decided to reach out and learn more. During a telephonic call or a discussion in person during a clinical examination, 107 women were asked about their experiences with black cohosh, who also underwent blood tests to check for liver disease. The researchers failed to find any connection between black cohosh and liver problems commenting that "in all of the patients, there was no sign of hepatic disease, or worsening of already altered but stable parameters."[11]

NOTES

1. Jiang, K., Y. Jin, L. Huang, et al. "Black Cohosh Improves Objective Sleep in Postmenopausal Women with Sleep Disturbance." *Climacteric* 18 (2015): 559–567.

2. Fritz, Heidi, Dugald Seely, Jessie McGowan, et al. "Black Cohosh and Breast Cancer: A Systematic Review." *Integrative Cancer Therapies* 13, no. 1 (2014): 12–29.

3. Sun, Y., Q. Yu, Q. Shen, et al. "Black Cohosh Ameliorates Metabolic Disorders in Female Ovariectomized Rats." *Rejuvenation Research* 19, no. 3 (June 2016): 204–214.

4. Shams, T., M. S. Setia, R. Hemmings, et al. "Efficacy of Black Cohosh-Containing Preparations on Menopausal Symptoms: A Meta-Analysis." *Alternative Therapies in Health and Medicine* 16, no. 1 (January–February 2010): 36–44.

5. Geller, Stacie E., Lee P. Shulman, Richard B. van Breeman, et al. "Safety and Efficacy of Black Cohosh and Red Clover for the Management of Vasomotor Symptoms: A Randomized Controlled Trial." *Menopause* 16, no. 6 (2009): 1156–1166.

6. Ross, Stephanie Maxine. "Efficacy of a Standardized Isopropanolic Black Cohosh (*Actaea Racemosa*) Extract in Treatment of Uterine Fibroids in Comparison with Tibolone Among Patients with Menopausal Symptoms." *Holistic Nursing Practice* 28, no. 6 (November–December 2014): 386–391.

7. Liu, S., K. Niu, Y. Da, et al. "Effects of Standardized Isopropanolic Black Cohosh and Estrogen on Salivary Function in Ovariectomized Rats." *Biomedicine & Pharmacotherapy* 97 (2018): 1438–1444.

8. Blitz, Matthew J., Michelle Smith-Levitin, and Burton Rochelson. "Severe Hyponatremia Associated with Use of Black Cohosh During Prolonged Labor and

Unsuccessful Home Birth." *American Journal of Perinatology Reports* 6, no. 1 (March 2016): e121–e124.

9. Adnan, Mohammed Muqeet, Muhammad Khan, Syed Hashmi, et al. "Black Cohosh and Liver Toxicity: Is There a Relationship?" *Case Reports in Gastrointestinal Medicine* 2014 (2014): Article ID 860614.

10. Vannacci, Alfredo, Francesco Lapi, Eugenia Gallo, et al. "A Case of Hepatitis Associated with Long-Term Use of *Cimicifuga racemosa.*" *Alternative Therapies in Health and Medicine* 15, no. 3 (May–June 2009): 62–63.

11. Firenzuoli, Fabio, Luigi Gori, and Paolo Roberti di Sarsina. "Black Cohosh Hepatic Safety: Follow-Up of 107 Patients Consuming a Special *Cimicifuga racemosa rhizome* Herbal Extract and Review of Literature." *Evidence-Based Complementary and Alternative Medicine* 2011 (2011): Article ID 821392.

REFERENCES AND FURTHER READING

Adnan, Mohammed Muqeet, Muhammad Khan, Syed Hashmi, et al. "Black Cohosh and Liver Toxicity: Is There a Relationship?" *Case Reports in Gastrointestinal Medicine* 2014 (2014): Article ID 860614.

Blitz, Matthew J., Michelle Smith-Levitin, and Burton Rochelson. "Severe Hyponatremia Associated with Use of Black Cohosh During Prolonged Labor and Unsuccessful Home Birth." *American Journal of Perinatology Reports* 6, no. 1 (March 2016): e121–e124.

Firenzuoli, Fabio, Luigi Gori, and Paolo Roberti di Sarsina. "Black Cohosh Hepatic Safety: Follow-Up of 107 Patients Consuming a Special *Cimicifuga racemosa rhizome* Herbal Extract and Review of Literature." *Evidence-Based Complementary and Alternative Medicine* 2011 (2011): Article ID 821392.

Fritz, Heidi, Dugald Seely, Jessie McGowan, et al. "Black Cohosh and Breast Cancer: A Systematic Review." *Integrative Cancer Therapies* 13, no. 1 (2014): 12–29.

Geller, Stacie E., Lee P. Shulman, Richard B. van Breemen, et al. "Safety and Efficacy of Black Cohosh and Red Clover for the Management of Vasomotor Symptoms: A Randomized Controlled Trial." *Menopause* 16, no. 6 (2009): 1156–1166.

Jiang, K., Y. Jin, L. Huang, et al. "Black Cohosh Improves Objective Sleep in Postmenopausal Women with Sleep Disturbance." *Climacteric* 18 (2015): 559–567.

Liu, Shuya, Kaiyu Niu, Yummeng Da, et al. "Effects of Standardized Isopropanolic Black Cohosh and Estrogen on Salivary Function in Ovariectomized Rats." *Biomedicine & Pharmacotherapy* 97 (2018): 1438–1444.

Ross, Stephanie Maxine. "Efficacy of a Standardized Isopropanolic Black Cohosh (*Actaea racemosa*) Extract in Treatment of Uterine Fibroids in Comparison with Tibolone Among Patients with Menopausal Symptoms." *Holistic Nursing Practice* 28, no. 6 (November–December 2014): 386–391.

Shams, T., M. S. Setia, R. Hemmings, et al. "Efficacy of Black Cohosh-Containing Preparations on Menopausal Symptoms: A Meta-Analysis." *Alternative Therapies in Health and Medicine* 16, no. 1 (January–February 2010): 36–44.

Sun, Y., Q. Yu, Q. Shen, et al. "Black Cohosh Ameliorates Metabolic Disorders in Female Ovariectomized Rats." *Rejuvenation Research* 19, no. 3 (June 2016): 204–214.

Vannacci, Alfredo, Francesco Lapi, Eugenia Gallo, et al. "A Case of Hepatitis Associated with Long-Term Use of *Cimicifuga racemosa.*" *Alternative Therapies in Health and Medicine* 15, no. 3 (May–June 2009): 62–63.

Branched-Chain Amino Acids

The 20 amino acids, which are the building blocks of proteins, make up thousands of different proteins in the human body. Nine of these are considered essential amino acids or those that cannot be made by the human body, and must be obtained through food or supplements. Of these nine, three are branched-chain amino acids (BCAAs)—leucine, isoleucine, and valine. The term branched-chain refers to the chemical structure of BCAAs, which are found in protein-rich foods such as eggs, meat, and dairy products. Although BCAA supplements are widely used among body builders and athletes, they are popular supplements that can be taken by people with varying athletic interests and abilities.

In humans, BCAAs account for 35% of the essential amino acids found in muscle proteins; they account for 40% of the total amino acids required by the body. Amino acids and proteins play a vital role in metabolism.

It should be parenthetically noted that branched-chain amino acids and branched-chain amino acid appear interchangeably in the literature. Therefore, they will be used in this entry interchangeably.

HEALTH BENEFITS AND RISKS

BCAAs are thought to build muscle, decrease overall fatigue and muscle fatigue, improve athletic performance, improve concentration, and alleviate muscle soreness. BCAAs may decrease muscle soreness by reducing damage to exercised muscles. Leucine is believed to activate a pathway in the body that stimulates the synthesis of muscle protein, the process of making muscle. BCAA supplementation may prevent the muscle wasting triggered by illnesses, such as cancer and malnutrition, and they may be useful for the natural muscle wasting associated with aging. In addition, BCAAs may be helpful in cirrhosis, a chronic disease in which the liver does not function properly. About half of the people with cirrhosis develop hepatic encephalopathy, a loss of brain function caused by the inability of the liver to remove toxins from the blood. Liver cirrhosis is a major risk for liver cancer.

Potential side effects of BCAAs include fatigue, loss of coordination, nausea, vomiting, diarrhea, and bloating. In rare instances, BCAAs may cause high blood pressure, headache, and skin whitening. It is not known if it is safe to take BCAAs during pregnancy or while breastfeeding. Because BCAAs may interfere with blood sugar levels, they may compromise medications for diabetes, and should not be combined with levodopa, a medication commonly used in Parkinson's disease. BCAAs should be discontinued at least 2 weeks before scheduled surgery.

HOW IT IS SOLD AND TAKEN

BCAAs are generally sold as a powder, capsule, or softgel; however, they may be administered intravenously by medical providers primarily for people with brain conditions associated with liver disease.

Dosing recommendations vary widely. Although the average requirement of BCAAs is 68 mg per day (34 mg leucine, 15 mg isoleucine, and 19 mg valine), higher doses, such as 144 mg, may be advised.

RESEARCH FINDINGS

BCAA Supplementation Helps People Undergoing Strenuous Exercise

In a clinical trial published in 2013 in the *Journal of Exercise Nutrition & Biochemistry*, researchers from Korea investigated the effects of BCAA supplementation on fatigue, muscle damage, and energy metabolism in people undergoing endurance exercise. Twenty-six male college students were randomly divided into a BCAA supplement group and a placebo group; there were 13 students in each group. After taking the supplement or placebo, they began cycling. Assessments were conducted before ingesting the supplement or placebo, 10 min before exercise began, 30 min into exercise, immediately after exercise stopped, and 30 min after exercise. The researchers learned that the serotonin levels in the BCAA group were lower. Serotonin is an important brain chemical that plays a role in exercise fatigue. The supplement also improved energy metabolism and lowered the levels of substances that indicate muscle damage, such as creatine and lactate dehydrogenase. The researchers concluded that "the intake of the BCAA is presumed to help contribute to enhancing exercise performance by exerting its influence on fatigue substances, muscle damage substances, and energy metabolism substances."[1]

BCAAs May or May Not Alleviate Exercise-Induced Muscle Damage

In a systematic review published in 2017 in the journal *Nutrients*, researchers from France examined studies on the ability of BCAAs to be useful for exercise-induced muscle damage or muscle injury. The researchers identified 11 studies that met their criteria; all included studies had 30 participants or less. Hence, they were relatively small in size. The researchers found large heterogeneity in both supplement strategies and exercise modalities resulting in considerable variability in the extent of damage. Yet, in general, the amount of muscle damage was low. Fifty-five percent of the studies found that BCAAs alleviated muscle damage; 27% found no noticeable differences; and 18% observed a negative effect. The studies tended to be short; more than half of the studies lasted 3 days or less. Nevertheless, positive effects were mostly observed with higher amounts of BCAA supplementation (over 200 mg per day), taken longer than 10 days, and started at least 7 days before the damaging exercises. The researchers concluded that "in specific conditions, BCAAs supplementation seems to diminish the outcomes of EIMD [exercise-induced muscle damage]."[2]

In a meta-analysis published in 2017 in the journal *Nutrition*, researchers from Iran examined the ability of BCAA supplementation to help recovery from exercise-induced muscle damage. Initially, the researchers identified eight trials. However, data from some of these trials were not accessible. As a result, only five randomized controlled trials were included in their analyses. There were a total of 70 healthy men with a mean age of 23 years. All the trials had multiple follow-up observations for each outcome. The researchers determined that the use of BCAA supplementation was better than passive recovery or rest after different exhaustive and damaging exercises. The researchers commented that "the advantages related to a reduction in muscle soreness and ameliorated muscle function because of an attenuation of muscle strength and muscle power loss after exercise."[3]

Taking BCAA Supplementation in Isolation Does Not Appear to Optimize Muscle Growth

In a trial published in 2017 in the journal *Frontiers in Physiology*, researchers from the United Kingdom and Davis, California (USA), investigated the ingestion of BCAAs without the ingestion of other essential amino acids following resistance training. Ten lower body resistance-trained men with an average age of 20.1 years completed two trials, separated by at least 3 weeks, drinking either 5.6 g of BCAAs or a placebo drink after resistance exercise. The researchers conducted various periodic assessments, such as muscle biopsies. As expected, the researchers found that BCAA supplements stimulated the muscle building response of the participants. However, on their own, BCAA supplements did not stimulate muscles as much as they did when combined with other essential amino acids. According to the researchers, taking BCAA supplements alone was not the best way to optimize muscle growth with weight training. Therefore, they concluded that "ingestion of BCAAs alone may not be the optimal nutritional regimen to stimulate a maximal MPS [muscle protein synthesis] response to resistance exercise training."[4]

BCAAs May Not Help Aerobic Performance in Untrained Males

In a trial published in 2011 in the *Journal of Strength and Conditioning Research*, researchers from Connecticut and Florida (USA) wanted to learn if BCAA supplementation would be useful for nine healthy but untrained males who performed three 90-min cycling routines. Before cycling and at the 60-min mark, the participants drank a beverage with BCAA supplements, an isocaloric carbohydrate–electrolyte drink, or a noncaloric drink; the participants were unaware of the beverage they drank. The only difference between the experimental trials was the beverage consumed. Assessments were conducted every 15 minutes, and each of the trials was separated by 8 weeks. At the end of each trial, the participants completed a 15-min trial in which they covered as much distance as possible. The researchers found that BCAA supplementation did not affect performance during this long endurance exercise. Yet, when compared to those who drank the noncaloric beverage, participants who drank the BCAA drink had reduced ratings of perceived exertion at the 75 and 90-min mark. The researchers suggested that BCAAs be combined with an isocaloric carbohydrate beverage during aerobic exercises.[5]

BCAA Supplementation May Benefit People with Advanced Liver Disease

In a retrospective, observational, multicenter trial published in 2017 in the journal *Medicine*, researchers from Korea wanted to learn if the long-term use of BCAA supplementation would help people dealing with the symptoms associated with advanced liver disease, such as malnutrition and the wasting of the body. The cohort consisted of 307 patients with advanced liver disease; for 6 months, 166 patients took BCAA supplementation and 141 were in the control group. The BCAA group was divided into three subgroups, with patients consuming 4.15 g, 8.3 g, or 12.45 g of BCAAs per day. Compared to the control group, the patients treated with 12.45 g of BCAAs had significant improvements in their model for end-stage liver disease (MELD) scores. Only marginal results were seen in patients treated with the lowest dose. As a result, the researchers concluded that "optimizing the dose of BCAA supplementation is important for maximizing the beneficial effects." Further, they added that there is a need for "a large-scale prospective study . . . for optimizing the dose of BCAA supplementation in patients with liver cirrhosis."[6]

BCAAs Combined with Exercise May Be Useful for Frail and Prefrail Elders

In a single-blind, randomized, crossover trial published in 2016 in the journal *Applied Physiology, Nutrition, and Metabolism*, researchers from Japan wanted to learn if a combination of BCAA supplementation and exercise would be useful for frail and prefrail elderly people who require long-term care. The cohort consisted of 52 frail and prefrail elders who received outpatient rehabilitation at a health service facility for the elderly. There were two periods of exercise and supplementation lasting 3 months which were separated by a 1-month washout period of exercise without supplementation. Twenty-seven participants ingested BCAA supplement in the first cycle and maltodextrin in the second cycle, and 25 ingested maltodextrin in the first cycle and BCAA supplement in the second cycle. The researchers learned that the addition of BCAA supplement to exercise improved gross lower limb muscle strength and dynamic balance ability. Although 95% of the participants in the control group were compliant with the exercise routine, they had minimal improvement in the gross muscle strength of their limbs. The researchers concluded that "the combination of BCAA intake and exercise therapy yielded significant improvement in gross lower limb muscle strength and dynamic balance ability."[7]

BCAAs May Improve Athletic Performance in People Competing for Two Consecutive Days

In a double-blind, randomized, crossover trial published in 2015 in the online journal *PLoS ONE*, researchers from Taiwan investigated the combined effects of BCAA and arginine supplementation on intermittent sprint performance in simulated handball games over two consecutive days. Fifteen male and seven female handball players, who had competed at the national or international level, consumed either the supplement or a placebo 1 h before two 60-min simulated handball games on consecutive days. The simulated games were designed to adhere to the activity patterns of real handball competitions. After a seven to 14-day washout period, the men and women completed the same testing with the alternative supplement option. The researchers learned that the combination supplement induced a small but significant improvement in performance on the second day in "well-trained subjects." The researchers concluded that their findings "have significant practical applications because the athletes of team sports frequently compete on consecutive days in tournaments."[8]

BCAAs Appear to Benefit People with Hepatic Encephalopathy

In a systematic review published in 2017 in the *Cochrane Database of Systematic Reviews*, researchers from Denmark, Spain, and Italy evaluated the beneficial and harmful effects of BCAAs on people with hepatic encephalopathy. The researchers identified 16 relevant trials with 827 participants. Eight trials assessed oral BCAAs and seven trials assessed intravenous BCAAs. In 15 trials, all the participants had liver cirrhosis. Seven trials were thought to be at low risk for bias, and nine trials were deemed at high risk of bias, primarily due to a lack of blinding or for-profit funding. The researchers determined that, although BCAAs had beneficial effects on hepatic encephalopathy, further research is needed before determinations are made on mortality, quality of life, or nutritional parameters.[9]

BCAAs May or May Not Be Useful for Adults and Children with Liver Cirrhosis

In a systematic review published in 2018 in the journal *Clinical Nutrition ESPEN*, researchers from Alberta, Canada wanted to learn if adults and children with liver cirrhosis would benefit from BCAA supplementation. Low levels of serum BCAA "is a hallmark feature" of people with liver cirrhosis. They wanted to determine if BCAA supplementation would improve body composition, muscle strength, liver biomarkers, medical and hepatic complications, patient care outcomes, health-related quality of life, and length of hospitalizations. A total of 40 articles published between 1989 and 2017 met the criteria for inclusion. Two of the 40 studies were conducted on children; the remaining 38 included only adults. The majority of the adult studies were prospective, and more than half were randomized controlled trials. Sample sizes ranged from six to 622, and the BCAA doses ranged from 5.5 to 30 g per day. There was "substantial variability" in the ratio of individual BCAAs provided to the participants. The researchers determined that BCAA supplementation may be beneficial in improving muscle strength, edema, hepatic complications, and fluid accumulation in the peritoneal cavity (ascites). In children with end-stage liver disease, BCAA supplementation improved certain factors such as body weight and fat mass. Little or no effects were seen in other factors, such as lean body mass and serum concentrations of certain liver biochemistries. The researchers commented that the "heterogeneity of study findings attributed to variability in BCAA dose (total, relative proportions), duration, disease severity and lack of uniformity in tools used for assessing patient outcomes limit overall conclusions." They underscored the need for more longitudinal studies.[10]

BCAA Supplementation May Not Be Useful for People with Heart Failure

In a randomized clinical trial published in 2016 in the journal *Clinical Nutrition*, researchers based in Mexico City, Mexico evaluated the ability of BCAA supplementation and a resistance exercise program to help people with stable heart failure. (Heart failure occurs when the heart has structural or functional alterations that make it unable to respond adequately to physiological demands.) The initial cohort consisted of 66 patients from a heart failure clinic in Mexico City. The patients were divided into a group that consumed 10 g per day of BCAA supplementation and participated in a resistance exercise program and a second group that only participated in the exercise program. The exercise sessions were held twice each week and lasted for an hour. For 12 weeks, various assessments were periodically conducted. Twenty-nine patients in the BCAA group and 26 in the control group completed the trial. The researchers learned that the exercise program resulted in clinical and physical improvements, which was accomplished without the help of BCAA supplementation. The researchers concluded that the "improvements in physical and functional capacities are attributed to resistance exercise program but not to BCAA supplementation."[11]

BCAA Supplementation May Be Useful for Recovery from Muscle Damage Caused by a Single Bout of Bulking Exercise in Resistance-Trained Athletes

In a double-blind, matched-pair design trial published in 2017 in the journal *Applied Physiology, Nutrition, and Metabolism*, researchers from the United

Kingdom and Australia wanted to learn if BCAA supplementation would help the recovery of muscle damage among experienced resistance-trained athletes. The cohort consisted of 14 males and two females who had routinely participated in resistance training for at least 3 years. Eight were randomly assigned to a BCAA supplement group, and eight were randomly assigned to a placebo group. All participants were placed on a specific diet plan. The participants performed six sets of ten full squats at "70 percent 1-repetition maximum" to induce muscle damage. The supplements (at a dosage of 0.087 g/kg body mass) or placebos were consumed 30 min before and after the muscle damage protocol. The researchers conducted various assessments and found that the BCAA supplement reduced the effects of the training session on isometric strength and increased the rate of recovery. The researchers concluded that "our findings support the suggestion that BCAA supplementation can increase the rate of recovery in muscle function among well-trained habitual weightlifters."[12]

When Combined with Walking, BCAA Supplementation May Help Prevent Muscle Wasting in People with Liver Cirrhosis

In a 3-month trial published in 2017 in the *European Journal of Gastroenterology & Hepatology*, researchers from Japan noted that people with chronic liver disease may suffer from a muscle wasting problem known as sarcopenia. They wanted to learn if a combination of BCAA supplementation and walking would help improve this medical problem. From December 2015 to July 2015, the researchers enrolled 33 Japanese patients with liver cirrhosis, with a median age of 67 years. Thirteen men and 20 women were included in the study, and none of them had a history of BCAA supplementation. All the patients consumed BCAA supplements as a late evening snack and walked 2000 more steps per day than they walked before the trial began. Assessments were conducted at baseline and at the end of the trial, which was completed by 31 patients. The researchers learned that only six patients, five of whom were women, showed no increasing ratio of muscle volume. They concluded that "the combination of BCAA supplementation as a nutritional approach with exercise might be an effective strategy for improving the muscle environment, and preventing progression of sarcopenia and presarcopenia."[13]

When Combined with Exercise, BCAA Supplementation May Benefit People with Osteoarthritis

In a single-blind, randomized trial published in 2018 in the *Hong Kong Physiotherapy Journal*, researchers from Japan wanted to learn if BCAA supplementation would be useful for people dealing with osteoarthritis. The initial cohort consisted of 43 women, with an average age of 64.2 years; all the women had osteoarthritis and were scheduled for a unilateral total hip arthroplasty to restore joint function. The women were randomized and divided into two groups. For 1 month, 21 women took BCAA supplementation and 22 women served as controls.

All the women participated in a hip abductor muscle exercise program. Ten minutes before exercising at home, they took their supplements or placebos. The researchers conducted various assessments. Four women did not complete the trial. The researchers concluded that the combination of BCAA supplements and exercise therapy resulted in "a significant improvement in hip abductor muscle strength of the contralateral side."[14]

NOTES

1. Kim, Dong-Hee, Seok-Hwan Kim, Woo-Seok Jeong, and Ha-Yan Lee. "Effect of BCAA Intake during Endurance Exercises on Fatigue Substances, Muscle Damage Substances, and Energy Metabolism Substances." *Journal of Exercise Nutrition & Biochemistry* 17, no. 4 (2013):169–180.

2. Fouré, Alexandra and David Bendahan. "Is Branched-Chain Amino Acids Supplementation a Efficient Nutritional Strategy to Alleviate Skeletal Muscle Damage? A Systematic Review." *Nutrients* 9, no. 10 (October 2017): 1047.

3. Rahimi, M. H., S. Shab-Bidar, M. Mollahosseini, and K. Djafarian. "Branched-Chain Amino Acid Supplementation and Exercise-Induced Muscle Damage in Exercise Recovery: A Meta-Analysis of Randomized Clinical Trials." *Nutrition* 42 (October 2017): 30–36.

4. Jackman, Sarah R., Oliver C. Witard, Andrew Philip, et al. "Branched-Chain Amino Acid Ingestion Stimulates Muscle Myofibrillar Protein Synthesis Following Resistance Exercise in Humans." *Frontiers in Physiology* 8 (June 2017): Article 390.

5. Greer, B. K., P. White, E. M. Arguello, and E. M. Haymes. "Branched-Chain Amino Acid Supplementation Lowers Perceived Exertion But Does Not Affect Performance in Untrained Males." *Journal of Strength and Conditioning Research* 25, no. 2 (February 2011): 539–544.

6. Park, Jung Gil, Won Young Tak, Soo Young Park, et al. "Effects of Branched-Chain Amino Acids (BSAAs) on the Progression of Advanced Liver Disease: A Korean Nationwide, Multicenter, Retrospective, Observational, Cohort Study." *Medicine* 96, no. 24 (June 2017): e6580.

7. Ikeda, Takashi, Junya Aizawa, Hiroshi Nagasawa, et al. "Effects and Feasibility of Exercise Therapy Combined with Branched-Chain Amino Acid Supplementation on Muscle Strengthening in Frail and Pre-Frail Elderly People Requiring Long-Term Care: A Crossover Trial." *Applied Physiology, Nutrition, and Metabolism* 41 (2016): 438–445.

8. Chang, Chen-Kang, Kun-Ming Chang Chien, Jung-Hsien Chang, et al. "Branched-Chain Amino Acids and Arginine Improve Performance in Two Consecutive Days of Simulated Handball Games in Male and Female Athletes: A Randomized Trial." *PLoS ONE* 10, no. 3 (2015): e0121866.

9. Gluud, L. L., G. Dam, I. Les, et al. "Branched-Chain Amino Acids for People with Hepatic Encephalopathy." *Cochrane Database of Systematic Reviews* 18, no. 5 (May 2017): CD001939.

10. Ooi, P. H., S. M. Gilmour, J. Yap, and D. R. Mager. "Effects of Branched Chain Amino Acid Supplementation on Patient Care Outcomes in Adults and Children with Liver Cirrhosis: A Systematic Review." *Clinical Nutrition ESPEN* 28 (2018): 41–51.

11. Pineda-Juárez, J. A., N. A. Sánchez-Ortiz, L. Castillo-Martinez, et al. "Changes in Body Composition in Heart Failure Patients After a Resistance Exercise Program and Branched Chain Amino Acid Supplementation." *Clinical Nutrition* 35, no. 1 (February 2016): 41–47.

12. Waldron, M., K. Whelan, O. Jeffries, et al. "The Effects of Acute Branched-Chain Amino Acid Supplementation on Recovery from a Single Bout of Hypertrophy Exercise in Resistance-Trained Athletes." *Applied Physiology, Nutrition, and Metabolism* 42, no. 6 (June 2017): 630–636.

13. Hiraoka, A., K. Michitaka, D. Kiguchi, et al. "Efficacy of Branched-Chain Amino Acid Supplementation and Walking Exercise for Preventing Sarcopenia in Patients with Liver Cirrhosis." *Journal of Gastroenterology & Hepatology* 29, no 12 (December 2017): 1416–1423.

14. Ikeda, Takashi, Tetsuya Jinno, Tadashi Masuda, et al. "Effect of Exercise Therapy Combined with Branched-Chain Amino Acid Supplementation on Muscle Strengthening in Persons with Osteoarthritis." *Hong Kong Physiotherapy Journal* 38, no. 1 (2018): 23–31.

REFERENCES AND FURTHER READING

Chang, Chen-Kang, Kun-Ming Chang Chien, Jung-Hsien Chang, et al. "Branched-Chain Amino Acids and Arginine Improve Performance in Two Consecutive Days of Simulated Handball Games in Male and Female Athletes: A Randomized Trial." *PLoS ONE* 10, no. 3 (2015): e0121866.

Fouré, Alexandre, and David Bendahan. "Is Branched-Chain Amino Acids Supplementation as Efficient Nutritional Strategy to Alleviate Skeletal Muscle Damage? A Systematic Review." *Nutrients* 9, no. 10 (October 2017): 1047.

Gluud, L. L., G. Dam, I. Les, et al. "Branched-Chain Amino Acids for People with Hepatic Encephalopathy." *Cochrane Database of Systematic Reviews* 18, no. 5 (May 2017): CD001939.

Greer, B. K., J. P. White, E. M. Arguello, and E. M. Haymes. "Branched-Chain Amino Acid Supplementation Lower Perceived Exertion But Does Not Affect Performance in Untrained Males." *Journal of Strength and Conditioning Research* 25, no. 2 (February 2011): 539–544.

Hiraoka, A., K. Michitaka, D. Kiguchi, et al. "Efficacy of Branched-Chain Amino Acid Supplementation and Walking Exercise for Preventing Sarcopenia in Patients with Liver Cirrhosis." *European Journal of Gastroenterology & Hepatology* 29, no. 12 (December 2017): 1416–1423.

Ikeda, Takashi, Junya Aizawa, Hiroshi Nagasawa, et al. "Effects and Feasibility of Exercise Therapy Combined with Branch-Chain Amino Acid Supplementation on Muscle Strengthening in Frail and Pre-Frail Elderly People Requiring Long-Term Care: A Crossover Trial." *Applied Physiology, Nutrition, and Metabolism* 41 (2016): 438–445.

Ikeda, Takashi, Tetsuya Jinno, Tadashi Masuda, et al. "Effect of Exercise Therapy Combined with Branched-Chain Amino Acid Supplementation on Muscle Strengthening in Persons with Osteoarthritis." *Hong Kong Physiotherapy Journal* 38, no. 1 (2018): 23–31.

Jackman, Sarah R., Oliver C. Witard, Andrew Philip, et al. "Branched-Chain Amino Acid Ingestion Stimulates Muscle Myofibrillar Protein Synthesis Following Resistance Exercise in Humans." *Frontiers in Physiology* 8 (June 2017): Article 390.

Kim, Dong-Hee, Seok-Hwan Kim, Woo-Seok Jeong, and Ha-Yan Lee. "The Effect of BCAA during Endurance Exercises on Fatigue Substances, Muscle Damage Substances, and Energy Metabolism Substances." *Journal of Exercise Nutrition & Biochemistry* 17, no. 4 (2013): 169–180.

Ooi, P. H., S. M. Gilmour, J. Yap, and D. R. Mager. "Effects of Branched-Chain Amino Acid Supplementation on Patient Care Outcomes in Adults and Children with

Liver Cirrhosis: A Systematic Review." *Clinical Nutrition ESPEN* 28 (December 2018): 41–51.

Park, Hung Gil, Won Young Tak, Soo Young Park, et al. "Effects of Branched-Chain Amino Acids (BCAAs) on the Progression of Advanced Liver Disease: A Korean Nationwide, Multicenter, Retrospective, Observational Cohort Study." *Medicine* 96, no. 24 (June 2017): e6580.

Pineda-Juárez, J. A., N. A. Sánchez-Ortiz, L. Castillo-Martinez, et al. "Changes in Body Composition in Heart Failure Patients After a Resistance Exercise Program and Branched-Chain Amino Acid Supplementation." *Clinical Nutrition* 35, no. 1 (February 2016): 41–47.

Rahimi, M. H., S. Shab-Bidar, M. Mollahosseini, and K. Djafarian. "Branched-Chain Amino Acid Supplementation and Exercise-Induced Muscle Damage in Exercise Recovery: A Meta-Analysis of Randomized Clinical Trials." *Nutrition* 42 (2017): 30–36.

Waldron, M., K. Whelan, O. Jeffries, et al. "The Effects of Acute Branched-Chain Amino Acid Supplementation on Recovery from a Single Bout of Hypertrophy Exercise in Resistance-Trained Athletes." *Applied Physiology, Nutrition, and Metabolism* 42, no. 6 (June 2017): 630–636.

Chia

Chia is an edible seed that comes from the desert plant *Salvia hispanica*, a member of the mint family that grows abundantly in southern Mexico and Central America. Chia seeds are the most important part of the plant. Historically, they were a major part of the Aztec and Mayan diets. In the United States, they were grown in the southwest, where they were primarily consumed by the Native Americans.

Despite their small size, chia seeds are rich in essential fatty acids, omega-3 fatty acids, and omega-6 fatty acids. They are also rich in calcium, phosphorus, magnesium, manganese, copper, iron, molybdenum, niacin, potassium, vitamins B1, B2, and B3, and zinc. Chia seeds have high amounts of antioxidants, which help prevent cell damage, and high amounts of fiber and quality protein. Yet, a tablespoon of chia seeds has only approximately 70 calories.

HEALTH BENEFITS AND RISKS

Because they expand dramatically when combined with a fluid, chia seeds are believed to be useful in weight loss. People who feel fuller are less likely to overeat and snack on unhealthy options. Likewise, because they are high in omega-3 fatty acids, chia seeds are thought to support cardiovascular health. They appear to improve cardiovascular risk factors, such as lowering cholesterol, triglycerides, and blood pressure. Because they contain important bone nutrients, chia seeds also support bone health. Moreover, chia seeds may be useful for people with type 2 diabetes, who often need to lose weight and benefit from cardiovascular support.

The omega-3 fatty acids in chia seeds give them blood-thinning properties. As a result, they should not be eaten before surgical procedures as they may increase bleeding. Until more is known about chia, it is probably best for pregnant women and nursing mothers to avoid chia supplementation.

HOW IT IS SOLD AND TAKEN

Chia is sold as seeds, ground seeds, and ground flour, and may be added to baked goods, such as breads and muffins. In vegan baking, chia may replace eggs. These seeds may be eaten raw or added to other foods, such as cereal, rice, yogurt, or vegetables. Chia seeds are highly absorbent and develop a gelatin-type texture when soaked in water. Chia may be purchased in capsules with seeds and in capsules that contain chia seed oil. Chia is often added to other products such as bars and cereals. There are no clear dosage guidelines for chia. In general, people seem to recommend between one to three tablespoons per day. However, there is insufficient information to know how much to consume. Check relevant directions on the label of any chia product.

RESEARCH FINDINGS

Adding Chia to Bread Dough Increases the Nutritional Quality of the Bread

In an article published in 2013 in the journal *European Food Research and Technology*, researchers from Valencia, Spain wanted to learn what would happen to bread if they replaced wheat flour with 5% chia seeds, 5% whole chia flour, 5% chia semi-defatted flour, or 5% low-fat chia flour. In addition, the researchers prepared a control bread that contained wheat flour, compressed yeast, sodium salt, tap water, and ascorbic acid. The researchers determined that the breads containing chia had significantly higher amounts of lipids, protein, minerals, and dietary fiber than the control bread. In addition, the bread tasters had a "high acceptance" of the chia breads. In fact, the bread with chia seeds showed 97.8% acceptance, and the breads with chia flours had acceptance rates ranging from 90.2% to 95.13%. Meanwhile, the control bread had an almost 70% acceptance. The researches concluded that "the inclusion of chia seeds or flours had a positive effect on the technological and sensory value of the bread products, and therefore its inclusion is recommended, even at levels greater than 5%."[1]

Chia Seed May Be Useful for People with Metabolic Syndrome

In a single-center, randomized, placebo-controlled, double-blind, parallel-arm trial published in 2012 in *The Journal of Nutrition*, researchers from Mexico wanted to learn if a mixture containing chia seeds, nopal, soy protein, and oats would help people with metabolic syndrome. (Metabolic syndrome is a condition characterized by central obesity, hypertension, and disturbed glucose and insulin metabolism. The syndrome has been linked to an increased risk of type 2 diabetes and cardiovascular disease.) Chia seeds were included because they contain fatty acids and antioxidants, and are believed to reduce inflammation. Initially, the cohort consisted of 97 participants, but only 67 completed the study; there were 35 participants in the control group and 32 in the intervention group. The trial was conducted in two phases. During the first 2 weeks, the participants were told to eat a low-energy diet that was low in saturated fat and cholesterol. During the second stage of the trial, which continued for 2 months, the participants ate a low-energy diet and consumed the supplemental mixture or a placebo. All participants lost weight and had reductions in body mass index and waist circumference. The participants consuming the chia seed mixture also had reduced triglycerides, C-reactive protein, and insulin levels. The researchers commented that "this type of dietary intervention could be adapted to different ethnic groups by incorporating native foods."[2]

Chia Flour May Be Useful for People with High Blood Pressure

In a randomized, double-blind, experimental, placebo-controlled trial published in 2014 in the journal *Plant Foods for Human Nutrition*, researchers from Brazil investigated the effect of chia flour on blood pressure in obese people with elevated levels of blood pressure, a condition known as hypertension. The participants were assigned to one of three groups—ten in a hypertensive drug-treated group, nine in a hypertensive untreated group, and seven were in a placebo group. For 12 weeks, the participants consumed 35 g per day of either chia flour or a placebo. The participants were clinically assessed 24 h before the beginning of the intervention, every 4 weeks during the intervention, and 48 h after the trial ended. While researchers found no change in the blood pressure levels of the participants in the placebo group, both chia groups experienced reductions in blood pressure. The reduction in the treated chia group was significant, whereas that in the untreated chia group was not. The researchers commented that their findings "not only give credibility to the antihypertensive power of chia but also reinforce the recommendations that antihypertensive treatment is much more [effective] when drug therapy is used in combination with other interventions."[3]

Adding Chia Seed to Yogurt May Reduce Short-Term Food Intake and Improve Mid-Morning Satiety

In a study published in 2017 in the journal *Nutrition Research and Practice*, researchers from Turkey wanted to learn if adding chia seeds to a mid-morning yogurt snack would reduce short-term food intake and improve satiety. The cohort consisted of 24 females between the ages of 19 and 25 years who were in good health. None of the participants was on a medication known to alter appetite or weight. The trial was conducted on three separate days with a 1-week washout period between each study. On each test day, the participants were randomly assigned to eat 180 g of yogurt without chia seeds, 140 g of yogurt with 7 g of chia seeds, or 100 g of yogurt with 14 g of chia seeds. After 2 h, they ate as much lunch as they wanted. The researchers used various methods to assess the amount of food that the women consumed. The researchers found that scores were significantly influenced by the amount of chia seed consumed in the yogurt. On the days they ate yogurt with 7 and 14 g of chia seeds, the participants reported significantly lower scores for hunger, prospective food consumption, amounts of food that could be consumed, desire for sugary foods, and higher scores for satiety. The women consumed almost 25% less lunch on the days they had a mid-morning snack of yogurt with chia seed. The researchers concluded that "these results suggest that chia seed consumption can be a useful dietary strategy in the prevention of overweight and obesity status in healthy individuals."[4]

People Who Include Chia Seed in Their Diet May Be More Satisfied Than Those Who Include Flax

In a trial published in 2017 in the *European Journal of Clinical Nutrition*, researchers based in Canada compared the effects of postprandial glycemia (glucose levels in the blood after eating a meal) and satiety scores of chia and flax seeds. Chia and flax have similar nutritional profiles, and people tend to use them in the same manner. On three separate occasions, five healthy men and ten healthy women received a 50 g glucose challenge alone or supplemented with either 25 g ground chia seeds or 31.5 g flax seeds. Blood samples were taken and satiety ratings were noted. The researchers learned that both the chia and flax drinks reduced blood glucose levels. However, people who consumed the drink containing chia were more satisfied than those who consumed the drink containing flax. The researchers suggested that this is possibly because chia is thicker than flax. Apparently, this viscosity delays the rate of absorption in the gut and increases satiety. The researchers commented that further studies should attempt "to establish whether the findings reported from this acute study would extend over longer intervention periods with respect to improved glycemic control, reduction in food intake and body weight management."[5]

Chia Seed Oil May Not Improve Running Performance in Humans

In a study published in 2015 in the journal *Nutrients*, researchers from North Carolina (USA) wanted to learn if chia seed oil would improve the performance of runners. (The lead author of the study is a marathon runner.) The cohort consisted of 16 male and 8 female runners between the ages of 24 and 55 years. After overnight fasting, the runners reported to the lab twice, at least 2 weeks apart. They provided blood samples and then drank either 0.5 L of flavored water alone or 0.5 L of water with chia seed oil. After 30 min, the runners provided a second blood sample and ran to exhaustion on treadmills at a marathon pace. More blood was drawn after they finished running. The blood tests revealed that the runners who consumed chia seed oil had high levels of alpha-linolenic acid in their blood, which is not surprising because chia is a rich source of this essential omega-3 fatty acid. However, regarding other factors, such as performance indicators and exercise-induced inflammation, there was no difference between those who consumed the two different drinks. Although the researchers had hypothesized that the runners who consumed chia seed oil would have an advantage over those who consumed flavored water, water with chia seed oil failed to improve the running time. The researchers concluded that intake of chia seed oil before running "provided no discernable benefits for the athletes in this study."[6]

Chia Seeds May Be Useful for Weight Loss

In a double-blind, randomized controlled trial published in 2017 in the journal *Nutrition, Metabolism and Cardiovascular Diseases*, researchers from Canada and Croatia investigated the ability of chia seeds to support weight loss in people with type 2 diabetes. The cohort, which consisted of 77 overweight or obese people with type 2 diabetes, was divided into two groups. For 6 months, the participants in both groups followed a calorie-restricted diet. The participants in one group also consumed ground chia seed supplementation daily; the participants in the other group consumed an oat-bran supplement. Fifty-eight participants were included in the final analysis. The researchers determined that the participants consuming chia seeds had a small but significant weight loss, which was accompanied by reductions of 3.5 cm in waist circumference. These reductions started near the beginning of the intervention and were sustained until the end, which suggests that more reductions might have occurred if the trial had lasted for a longer period of time. The researchers concluded that "supplementation of Salba-chia may be a useful dietary addition to conventional therapy in the management of obesity in diabetes."[7]

Then Again, Chia Seeds May Not Support Weight Loss

In a trial published in 2009 in the journal *Nutrition Research*, researchers from North Carolina (USA) assessed the ability of chia seeds to promote weight loss and alter disease risk factors in overweight adults. The initial cohort consisted of 90 men and women between the ages of 20 and 70 years who were overweight or obese. For 12 weeks, the participants took either two daily doses of a 25 g chia seed supplement or a placebo. Seventy-six participants (28 men and 48 women) completed the trial. By the end of the trial, there were no significant differences between the two groups. Neither body mass nor body composition changed in either group. There were also no changes in serum lipoprotein, serum glucose, and systolic blood pressure. The researchers concluded that the ingestion of 50 g per day of chia seed by overweight or obese men and women "had no influence on body mass composition or various disease risk factor measures."[8]

Athletes May Use Chia Seeds for "Carb Loading"

In a study published in 2011 in the *Journal of Strength & Conditioning Research*, researchers from Alabama (USA) investigated the carb loading ability of chia seeds. The researchers recruited six "highly trained" men and assigned them to carb load with either Gatorade (100% of the calories) or an equal caloric mix of Gatorade and omega-3 chia seeds. After carb loading with a beverage, the men ran for 1 h at about 65% of their maximum performance levels on a treadmill, which was followed by a 10-km (10K) trial run on a track. Two weeks after the first test, the participants were crossed over to the other carb loading test. The researchers found that there was no significant difference between the two groups. The mean 10K time for the Gatorade/chia group was 37 min and 49 s, whereas the mean 10K time for the Gatorade only group was 37 min and 43 s. By adding chia seeds to half the amount of Gatorade, the runners were able to decrease their sugar intake while increasing their intake of omega-3 fatty acids. However, the Gatorade/chia drink offered no performance advantages. The researchers concluded that the Gatorade/chia drink was a "viable option" for lower sugar carb loading prior to vigorous exercise of more than 90 min.[9]

Eating Raw Chia Seeds May Be Dangerous

In a report published on the website of WBUR, a public radio station based in Boston, Massachusetts (USA), described a 39-year-old man from North Carolina

(USA) who ate more than a tablespoon of dry chia seeds. Rebecca Rawl, MD, outlined the case in a poster presentation at the 2014 annual meeting of the American College of Gastroenterology in Philadelphia, Pennsylvania (USA). She noted that the man arrived at the hospital with pain at the top of his stomach, with an inability to swallow anything. After he had an upper endoscopy, the physicians located the culprit—chia seeds. Dr. Rawl said that she initially attempted to remove the seeds with an adult endoscope: "We tried to push the mass or gel of chia seeds through the stomach. But because of the consistency, the seeds would just go around the scope." Eventually, Dr. Rawl switched to a neonatal or baby endoscope: "We were able to get past the obstruction to see what was ahead and we used the tip of instrument to push a few seeds at a time into the stomach." Over several hours, medical providers cleared the man's esophagus: "Afterwards, he was fine." According to Dr. Rawl, people should not eat dry chia seeds: "Let them expand fully in some kind of liquid first—especially for people who have this sensation of food getting stuck. Chia seeds are tiny, so people would not necessarily think there are problems, but some people do have underlying 'strictures' or narrowing of the esophagus."[10]

NOTES

1. Iglesias-Puig, Esther, and Monika Haros. "Evaluation of Performance of Dough and Bread Incorporating Chia (*Salvia hispanica* L.)." *European Food Research and Technology* 237, no. 6 (December 2013): 865–874.

2. Guevara-Cruz, Martha, Armando R. Tovar, Carlos A. Aguilar-Salinas, et al. "A Dietary Pattern Including Nopal, Chia Seed, Soy Protein, and Oat Reduces Serum Triglycerides and Glucose Intolerance in Patients with Metabolic Syndrome." *The Journal of Nutrition* 142, no. 1 (January 2012): 64–69.

3. Toscano, L. T., C. S. O. Silva, L. T. Toscano, et al. "Chia Flour Supplementation Reduces Blood Pressure in Hypertensive Subjects." *Plant Foods for Human Nutrition* 69 (2014): 392–398.

4. Ayaz, A., A. Akyol, E. Inan-Eroglu, et al. "Chia Seed (*Salvia Hispanica* L.) Added Yogurt Reduces Short-Term Food Intake and Increases Satiety: Randomised Controlled Trial." *Nutrition Research and Practice* 11, no. 5 (October 2017): 412–418.

5. Vuksan, V., L. Choleva, E. Jovanovski, et al. "Comparison of Flax (*Linum usitatissimum*) and Salba-Chia (*Salvia hispanica* L.) Seeds on Postprandial Glycemia and Satiety in Healthy Individuals: A Randomized, Controlled, Crossover Study." *European Journal of Clinical Nutrition* 71 (2017): 234–238.

6. Nieman, David C., Nicolas D. Gillitt, May Pat Meaney, and Dustin A. Dew. "No Positive Influence of Ingesting Chia Seed Oil on Human Running Performance." *Nutrients* 7 (2015): 3666–3676.

7. Vuksan, V., A. L. Jenkins, C. Brissette, et al. "Salba-Chia (*Salvia hispanica* L.) in the Treatment of Overweight and Obese Patients with Type 2 Diabetes: A Double-Blind Randomized Controlled Trial." *Nutrition, Metabolism and Cardiovascular Diseases* 27, no. 2 (February 2017): 138–146.

8. Nieman, D. C., E. J. Cayea, M. D. Austin, et al. "Chia Seed Does Not Promote Weight Loss or Alter Disease Risk Factors in Overweight Adults." *Nutrition Research* 29, no. 6 (June 2009): 414–418.

9. Illian, T. G., J. C. Casey, and P. A. Bishop. "Omega 3 Chia Seed Loading as a Means of Carbohydrate Loading." *Journal of Strength & Conditioning Research* 25, no. 1 (January 2011): 61–65.

10. Zimmerman, Rachel. "Chia Seed Alert: Superfood, Yes, But They Landed One Man in the ER." October 24, 2014. http://www.wbur.org.

REFERENCES AND FURTHER READING

Ayaz, A., A. Akyol, E. Inan-Eroglu, et al. "Chia Seed (*Salvia Hispanica* L.) Added Yogurt Reduces Short-Term Food Intake and Increases Satiety; Randomised Controlled Trial." *Nutrition Research and Practice* 11, no. 5 (October 2017): 412–418.

Guevara-Cruz, Martha, Armando R. Tovar, Carlos A. Aguilar-Salinas, et al. "A Dietary Pattern Including Nopal, Chia Se, Soy Protein, and Oat Reduces Serum Triglycerides and Glucose Intolerance in Patients with Metabolic Syndrome." *The Journal of Nutrition* 142, no. 1 (January 2012): 64–69.

Iglesias-Puig, Esther, and Monika Haros. "Evaluation of Performance of Dough and Bread Incorporating Chia (*Salvia hispanica* L.)." *European Food Research and Technology* 237, no. 6 (December 2013): 865–874.

Illian, T. G., J. C. Casey, and P. A. Bishop. "Omega 3 Chia Seed Loading as a Means of Carbohydrate Loading." *Journal of Strength & Conditioning Research* 25, no. 1 (January 2011): 61–65.

Nieman, David C., E. J. Cayea, M. D. Austin, et al. "Chia Seed Does Not Promote Weight Loss or Alter Disease Risk Factors in Overweight Adults." *Nutrition Research* 29, no. 6 (June 2009): 414–418.

Nieman, David C., Nicolas D. Gillitt, Mary Pat Meaney, and Dustin A. Dew. "No Positive Influence of Ingesting Chia Seed Oil on Human Running Performance." *Nutrients* 7 (2015): 3666–3676.

Toscano, L. T., C. S. O. da Silva, L. T. Toscano, et al. "Chia Flour Supplementation Reduces Blood Pressure in Hypertensive Subjects." *Plant Foods for Human Nutrition* 69 (2014): 392–398.

Vuksan, L., L. Choleva, E. Jovanovski, et al. "Comparison of Flax (*Linum usitatissimum*) and Salba-Chia (*Salvia hispanica* L.) Seeds on Postprandial Glycemia and Satiety in Healthy Individuals: A Randomized, Controlled, Crossover Study." *European Journal of Clinical Nutrition* 71 (2017): 234–238.

Vuksan, V., A. L. Jenkins, C. Brisssette, et al. "Salba-Chia (*Salvia hispanica* L.) in the Treatment of Overweight and Obese Patients with Type 2 Diabetes: A Double-Blind Randomized Controlled Trial." *Nutrition, Metabolism and Cardiovascular Diseases* 27, no. 2 (February 2017): 138–146.

WBUR. http://www.wbur.org.

Cinnamon

For thousands of years, cinnamon has been harvested from the inner bark of *Cinnamomum* trees. In fact, the use of cinnamon dates as far back as ancient Egypt, where it was a rare and expensive spice. Cinnamon has also been mentioned in the Bible many times. It was thought to be a treatment for a wide variety of illnesses.

While approximately 250 species of cinnamon have been identified, there are two main types—Ceylon cinnamon and Cassia cinnamon—which come from different but related trees. Ceylon cinnamon, which is grown in Sri Lanka and southern India, is harder to find and more costly. Cassia cinnamon, which is grown in China, Indonesia, and Vietnam, is less expensive and more readily available. Most of the research studies have been conducted on Cassia cinnamon.

HEALTH BENEFITS AND RISKS

Cinnamon is known to contain high amounts of antioxidants and anti-inflammatory compounds, which are believed to offer numerous health benefits, such as improving cardiovascular health, reducing inflammation, and fighting bacteria. Cinnamon also has antimicrobial and antifungal properties. In addition, it may lower glucose levels in people with type 2 diabetes, and its antioxidant properties may fight against cell damage from free radicals. Cinnamon has been used to treat sore throat, cough, indigestion, abdominal cramps, intestinal spasms, nausea, flatulence, and diarrhea.[1] Whether these claims are true is hard to know. There have been few studies among humans investigating the health benefits of cinnamon.

Cinnamon supplements appear to be safe for most people, especially if used for a relatively short period of time. However, in higher doses, cinnamon has the potential to become toxic, and may cause sores in the mouth and lips. It is important to never exceed the recommended dose. Pregnant or breastfeeding women and people with diabetes or liver disease should use cinnamon supplementation with caution, if at all. Before using cinnamon essential oil, it is best to do a patch test on a small amount of skin.

Cinnamon contains the natural flavoring known as coumain. Consuming excessive amounts of coumain may cause liver damage and alter coagulation. People with liver damage or those on anticoagulating medications should not take cinnamon supplementation without first discussing with a medical provider.

HOW IT IS SOLD AND TAKEN

Most often, cinnamon is sold as a powder, in capsules, and in sticks. Some recommend half to one teaspoon per day, while others recommend up to 1.2 teaspoons per day. However, there are no specific guidelines. Cinnamon may also be added to baked goods, such as cinnamon buns and cinnamon raisin bread, as well as other products. Although cinnamon essential oil may be applied topically, it requires dilution to avoid skin irritation. It is important to carefully read the directions on the label and to only use it externally.

RESEARCH FINDINGS

Cinnamon May Have Lipid-Lowering Properties

In a study published in 2013 in the *Journal of Enam Medical College*, researchers from Bangladesh wanted to determine if cinnamon had lipid-lowering properties. In the first part of their study, the researchers divided 12 rats into two groups. For 35 days, six rats were fed a normal diet, and six rats were fed a normal diet supplemented with cinnamon. In the second part of the study, 18 rats were fed a diet designed to increase lipid levels. These rats were then divided into three groups of six rats. For 35 days, one group took supplemental cinnamon; one group took atorvastatin, a medication to lower cholesterol; and one group served as the control. The control rats had elevated levels of serum total cholesterol, serum low-density lipoprotein (LDL) or "bad" cholesterol, and serum triglycerides. The researchers determined that the rats on high-fat diet and cinnamon had reduced total cholesterol, triglycerides, and LDL. The results were similar to those obtained with atorvastatin. The researchers concluded that "cinnamon might have a direct role in lipid metabolism and prevent hypercholesterolemia and hypertriglyceridemia and lower free fatty acids by its strong lipolytic activity."[2]

Cinnamon Supplementation May Be Useful for People with Type 2 Diabetes

In a meta-analysis and systematic review, researchers from California and Connecticut (USA) evaluated the effect of cinnamon supplementation on glycemia (glucose in the blood) and lipid levels in people with type 2 diabetes. The cohort consisted of ten randomized controlled trials that included a total of 543 participants. After conducting various analyses, the researchers determined that cinnamon was associated with statistically significant reductions in levels of fasting plasma glucose, total cholesterol, LDL, and triglycerides. In addition, there were statistically significant increases in high-density lipoprotein (HDL) or "good" cholesterol. However, because the preferred dose and duration of therapy varied widely, "the ability to apply these results to patient care" are limited.[3]

Cinnamon May Also Be Useful for People with Type 2 Diabetes Who Are Overweight

In a study published in 2014 in the *Journal of Intercultural Ethnopharmacology*, researchers from Egypt investigated the treatment of overweight, diabetic rats with cinnamon or ginger. They randomly divided 42 male Sprague–Dawley rats into six equal groups of seven. While the rats in the first group served as negative controls, those in the other five groups were fed a high-fat diet for 4 weeks. The obese rats were then injected with alloxan for 5 days to induce diabetes. The second group was the positive control. The other four groups received supplemental cinnamon and ginger in two different doses for 6 weeks. The researchers learned that supplementation with cinnamon and ginger reduced body weight and body fat mass, normalized serum levels of liver enzymes, decreased blood glucose, improved lipid profile, and increased insulin serum levels. The researchers concluded that their findings "affirm the traditional use of cinnamon and ginger for treating patients suffering from obesity and diabetes."[4]

When Combined with Chromium and Carnosine, Cinnamon May Be Useful for Overweight and Obese Prediabetic Patients

In a randomized, double-blind, single-center, placebo-controlled trial published in 2015 in the online journal *PLoS ONE*, researchers from Paris, France evaluated the effects of a 4-month treatment of a supplement containing cinnamon, chromium, and carnosine on overweight or obese prediabetic participants. The initial cohort consisted of 62 participants between the ages of 25 and 65 years who were unwilling to change their dietary and physical activity habits. There were 40 women and 22 men in the study. The trial was completed between November 2011 and August 2012. For 4 months, the participants consumed either the supplement or the placebo; the capsules were identical in color, form, and smell. Follow-ups were scheduled at 2, 4, and 6 months. Fifty-two participants completed all the requirements and were included in the final analysis. The researchers learned that the participants taking the supplement had reduced fasting plasma glucose. No such changes were observed in the placebo group. The participants with higher fasting plasma glucose benefited most from the supplement. The participants on the supplement also had increased fat free mass. The researchers concluded that "whether the dietary supplement tested in this study can prevent the risk of T2D [type 2 diabetes] and related complications remains to be established in larger studies with longer treatment and follow-up durations, using clinical endpoints."[5]

Cinnamon Appears to Be Useful against *Helicobacter pylori*

In a randomized open-label trial published in 2012 in the *Prime Journal of Microbiology Research*, a researcher from Egypt wanted to learn if a supplement containing cinnamon or ginger would be useful for people dealing with *Helicobacter pylori*, the gram-negative bacterium associated with gastritis and peptic ulcer disease. The cohort consisted of 52 men and eight women between the ages of 24 and 56 years who were diagnosed with *H. pylori*. They were divided into three groups of 20. The participants in one group consumed cinnamon and omeprazole, a medication to treat peptic ulcer disease; the participants in another group consumed ginger and omeprazole; and the participants in the third group consumed cinnamon, ginger, and omeprazole. The trial continued for 14 days, and the findings were notable. Fifty percent of the participants consuming cinnamon and omeprazole were successfully treated; 70% of those taking ginger and omeprazole were successfully treated; and 80% of those on cinnamon, ginger, and omeprazole experienced complete eradication of the disease. In addition, only hours after the treatment began, all the regimens reduced the associated symptoms. Hence, the researchers concluded that "ginger and cinnamon preparations traditionally used for the treatment of gastrointestinal disorders are effective as components of *H. pylori* eradication regimens with little or no adverse reactions."[6]

Cinnamon May Lower Blood Pressure for a Brief Period of Time

In an article published in 2013 in the journal *Nutrition*, researchers from Canada and the United Kingdom conducted a comprehensive literature review of the association between cinnamon supplementation and blood pressure. They included three randomized clinical trials published between January 2000 and September 2012. Two of the trials included people with diabetes, and one included people with prediabetes. All studies lasted 12 weeks, with cinnamon doses ranging from 500 mg to 2.4 g per day. After data analysis, the researchers found that cinnamon significantly reduced systolic and diastolic blood pressure. If the trials had continued for longer periods of time, would cinnamon continue to lower blood pressure? It remains unknown. According to the researchers, "although cinnamon shows hopeful effects on BP [blood pressure]-lowering potential, it would be premature to recommend cinnamon for BP control because of the limited number of studies available."[7]

Cinnamon Oil Appears to Have Antifungal Properties

In a study published in 2012 in the *Journal of Traditional Chinese Medicine*, researchers from China wanted to learn more about the antifungal properties of cinnamon oil both in the laboratory and in patients suffering from intestinal candida, a fungal infection. In the laboratory, researchers treated three species of candida cells with cinnamon oil combined with pogostemon oil. They found that the oils had strong antifungal activity against the three fungal strains. The researchers noted that "irregular hollows appeared on the surfaces, inside organelles were destroyed and the cells burst after treatment." Interestingly, when the researchers tested fluconazole, an antifungal medication, against these strains of candida, it was effective against two strains, but not very effective against the third strain. During the clinical portion of the study, the study cohort consisted of 100 participants infected with candida displaying symptoms, such as chronic diarrhea and abdominal pain. For 14 days, 60 participants were treated with capsules containing cinnamon oil and pogostemon oil, and the remaining 40 were treated with fluconazole. The researchers determined that both treatment types had strong antifungal properties. The findings on the combination oil treatment were especially notable. Seventy-two percent of the participants had no candida in their stool, and the remaining 28% had a significant reduction. The researchers concluded "that the use of cinnamon oil in the treatment of deep candida infection may provide a valid treatment option."[8]

Cinnamon Supplementation Has the Potential to Cause Acute Hepatitis

In a case report published in 2015 in the *American Journal of Case Reports*, medical providers from Southfield, Michigan (USA), described the case of a 73-year-old woman who was seen in an emergency department. Since starting a cinnamon supplement regimen about a week before the hospital visit, she had been experiencing abdominal pain with vomiting and diarrhea. She had hoped cinnamon would help manage her diabetes. The woman also took a statin to treat coronary artery disease and a host of other medications to treat her several medical problems. Laboratory and imaging studies confirmed a diagnosis of acute hepatitis. Her medical providers temporarily discontinued the statin medication and instructed the woman to stop taking cinnamon supplementation. Moreover, they concluded that "the combination of cinnamon supplementation and a high dose statin therapy was the likely etiology of the patient's acute hepatitis." Therefore, "patients should be warned against the use of these medications in combination." After her hospitalization, the patient was discharged, and she continued her recovery at home.[9]

Cinnamon Flavor May Cause Problems in the Mouth

In an article published in 2015 in *The Open Dentistry Journal*, dentists from Brazil described the case of a 64-year-old white woman who was referred to their clinic for symptomatic oral lesions that had been present for 3 days. The woman complained that she had "a constant burning sensation along with roughness and thickness on the oral mucosa." Upon further discussion with the woman, the dentists learned that she had recently changed the flavor of her mints to cinnamon. The dentists advised the woman to discontinue the use of those mints. Soon after discontinuation, she had relief from her symptoms, and in 3 weeks, she was completely healed. To confirm this sensitivity, the woman once again used the mints and had a similar reaction. At that point, she stopped using the mints. The researchers commented that "clinicians should suspect this condition whenever patients report use of cinnamon products."[10]

Another article, published in 2010 in *Journal of Dermatological Case Reports*, described the case of a 20-year-old female in Athens, Greece who had a "burning tongue" and white elevated mucosal patches in the right lateral board of the tongue. Her medical history was unremarkable, and she had good oral hygiene. However, she reported frequent use of a chewing gum with a cinnamon flavor, which she held on the right side of her mouth. The dermatologist diagnosed cinnamon contact stomatitis (CCS), a rare reaction to the use of products containing artificial cinnamon-flavored ingredients. The patient was told to avoid all use of cinnamon-flavored chewing gums. Once the patient stopped using the gum, the tongue returned to a normal appearance. The researchers concluded that "clinicians who treat patients with oral conditions should be aware of CCS in order to be able to correctly diagnose and manage this condition."[11]

People Should Be Aware of the Dangers of the "Cinnamon Challenge"

An article published in 2013 in the journal *Pediatrics* described the practice known as the "Cinnamon Challenge." The challenge entails swallowing a tablespoon of ground cinnamon in 60 seconds without drinking any fluids. According to the website, www.cinnamonchallenge.com, this challenge is practically impossible, decidedly unpleasant, and potentially harmful. Still, videos of the challenge are frequently posted on the Internet. The researchers noted that "typically, the video reveals a group of adolescents watching as someone taking the challenge begins coughing and choking when the spice triggers a severe gag reflex in response to a caustic sensation in the mouth and throat." Most of the millions of people who watch these videos are predominantly between the ages of 13 and 24 years. While most of the effects are temporary, there are concerns about choking, aspiration, and pulmonary damage. The authors of the article underscored the need for parents and medical providers to raise awareness about this hazard, especially among tweens, teens, and young adults who have cinnamon hypersensitivity, asthma, pulmonary cystic fibrosis, and chronic lung disease. These discussions will help young people "weigh the risk and rewards of yielding to peer pressure when considering senseless and risky behaviors."[12]

NOTES

1. Hamidpour, Rafie, Mohsen Hamidpour, Soheila Hamidpour, and Mina Shahlari. "Cinnamon from the Selection of Traditional Applications to Its Novel Effects on the Inhibition of Angiogenesis in Cancer Cells and Prevention of Alzheimer's Disease, and a Series of Functions Such as Antioxidant, Anticholesterol, Antidiabetes, Antibacterial, Antifungal, Nematicidal, Acaracidal, and Repellent Activities." *Journal of Traditional and Complementary Medicine* 5, no. 2 (April 2015): 66–70.

2. Rahman, Sonia, Halima Begum, Zaida Rahman, et al. "Effect of Cinnamon (*Cinnamomum cassia*) as a Lipid Lowering Agent on Hypercholesterolemic Rats." *Journal of Enam Medical College* 3, no. 2 (July 2013): 94–98.

3. Allen, Robert W., Emmanuelle Schwartzman, William L. Baker, et al. "Cinnamon Use in Type 2 Diabetes: An Updated Systematic Review and Meta-Analysis." *Annals of Family Medicine* 11, no. 5 (September/October 2013): 452–459.

4. Shalaby, Mostafa Abbas, and Hamed Yahya Saifan. "Some Pharmacological Effects of Cinnamon and Ginger Herbs in Obese Diabetic Rats." *Journal of Intercultural Ethnopharmacology* 3, no. 4 (2014): 144–149.

5. Liu, Yuejun, Aurélie Cotillard, Camille Vatier, et al. "A Dietary Supplement Containing Cinnamon, Chromium and Carnosine Decreases Fasting Plasma Glucose and Increases Lean Mass in Overweight or Obese Pre-Diabetic Subjects: A Randomized, Placebo-Controlled Trial." *PLoS ONE* 10, no. 9 (September 25, 2015): e0138646.

6. Ali, Ahmed M. "Efficacy of Ginger and Cinnamon Pharmaceutical Preparations in Patients with *Helicobacter pylori*–Associated Functional Dyspepsia." *Prime Journal of Microbiology Research* 2, no. 1 (2012): 67–72.

7. Akilen, R., Z. Pimlott, A. Tsiami, and N. Robinson. "Effects of Short-Term Administration of Cinnamon on Blood Pressure in Patients with Prediabetes, and Type 2 Diabetes." *Nutrition* 29, no. 10 (October 2013): 1192–1196.

8. Weng, Gang-sheng, Jie-hua Deng, Yao-hui Ma, et al. "Mechanisms, Clinical Curative Effects, and Antifungal Activities of Cinnamon Oil and Pogostemon Oil Complex Against Three Species of Candida." *Journal of Traditional Chinese Medicine* 32, no. 1 (March 2012): 19–24.

9. Brancheau, D., B. Patel, and M. Zughaib. "Do Cinnamon Supplements Cause Acute Hepatitis?" *American Journal of Case Reports* 16 (April 29, 2015): 250–254.

10. Vivas, Ana P. M., and Dante A. Migliari. "Cinnamon-Induced Oral Mucosal Contact Reaction." *The Open Dentistry Journal* 9 (2015): 257–259.

11. Georgakopoulou, Eleni A. "Cinnamon Contact Stomatitis." *Journal of Dermatological Case Reports* 2 (2010): 28–29.

12. Grant-Alfieri, Amelia, Judy Schaechter, and Steven E. Lipshultz. "Ingesting and Aspirating Dry Cinnamon by Children and Adolescents: The 'Cinnamon Challenge.'" *Pediatrics* 131, no. 5 (My 2013): 833–835.

REFERENCES AND FURTHER READING

Akilen, R., Z. Pimlott, A. Tsiami, and N. Robinson. "Effect of Short-Term Administration of Cinnamon on Blood Pressure in Patients with Prediabetes and Type 2 Diabetes." *Nutrition* 29, no. 10 (October 2013): 1192–1196.

Ali, Ahmed M. "Efficacy of Ginger and Cinnamon Pharmaceutical Preparations in Patients with *Helicobacter pylori*–Associated Functional Dyspepsia." *Prime Journal of Microbiology Research* 2, no. 1 (2012): 67–72.

Allen, Robert W., Emmanuelle Schwartzman, William L. Baker, et al. "Cinnamon Use in Type 2 Diabetes: An Updated Systematic Review and Meta-Analysis." *Annals of Family Medicine* 11, no. 5 (September/October 2013): 452–459.

Brancheau, D., B. Patel, and M. Zughaib. "Do Cinnamon Supplements Cause Acute Hepatitis?" *American Journal of Case Reports* 16 (April 29, 2015): 250–254.

Georgakopoulou, Eleni A. "Cinnamon Contact Stomatitis." *Journal of Dermatological Case Reports* 2 (2010): 28–29.

Grant-Alfieri, Amelia, Judy Schaechter, and Steven E. Lipshultz. "Ingesting and Aspirating Dry Cinnamon by Children and Adolescents: The 'Cinnamon Challenge.'" *Pediatrics* 131, no. 5 (May 2013): 833–835.

Hamidpour, Rafie, Mohsen Hamidpour, Scheila Hamidpour, and Mina Shahlan. "Cinnamon from the Selection of Traditional Applications to Its Novel Effects on the Inhibition of Angiogenesis in Cancer Cells and Prevention of Alzheimer's Disease, and a Series of Functions Such as Antioxidant, Anticholesterol Antidiabetes, Antibacterial, Antifungal, Nematicidal, Acaracidal, and Repellent Activities." *Journal of Traditional and Complementary Medicine* 5, no. 2 (April 2015): 66–70.

Liu, Yuejun, Aurélie Cotillard, Camille Vatier, et al. "A Dietary Supplement Containing Cinnamon, Chromium and Carnosine Decreases Fasting Plasma Glucose and Increases Lean Mass in Overweight or Obese Prediabetic Subjects: A Randomized, Placebo-Controlled Trial." *PLoS ONE* 10, no. 9 (September 25, 2015): e0138646.

Rahman, Sonia, Halima Begum, Zaida Rahman, et al. "Effect of Cinnamon (*Cinnamomum cassia*) as a Lipid Lowering Agent on Hypercholesterolemic Rats." *Journal of Enam Medical College* 3, no. 2 (July 2013): 94–98.

Shalaby, Mostafa Abbas, and Hamed Yahya Saifan. "Some Pharmacological Effects of Cinnamon and Ginger Herbs in Obese Diabetic Rats." *Journal of Intercultural Ethnopharmacology* 3, no. 4 (2014): 144–149.

Vivas, Ana P. M., and Dante A. Migliari. "Cinnamon-Induced Oral Mucosal Contact Reaction." *The Open Dentistry Journal* 9 (2015): 257–259.

Wang, Gang-sheng, Jie-hua Deng, Yao-hui Ma, et al. "Mechanisms, Clinically Curative Effects, and Antifungal Activities of Cinnamon Oil and Pogostemon Oil Complex Against Three Species of Candida." *Journal of Traditional Chinese Medicine* 32, no. 1 (March 2012): 19–24.

Cod Liver Oil

Derived from the liver of the codfish, cod liver oil is a nutrient-dense source of essential vitamins including vitamins A and D. It also contains high levels of omega-3 fatty acids, which have anti-inflammatory properties.

The medical use of cod liver oil may be traced to the late eighteenth century when a physician in England used the oil to treat rheumatism. A few decades later, cod liver oil was considered to be a remedy for rickets. By the 1930s, it was often a part of the daily supplement regimen given to children in the United States, and was considered an important component for improving the overall health of children.

There is a difference between cod liver oil and regular fish oils. While regular fish oils are extracted from the tissue of deep-sea oily fish, cod liver oil is derived only from the liver of the codfish.

HEALTH BENEFITS AND RISKS

Because of high amounts of vitamins A and D and the abundance of omega-3 fatty acids, cod liver oil is believed to have numerous health benefits. These benefits include cardiovascular support, maintaining bone health and reducing the risk of osteoporosis, treating depression, healing skin wounds, and protecting eyesight. In addition, cod liver oil is believed to be useful for arthritis conditions. On consuming cod liver oil, people with arthritis report reductions in pain, joint stiffness, and swelling. Furthermore, there is some evidence that cod liver oil improves brain function.

On oral consumption, some people experience belching, bad breath, loose stools, nosebleeds, heartburn, and nausea from cod liver oil. Consuming cod liver oil with a meal tends to diminish these side effects.

The omega-3 fatty acids present in cod liver oil give it blood-thinning properties. Hence, people on anticoagulant medication should not consume cod liver oil without discussing with a medical provider. It is a good idea to discontinue cod liver oil supplementation before any surgery as it may increase the risk of bleeding. Likewise, people on high blood pressure medication should use cod liver oil with caution as it may lower blood pressure significantly. Consuming large amounts of cod liver oil supplementation places people at risk of an excess intake of vitamin A. Symptoms of excessive vitamin A include dizziness, nausea, headaches, coma, and even death.

It is best to avoid consuming cod liver oil during pregnancy and breastfeeding as there is insufficient information to determine if it is safe for both the mother and the child.

HOW IT IS SOLD AND TAKEN

Because each brand of cod liver oil contains varying amounts of vitamins A and D and omega-3 fatty acids, it is impossible to provide dosing recommendations. Moreover, many brands contain fillers or synthetic ingredients. Nevertheless, the suggested dosing for regular cod liver oil is often two teaspoons, and the suggested dosing for high-vitamin cod liver oil is often one teaspoon. It is best to have a trusted medical provider suggest a specific brand. If this is not possible, select a preferred brand that contains astaxanthin or some other antioxidant to keep the oil from oxidizing. Cod liver oil is sold as a liquid in bottles and in capsules and gummies.

RESEARCH FINDINGS

There May Be an Association between Cod Liver Oil and Multiple Sclerosis

In a study published in 2015 in *Multiple Sclerosis Journal*, researchers from Boston, Massachusetts (USA), and Norway investigated the possible association between multiple sclerosis and the use of cod liver oil. Apparently, low levels of vitamin D have been "consistently associated with multiple sclerosis." Data were obtained from the Norwegian component of the multinational case-control study Environmental Factors in Multiple Sclerosis (EnvIMS). The study included 953 multiple sclerosis patients with maximum disease duration of 10 years and 1717 controls. All participants reported their cod liver oil use from childhood to adulthood. Supplementation during childhood, adolescence, and adulthood was more common among participants born before 1962. The researchers learned that the self-reported use of cod liver oil between the ages of 13 and 18 years was associated with a reduced risk for multiple sclerosis; cod liver oil supplementation earlier in childhood or adulthood did not appear to alter the risk of multiple sclerosis. The researchers commented that their "findings suggest that adolescence might be an especially susceptible period for disease risk modification through dietary vitamin D." Perhaps, the researchers added, "higher doses of vitamin D may be needed during childhood and adulthood to reach the same degree of risk modification as during adolescence."[1]

Cod Liver Oil Appears to Support Bone Mineralization

In a study published in 2012 in the journal *Toxicology and Industrial Health*, researchers from Saudi Arabia explained that the lower levels of estrogen in postmenopausal women increase their risk for osteoporosis. Yet, hormone therapy, which supports bones, has numerous negative side effects. Therefore, it is important to find other ways to improve bone health. In this study, they investigated the ability of cod liver oil to support bone mineralization in ovariectomized female rats. The study began with 48 rats divided into four groups of 12 rats. One group of rats served as the control; the rats in the three other groups had ovariectomy surgery. A second group of rats only had the surgery. During the surgery, the rats in the third group received estrogen implants, and the rats in the fourth group took cod liver oil supplementation for 8 weeks. At the end of the study, the rats were sacrificed. The researchers found that the rats with estrogen implants and those on cod liver oil had increased levels of calcium in their femurs. The researchers concluded that "the positive effect of CLO [cod liver oil] in the treatment of osteoporosis to lower the estrogen needed and thus reduces the dangerous side effects of estrogen treatment."[2]

Cod Liver Oil Intake during Younger Years May or May Not Impact Bones of Older People

In a study published in 2008 in the *American Journal of Epidemiology*, researchers from Norway noted that it is not uncommon for cod liver oil supplementation to be recommended during the fall and winter months to prevent vitamin D deficiency and rickets. They wanted to determine if this supplementation would somehow interfere with bone mineral density or fractures in adult life. As part of a substudy of the population-based Nord-Trøndelag Health Study, in 2001, a total of 3052 Norwegian women, virtually all Caucasian, between the ages of 50 and 70 years, underwent forearm bone mineral density tests. The women were asked if they consumed cod liver oil during their childhood. There answers were reported as "never, irregularly, during the fall and winter, and throughout the year." The women were also asked about their current intake of cod liver oil. Cod liver oil intake during childhood was reported by more than 90% of the 2854 women who answered that question. Current intake of cod liver oil was reported by almost 60% of the women. The women who reported no childhood intake of cod liver oil had statistically significant higher bone mineral density than those with any ingestion of cod liver oil. There was no association between current intake of cod liver oil and bone mineral density. The researchers commented that "this unexpected result is paradoxical, considering the good bone health intentions behind the long-standing cod liver oil recommendations."[3]

On the other hand, in a study published in 2015 in the *British Journal of Nutrition*, researchers from Iceland and Bethesda, Maryland (USA), investigated the association between the lifelong consumption of cod liver oil and hipbone mineral density in old age. The researchers noted that cod liver oil is a traditional source of vitamin D in Iceland. The cohort consisted of the 4798 participants in the Age, Gene/Environment Susceptibility (AGES)-Reykjavik Study, in which the participants, aged 66–96 years, reported on their intake of cod liver oil during adolescence, midlife, and old age. The intake levels were divided into three groups—never or less than once per week, one to six times per week, or daily intake. The researchers learned that the intake of cod liver oil was fairly common. In fact, in the mid-twentieth century, when many of the participants were in their teens, cod liver oil was given to them in most schools. Yet, the researchers found no significant associations between retrospective cod liver oil intake and hipbone mineral density in old age. They concluded that there was "no evidence that cod liver oil intake at any age might be harmful to hip BMD [bone mineral density] in old age."[4]

The Consumption of Cod Live Oil during Adolescence and Midlife May Reduce the Risk of Coronary Heart Disease in Older Women

In a study published in 2016 in *Public Health Nutrition*, researchers based in Iceland examined the association between the consumption of fish and cod liver oil in adolescence and midlife and the risk of coronary heart disease in older women. Data were obtained from the AGES-Reykjavik Study of the Iceland Heart Association, which included 3326 women between the ages of 66 and 96 years. Because of missing data, 360 women were excluded. The final analysis included 2966 women. Coronary heart disease was identified in 234 women (7.9%). Compared to women with no intake of cod liver oil, women who consumed cod liver oil at least three times per week in adolescence and midlife had a decreased risk of coronary heart disease. The consumption of cod liver oil "from early life, may reduce the risk of CHD in older women." This association was not observed when cod liver oil consumption was replaced with the consumption of fish oil. The researchers concluded that "data did not show any protection by fish consumption against CHD [coronary heart disease], neither during the adolescent period not in midlife."[5]

Cod Liver Oil during the First Year of Life May Help Prevent Type 1 Diabetes

In a somewhat dated but intriguing study published in 2003 in the *American Journal of Clinical Nutrition*, researchers from Norway wanted to determine if cod liver oil (or other vitamin D supplements), either taken by the mother during pregnancy or by the child during the first year of life, was associated with a child's reduced risk for type 1 diabetes. The cohort consisted of 545 people who had childhood-onset type 1 diabetes and 1668 controls. The researchers found no association between the mother's use of cod liver oil or other vitamin D-containing supplements during pregnancy and type 1 diabetes diagnosis in children. On the other hand, the researchers found that the use of cod liver oil during a baby's first year of life was associated with a significantly lower risk of type 1 diabetes. This association was somewhat stronger among girls than boys. The researchers concluded that "cod liver oil or individual fatty acids such as DHA may be candidates for preventive interventional trials."[6]

Cod Liver Oil May Relieve the Symptoms of Rheumatoid Arthritis

In a dual-center, double-blind, placebo-controlled randomized trial published in 2008 in the journal *Rheumatology*, researchers from the United Kingdom attempted to determine if cod liver oil supplementation would enable people with rheumatoid arthritis to take less nonsteroidal anti-inflammatory drug (NSAID) pain medication. The initial cohort consisted of 97 patients aged 18 years or older with rheumatoid arthritis. They were placed on either a cod liver oil supplement or an identical looking placebo. The patients were assessed at baseline, 4 weeks, 12 weeks, 24 weeks, and 36 weeks. Thirty-two of the patients in the cod liver oil group and 26 in the placebo group completed the study. After 9 months, 19 patients in the cod liver oil group and five in the placebo group were able to reduce their intake of NSAID by more than 30%, "without worsening of disease activity." According to the researchers, their findings "suggest that cod liver oil supplements containing n-3 fatty acids can be used as NSAID-sparing agents in RA [rheumatoid arthritis] patients."[7]

Users of Cod Liver Oil and Other Supplements May Have Better Rates of Survival from Cancerous Tumors

In a study published in 2009 in the *International Journal of Cancer*, researchers from Norway wanted to learn if the use of cod liver oil and other supplements before a cancerous tumor diagnosis had any effect on the survival rates. The researchers used data obtained from the Norwegian Women and Cancer cohort study. Cod liver oil was the most frequently used dietary supplement, followed by multivitamin and mineral supplements. The cohort consisted of 68,518 women who answered a self-administered questionnaire. Their mean age at diagnosis was 58.4 years. The researchers learned that the consumption of cod liver oil daily for a year prior to diagnosis was associated with a 23% reduction in death among people with solid tumors, and a reduction of 44% among those with lung cancer. The researchers commented that they were unable to determine if these differences were "due to beneficial effects of supplements or differences between supplement users and nonusers."[8]

In Addition to Some Other Oils, Cod Liver Oil May Be Useful for Side Effects of Diabetes

In a study published in 2013 in the *Journal of Diabetes & Metabolic Disorders*, researchers from Saudi Arabia assessed the ability of several oils, including cod liver oil, to ameliorate problems associated with diabetes, such as serum glucose, liver function, and kidney function. The cohort consisted of 45 male albino rats; 40 rats were injected with streptozotocin to induce diabetes, and five rats were assigned to each of the nine groups. Different oils were fed to rats in seven groups. Each oil was added to the animals' diet at 10% level for 28 days. Cod liver oil was found to have numerous positive effects, including improving liver function and amelioration of renal dysfunction. None of the oils were able to curtail the increases in serum glucose caused by diabetes. The researchers commented that "the findings of this study strongly support the efficacy of vegetable and fish oils in the amelioration and even prevention of the side effects of type 2 diabetes mellitus."[9]

Cod Liver Intake May Be Associated with Increased Rates of Asthma

In a study published in 2013 in the journal *Thorax*, researchers from Norway, Canada, and Boston noted that before 1999 the cod liver formula in Norway contained high concentrations of vitamin A, which has been associated with several chronic diseases. Therefore, they examined the association between high intake of cod liver oil and the incidence of asthma in the previously mentioned Nord-Trøndelag Health Study. Their cohort consisted of 17,528 Norwegian adults, of which 18% consumed cod liver oil daily for 1 month or more during the previous year. The cumulative incidence of asthma over the 11-year follow-up was 4.4% among people who regularly consumed cod liver oil and 2.9% among people who did not. The consumption of cod liver oil was significantly associated with an increased incidence of asthma. Moreover, each 1-month daily intake of cod liver oil was significantly associated with incident asthma. The researchers concluded that the "intake of cod liver oil with high vitamin A content was significantly associated with increased incidence of adult-onset asthma."[10]

People May Have an Allergic Reaction to Cod Liver Oil

In a case report published in 2007 in the journal *Contact Dermatitis*, medical providers from Italy described the case of an 80-year-old woman with hepatitis C and post-thrombotic leg ulcers who experienced severe and intense itching on her right leg and back. The reaction appeared while using an emollient cream containing cod liver oil. After the cream was discontinued, the symptoms stopped. At a later date, the medical providers conducted patch testing of all the ingredients in the cream. The symptoms once again appeared in the cod liver oil areas. The medical providers concluded that people need to be aware of "the capacity of cod liver oil to induce contact sensitization considering its use for self-medication on compromised skin."[11]

NOTES

1. Cortese, Marianna, Trond Riise, Kjetil Bjornevik, et al. "Timing of Use of Cod Liver Oil, a Vitamin D Source, and Multiple Sclerosis Risk: The EnvIMS Study." *Multiple Sclerosis Journal* 21, no. 14 (2015): 1856–1864.

2. Moselhy, S. S., A. L. Al-Malki, T. A. Kumosani, and J. A. Jalal. "Modulatory Effect of Cod Liver Oil on Bine Mineralization in Overiectomized Female Sprague Dawley Rats." *Toxicology and Industrial Health* 28, no. 5 (June 2012): 387–392.

3. Forsmo, Siri, Sigurd Kjørstad, and Arnulf Langhammer. "Childhood Cod Liver Oil Consumption and Bone Mineral Density in a Population-Based Cohort of Peri- and Post-Menopausal Women: The Nord-Trøndelag Health Study." *American Journal of Epidemiology* 167, no. 4 (February 2008): 406–411.

4. Eysteinsdottir, T., T. I. Hallddorsson, I. Thorsdottir, et al. "Cod Liver Oil Consumption at Different Periods of Life and Bone Mineral Density in Old Age." *British Journal of Nutrition* 114, no. 2 (July 2015): 248–256.

5. Haraoldsdottir, Alfheidur, Johanna E. Torfadottir, Unnur A. Valdimarsdottir, and Thor Aspelund. "Fish and Fish-Live Oil Consumption in Adolescence and Midlife and

Risk of CHD in Older Women." *Public Health Nutrition* 19, no. 2 (February 2016): 318–325.

6. Stene, L. C., G. Joner, and Norwegian Childhood Diabetes Study Group. "Use of Cod Liver Oil during the First Year of Life Is Associated with Lower Risk of Childhood-Onset Type 1 Diabetes: A Large, Population-Based, Case-Control Study." *American Journal of Clinical Nutrition* 78, no. 6 (December 2003): 1128–1134.

7. Galarraga, B., M. Ho, H. M. Youssef, et al. "Cod Live Oil (n-3 Fatty Acids) as an Non-Steroidal Anti-Inflammatory Drug Sparing Agent in Rheumatoid Arthritis." *Rheumatology* 47, no. 5 (May 2008): 665–669.

8. Skeie, Guri, Tonje Braaten, Anette Hjartåker, et al. "Cod Liver Oil, Other Dietary Supplements and Survival among Cancer Patients with Solid Tumours." *International Journal of Cancer* 125, no. 5 (September 1, 2009): 1155–1160.

9. Al-Amoudi, N. S., and H. A. Abu Araki. "Evaluation of Vegetable and Fish Oils for the Amelioration of Diabetes Side Effects." *Journal of Diabetes & Metabolic Disorders* 12, no. 1 (February 21, 2013): 13.

10. Mai, X. M., A. Langhammer, Y. Chen, and C. A. Camargo Jr. "Col Live Oil Intake and Incidence of Asthma in Norwegian Adults–The HUNT Study." *Thorax* 68, no. 1 (January 2013): 25–30.

11. Foti, C., D. Bonamonte, A. Conserva, et al. "Allergic Contact Dermatitis to Cod Liver Oil Contained in a Topical Ointment." *Contact Dermatitis* 57, no. 4 (October 2007): 281–282.

REFERENCES AND FURTHER READING

Al-Amoudi, N. S., and H. A. Abu Araki. "Evaluation of Vegetable and Fish Oil Diets for the Amelioration of Diabetes Side Effects." *Journal of Diabetes & Metabolic Disorders* 12, no. 1 (February 21, 2013): 13.

Cortese, Marianna, Trond Riise, Kjetil Bjornevik, et al. "Timing of Use of Cod Liver Oil, a Vitamin D Source, and Multiple Sclerosis Risk: The EnvIMS Study." *Multiple Sclerosis Journal* 21, no. 14 (2015): 1856–1864.

Eysteinsdottir, T., T. I. Halldorsson, I. Thorsdottir, et al. "Cod Liver Oil Consumption at Different Periods of Life and Bone Mineral Density in Old Age." *British Journal of Nutrition* 114, no. 2 (July 2015): 248–256.

Forsmo, Siri, Sigurd Kjørstad Fjeldbo, and Arnulf Langhammer. "Childhood Cod Liver Oil Consumption and Bone Mineral Density in a Population-Based Cohort of Peri-and Postmenopausal Women: The Nord-Trøndelag Health Study." *American Journal of Epidemiology* 167, no. 4 (February 2008): 406–411.

Foti, C., D. Bonamonte, A. Conserva, et al. "Allergic Contact Dermatitis to Cod Liver Oil Contained in a Topical Ointment." *Contact Dermatitis* 57, no. 4 (October 2007): 281–282.

Galarraga, B., M. Ho, H. M. Youssef, et al. "Cold Live Oil (n-3 Fatty Acids) as an Non-Steroidal Anti-Inflammatory Drug Sparing Agent in Rheumatoid Arthritis." *Rheumatology* 47, no. 5 (May 2008): 665–669.

Haraldsdottir, Alfheidur, Johanna E. Torfadottir, Unnur A. Valdimarsdottir, and Thor Aspelund. "Fish and Fish-Liver Oil Consumption in Adolescence and Midlife and Risk of CHD in Older Women." *Public Health Nutrition* 19, no. 2 (February 2016): 318–325.

Mai, X. M., A. Langhammer, Y. Chen, and C. A. Camargo Jr. "Cod Liver Oil Intake and Incidence of Asthma in Norwegian Adults–The HUNT Study." *Thorax* 68, no. 1 (January 2013): 25–30.

Moselhy, S. S., A. L. Al-Malki, T. A. Kumosani, and J. A. Jalal. "Modulatory Effect of Cod Liver Oil on Bone Mineralization in Overiectomized Female Sprague Dawley Rats." *Toxicology and Industrial Health* 28, no. 5 (June 2012): 387–392.

Skeie, Guri, Tonje Braaten, Anette Hjartåker, et al. "Cod Liver Oil, Other Dietary Supplements and Survival among Cancer Patients with Solid Tumours." *International Journal of Cancer* 125, no. 5 (September 1, 2009): 1155–1160.

Stene, L. C., G. Joner, and Norwegian Childhood Diabetes Study Group. "Use of Cod Liver Oil during the First Year of Life Is Associated with Lower Risk of Childhood-Onset Type 1 Diabetes: A Large, Population-Based, Case-Control Study." *American Journal of Clinical Nutrition* 78, no. 6 (December 2003): 1128–1134.

Coenzyme Q10

Coenzyme Q10, also known as ubiquinone and CoQ10, is found in the mitochondria of almost every cell in the body. It helps convert food into energy, and is a powerful antioxidant. It fights particles in the body known as free radicals, which contribute to a number of chronic health problems such as heart disease and cancer. Antioxidants such as coenzyme Q10 neutralize free radicals and help prevent some of the damage they cause. In the human body, the highest amounts of coenzyme Q10 are found in the heart, liver, kidneys, and pancreas.

Dietary sources of coenzyme Q10 include oily fish such as salmon and tuna, and organ meats such as liver and whole grains. Because none of these sources contain large amounts of coenzyme Q10, food alone cannot significantly raise coenzyme Q10 levels in the body. However, the body synthesizes coenzyme Q10. Hence, while few foods contain larger amounts of this compound, in most cases, this is not a problem as the body creates what it needs.

HEALTH BENEFITS AND RISKS

Because it is an antioxidant, coenzyme Q10 is believed to be useful for a wide variety of medical problems, such as cardiovascular disease, heart failure, high blood pressure, high cholesterol, and diabetes. It may also be useful for gum disease, improving immunity, Parkinson's disease, and migraines. Because statin medications, used to lower cholesterol, tend to lower the levels of coenzyme Q10 in the body, people consuming statins may want to consider coenzyme Q10 supplementation.

Coenzyme Q10 supplementation has been associated with several side effects including stomach upset, diarrhea, loss of appetite, insomnia, increased liver enzymes, rashes, nausea, upper abdominal pain, dizziness, light sensitivity, irritability, headaches, heartburn, and fatigue. It is not yet known if it is safe to consume coenzyme Q10 during pregnancy and breastfeeding.

HOW IT IS SOLD AND TAKEN

Coenzyme Q10 supplementation is sold in various forms including capsules, soft gel capsules, hard shell capsules, oral spray, liquid, and tablets. Medical providers may also prescribe intravenous coenzyme Q10. Though there is no established ideal dose, the recommended dose for adults 19 years and older tends to range between 100 and 200 mg per day; however, some may recommend much higher doses. Because coenzyme Q10 is fat soluble, it should be taken with a meal that has some fat. Unless under the direction of a medical professional, children and teens should not consume coenzyme Q10.

RESEARCH FINDINGS

When Used in Conjunction with Vitamin B6, Coenzyme Q10 Appears to Reduce the Risk of Coronary Artery Disease

In a case-control study published in 2012 in the journal *Nutrition Research*, researchers from Taiwan wanted to learn more about the association between intake of coenzyme Q10 and vitamin B6 and coronary artery disease. The cohort consisted of 45 participants who had at least 50% stenosis of one major coronary artery, identified by cardiac catheterization, and 89 healthy controls who had normal blood biochemistry testing. The researchers determined that the participants with coronary artery disease had significantly lower plasma levels of coenzyme Q10 and vitamin B6 than the controls. The participants with the higher concentrations of coenzyme Q10 had significantly lower risk of coronary artery disease. In fact, the researchers observed that the participants with coronary artery disease were deficient in coenzyme Q10. The researchers commented that their findings "suggest that increasing the plasma coenzyme Q10 level may reduce the risk of CAD [coronary artery disease], and there may be a benefit in administering coenzyme Q10 combined with vitamin B-6 to CAD patients, especially the patients with a low coenzyme Q10 and Vitamin B-6 levels."[1]

Coenzyme Q10 May Be Useful for Elite Athletes

In a double-blind study published in 2008 in the *British Journal of Nutrition*, researchers from Japan wanted to learn if coenzyme Q10 would benefit elite athletes. Specifically, they wanted to determine if the supplement would reduce muscular injury and oxidative stress during exercise training. The cohort consisted of 18 male students who were elite modern martial arts (kendo) athletes. For 20 days, they randomly received either 300 mg per day of coenzyme Q10 (n = 10) or a placebo (n = 8). Both the supplement and placebo were identical in appearance. During the intervention period, the athletes had daily training session of 5½ h per day for six days. Blood tests determined that the athletes taking coenzyme Q10 had less muscle damage, injury, and oxidative stress. The researchers commented that their findings "indicated that muscular injury in these collegiate athletes was attenuated by CoQ10 supplementation."[2]

Coenzyme Q10 May Have Antifatigue Properties

In a double-blind, placebo-controlled, three crossover design trial published in 2008 in the journal *Nutrition*, researchers from Japan tested the ability of coenzyme Q10 supplementation to reduce fatigue during physical exercise. The cohort consisted of 17 healthy volunteers randomized to take 100 mg or 300 mg per day or a placebo for 8 days. All the participants participated in three interventions, with washout periods separating the 8-day studies. The researchers learned that physical performance, tested on a bicycle ergometer at fixed workloads, increased when the participants took the 300 mg per day dose of coenzyme Q10. In addition, those on the higher dose of coenzyme Q10 experienced subjective fatigue reduction and greater recovery. The researchers concluded that "oral administration of coenzyme Q10 improved subjective fatigue sensation and physical performance during fatigue-induced workload trials and might prevent unfavorable conditions as a result of physical fatigue."[3]

Coenzyme Q10 Does Not Appear to Be Useful for Fatigue in Newly Diagnosed Patients with Breast Cancer

In a randomized, double-blind, placebo-controlled trial published in 2013 in the *Journal of Supportive Oncology*, researchers based in North Carolina (USA) wanted to learn if coenzyme Q10 would be useful for the fatigue, depression, and quality of life issues experienced by some newly diagnosed breast cancer patients being treated with chemotherapy. The initial cohort consisted of 236 female patients who were enrolled between August 2004 and March 2009. The patients age ranged between 28 and 85 years, with a median age of 51 years. For 24 weeks, they took either coenzyme supplementation or a placebo. However, before completing the entire study, 97 patients withdrew. Still, the results were notable. The researchers learned that coenzyme supplementation did not significantly relieve any of the measures of fatigue, depression, or quality of life. In addition, there was no reason to believe that coenzyme Q10 would be useful for these conditions.[4]

When Combined with Selenium, Coenzyme Q10 Appears to Support Heart Health in the Elderly

In a 5-year, prospective, randomized, double-blind, placebo-controlled trial published in 2013 in the *International Journal of Cardiology*, researchers from Sweden tested the ability of a supplement containing coenzyme Q10 and selenium to improve cardiac function. The initial cohort consisted of 443 Swedish citizens between the ages of 70 and 88 years. Participants were assigned to receive either 200 mg per day of coenzyme Q10 capsules and 200 µg per day of organic selenium yeast tablets (n = 221) or a similar looking placebo (n = 222). Two hundred and twenty-eight participants completed the entire trial. The researchers learned that 5.9% of the participants in the supplement group and 12.6% of those in the placebo group died of cardiovascular disease. Moreover, a biomarker of tension in the heart wall (N-terminal proBNP) was also significantly lower in the supplement group. The researchers concluded that "long-term supplementation of selenium/coenzyme Q10 reduces cardiovascular mortality."[5]

Coenzyme Q10 May Be Useful for People with Heart Failure

In a study published in 2014 in the journal *JACC: Heart Failure*, researchers from multiple countries throughout the world but based in Denmark examined the effect of coenzyme supplementation on patients with moderate-to-severe heart failure (failure of the heart to function properly). Four hundred and twenty patients were from 17 European, Asian, and Australian medical centers, who were randomly assigned to consume coenzyme Q10 (n = 202) supplementation or a placebo (n = 218). After 3 months, the researchers learned that the levels of a heart failure biomarker were lower in the supplement group. At the end of 2 years, when the trial concluded, 14% of the participants taking coenzyme Q10 supplementation had a major adverse cardiovascular event, which was lower than the 25% noted in the placebo group. The participants in the supplement group also had lower rates of mortality and fewer hospitalizations. Eighteen participants died in the supplement group, and 36 died in the placebo group. The researchers concluded that treatment with coenzyme Q10 "in addition to standard therapy for patients with moderate to severe HF [heart failure] is safe, well-tolerated, and associated with a reduction in symptoms."[6]

In a meta-analysis published in 2013 in the *American Journal of Clinical Nutrition*, researchers from New Orleans, Louisiana (USA), wanted to determine if coenzyme Q10 would be useful for people with congestive heart failure. The researchers identified 13 relevant clinical trials, with 395 participants whose mean age ranged from 49.8 to 68 years. There were a total of seven crossover and six parallel-arm studies, 12 double-blind studies, and one single-blind study. The study duration ranged from 4 to 28 weeks, and the daily dosage of coenzyme Q10 was between 60 and 300 mg. The researchers found that coenzyme Q10 was associated with a 3.67% improvement in blood flow from the heart. However, the researchers underscored the need for more studies that "examine whether there is an effect when this supplementation is added to the current standard therapy for CHF [congestive heart failure] or whether there is a dose-response effect between the stage of CHF at baseline and the dose of CoQ10 required for an improvement to be seen."[7]

Coenzyme Q10 Supplementation May Be Useful Following Surgery for Liver Cancer

In a single-blind, randomized, parallel, placebo-controlled study published in 2016 in *Nutrition Journal*, researchers from Taiwan wanted to determine if coenzyme Q10 would benefit people recovering from liver cancer (hepatocellular carcinoma) surgery. The cohort consisted of 41 patients who had surgery for liver cancer. After surgery, the patients were assigned to consume coenzyme Q10 supplement (n = 21) or a placebo (n = 20) for 12 weeks. Twenty participants consuming coenzyme Q10 and 19 consuming placebo completed the study. The researchers determined that the patients on coenzyme Q10 supplementation had significantly reduced levels of oxidative stress and inflammatory markers, with significantly higher levels of antioxidant enzymes. The researchers concluded that coenzyme Q10 may be considered a complementary supplement for patients who have had liver cancer surgery, "particularly those under higher levels of oxidative stress and inflammation."[8]

Because Statin Medications Lower Levels of Coenzyme Q10, People on Statin Medications May Benefit from Coenzyme Q10 Supplementation

In a meta-analysis published in 2015 in the journal *Pharmacological Research*, researchers from many locations throughout the world reviewed studies concerning the impact of statin medications on the levels of serum coenzyme Q10. The cohort consisted of six randomly controlled trials. In total, 240 participants were in the statin group and 210 in the control group. The number of participants in these trials ranged from 19 to 120. The duration of the statin interventions ranged from 6 to 26 weeks. Four trials had a parallel-group design and two had a crossover design. The researchers found that treatment with statin medications caused a significant reduction in serum levels of coenzyme Q10. This reduction was observed in the trials that lasted less than 12 weeks and those lasting 12 weeks or longer. The researchers concluded that their "meta-analysis showed a significant reduction in plasma CoQ10 concentrations following treatment with statins."[9] People consuming statin medications may well benefit from coenzyme Q10 supplementation.

Coenzyme Q10 May or May Not Be Very Useful for People with High Blood Pressure and Metabolic Syndrome

In a randomized, double-blind, placebo-controlled crossover trial published in 2012 in the *American Journal of Hypertension*, researchers from New Zealand wanted to learn if people with high blood pressure and metabolic syndrome would benefit from coenzyme Q10 supplementation. The initial cohort consisted of 30 participants between the ages of 25 and 75 years, with metabolic syndrome and inadequately treated blood pressure. For 12 weeks, the participants took either coenzyme Q10 supplementation or a placebo. After a 4-week washout period, they were placed on the alternative supplement. Compared to placebo, the treatment with coenzyme Q10 was not associated with statistically significant reductions in systolic or diastolic blood pressure and heart rate, although daytime diastolic blood pressure was significantly lower with coenzyme supplementation. The researchers concluded that they "cannot rule out the possibility that coenzyme Q10 may have clinically useful antihypertensive effects in selected populations." Still, their data failed to "support a role in the routine management of patients with metabolic syndrome."[10]

When Combined with Riboflavin and Magnesium, Coenzyme Q10 and Small Amounts of Other Vitamins May Be Useful for Some Migraine Symptoms

In a randomized, double-blind, placebo-controlled trial published in 2015 in *The Journal of Headache and Pain*, researchers from Germany wanted to determine if a supplement containing coenzyme Q10, riboflavin, and magnesium, as well as small amounts of other vitamins would help people who suffer from migraines.

The researchers acknowledged that there are medications to treat migraines, but they have "potential side effects, sometimes of [a] severe nature." The initial cohort consisted of 130 adults between the ages of 18 and 65 years who have three or more migraine attacks per month. For 3 months, they took the supplement or a placebo. The participants were assessed at baseline and at the end of the trial. The final analysis included 55 participants in the treatment group and 57 in the placebo group. The researchers determined that migraine days in the treatment group dropped from 6.2 to 4.4 days per month. In the placebo group, it dropped from 6.2 to 5.2 days per month. The treatment group also experienced a significant reduction in the intensity of the migraine pain. The researchers observed that the "patients rated the efficacy of the treatment significantly superior to placebo."[11]

Coenzyme Q10 Supplementation May or May Not Improve Muscle Pain Associated with Statin Medication

In a review published in 2014 in the *Journal of the American Association of Nurse Practitioners*, researchers noted that muscle pain is the most common side effect of statin medications. As many as 10%–15% of people taking statins experience some degree of muscle pain. Therefore, the researchers wanted to learn if coenzyme Q10 would help reduce this pain. They examined seven relevant studies, which included participants aged 18 to 81 years. Several different types of statins were used at doses ranging from 10 to 40 mg per day. Doses of coenzyme Q10 ranged from 100 to 240 mg per day. The researchers found that in a few studies the muscle pain associated with statin decreased with coenzyme supplementation. One study showed no such benefit. The researchers concluded that "patients experiencing statin-related myopathy might benefit from supplementation with CoQ10." Further, they reported that clinicians may want to suggest a dose between 30 and 200 mg per day.[12]

On the other hand, in a 3-month study published in 2012 in the *American Journal of Cardiology*, researchers based at Fort Gordon, Georgia (USA), recruited 76 patients with statin-related muscle pain, primarily in their calves and thighs. The mean age of the participants was about 62 years. Forty patients were randomly assigned to take coenzyme supplementation, and 36 were randomly assigned to take a placebo. No significant pain differences were observed between the two groups. Coenzyme Q10 supplementation "was not more effective than placebo at decreasing muscle pain that was presumed to be statin induced." Moreover, both groups showed a substantial decrease in pain at one month, "suggesting a substantial placebo effect."[13]

In a systematic review and meta-analysis published in 2015 in the *Mayo Clinic Proceedings*, researchers from numerous locations throughout the world reviewed the same issue. Their analysis included six trials, and dosing varied from trial to trial—from 100 to 400 mg per day. All 302 participants were 18 years or older. The duration of supplementation ranged from 30 days to 3 months. The researchers found that coenzyme Q10 had no significant effect on muscle pain, at least in the doses they studied. The researchers acknowledged that other researchers, in smaller studies, have found that coenzyme Q10 may be useful for statin-related pain. However, they were unable to confirm that finding. According to their meta-analysis, there does not appear to be "any significant benefit of CoQ10 supplementation in improving statin-induced myopathy." They stressed on the need for more studies with higher doses of coenzyme Q10.[14]

Coenzyme Q10 Does Not Appear to Be Helpful for High-Altitude Cardiac Alterations

In a study published in 2014 in the journal *High Altitude Medicine & Biology*, researchers from the United Kingdom, Reno, Nevada (USA), and Australia investigated the ability of coenzyme Q10 to attenuate cardiac alterations caused by high altitudes. The cohort consisted of ten male and 13 female volunteers with an average age of 46 years. Recruited from the 2009 Caudwell Xtreme Everest Research Treks, the participants were studied before and within 48 hours of return from a 17-day trek to Everest Base Camp. After their baseline testing, the participants were randomly allocated to receive no intervention or coenzyme Q10 (300 mg per day) throughout the trek. All the participants successfully completed the trek and did not require supplemental oxygen. The researchers determined that the high-altitude trek "led to decreased cardiac mass and alternations in diastolic parameters" in both groups. Coenzyme Q10 did not alter any of the frequently occurring changes triggered by high altitudes.[15]

NOTES

1. Lee, Bor-Jen, Chi-Hua Yen, Hui-Chen Hsu, et al. "A Significant Correlation between the Plasma Levels of Coenzyme Q10 and Vitamin B-6 and a Reduced Risk of Coronary Artery Disease." *Nutrition Research* 32 (2012): 751–756.

2. Kon, Michihiro, Kai Tanabe, Takayuki Akimoto, et al. "Reducing Exercise-Induced Muscular Injury in *Kendo* Athletes with Supplementation of Coenzyme Q10." *British Journal of Nutrition* 100 (2008): 903–909.

3. Mizuno, K., M. Tanaka, S. Nozaki, et al. "Antifatigue Effects of Coenzyme Q10 during Physical Fatigue." *Nutrition* 24, no. 4 (April 2008): 293–299.

4. Lesser, G. J., D. Case, N. Stark, et al. "A Randomized, Double-Blind, Placebo-Controlled Study of Oral Coenzyme Q10 to Relieve Self-Reported Treatment-Related Fatigue in Newly Diagnosed Patients with Breast Cancer." *Journal of Supportive Oncology* 11, no. 1 (March 2013): 31–42.

5. Alehagen, Urban, Peter Johansson, Mikael Björnstedt, et al. "Cardiovascular Mortality and N-Terminal-proBNP Reduced after Combined Selenium and Coenzyme Q10 Supplementation: A 5-Year Prospective Randomized Double-Blind Placebo-Controlled Trial among Elderly Swedish Citizens." *International Journal of Cardiology* 167 (2013): 1860–1866.

6. Mortensen, S. A., F. Rosenfeldt, A. Kumar, et al. "The Effect of Coenzyme Q10 on Morbidity and Mortality in Chronic Heart Failure: Results from Q-SYMBIO: A Randomized Double-Blind Trial." *JACC: Heart Failure* 2, no. 6 (December 2014): 641–649.

7. Fotino, A. Domnica, Angela M. Thompson-Paul, and Lydia A. Bazzano. "Effect of Coenzyme Q10 Supplementation on Heart Failure: A Meta-Analysis." *American Journal of Clinical Nutrition* 97, no. 2 (February 2013): 268–275.

8. Liu, Hsiao-Tien, Yi-Chia Huang, Shao-Bin Cheng, et al. "Effects of Coenzyme Q10 Supplementation on Antioxidant Capacity and Inflammation in Hepatocellular

Carcinoma Patients after Surgery: A Randomized, Placebo-Controlled Trial." *Nutrition Journal* 15 (2016): 85–93.

9. Banach. M., C. Serban, S. Ursoniu, et al. "Statin Therapy and Plasma Coenzyme Q10 Concentrations—A Systematic Review and Meta-Analysis of Placebo-Controlled Trials." *Pharmacological Research* 99 (September 2015): 329–336.

10. Young, J. M., C. M. Florkoeski, S. L. Molyneux, et al. "A Randomized, Double-Blind, Placebo-Controlled Crossover Study of Coenzyme Q10 Therapy in Hypertensive Patients with the Metabolic Syndrome." *American Journal of Hypertension* 25, no. 2 (February 2012): 261–270.

11. Gaul, C., H. C. Diener, U. Danesch and on behalf of the Migravent® Study Group."Improvement of Migraine Symptoms with a Proprietary Supplement Containing Riboflavin, Magnesium and Q10: A Randomized, Double-Blind, Multicenter Trial." *The Journal of Headache and Pain* 16 (2015): 32–39.

12. Littlefield, N., R. L. Beckstrand, and K. E. Luthy. "Statins' Effect on Plasma Levels of Coenzyme Q10 and Improvement in Myopathy with Supplementation." *Journal of the American Association of Nurse Practitioners* 26, no. 2 (February 2014): 85–90.

13. Bookstaver, David A., Nancy A. Burkhalter, and Christos Hatzigeorgiou. "Effect of Coenzyme Q10 Supplementation on Statin-Induced Myalgias." *American Journal of Cardiology* 110, no. 4 (August 2012): 526–529.

14. Banach, M. C. Serban, A. Sahebkar, et al. "Effects of Coenzyme Q10 on Statin-Induced Myopathy: A Meta-Analysis of Randomized Controlled Trials." *Mayo Clinic Proceedings* 90, no. 1 (January 2015): 24–34.

15. Holloway, C. J., A. J. Murray, K. Mitchell, et al. "Oral Coenzyme Q10 Supplementation Does Not Prevent Cardiac Alternations during a High Altitude Trek to Everest Base Camp." *High Altitude Medicine & Biology* 15, no. 4 (December 2014): 459–467.

REFERENCES AND FURTHER READING

Alehagen, Urban, Peter Johansson, Mikael Björnstedt, et al. "Cardiovascular Mortality and N-Terminal-proBNP Reduced After Combined Selenium and Coenzyme Q10 Supplementation: A 5-Year Prospective Randomized Double-Blind Placebo-Controlled Trial among Elderly Swedish Citizens." *International Journal of Cardiology* 167 (2013): 1860–1866.

Banach, M., C. Serban, A. Sahebkar, et al. "Effects of Coenzyme Q10 on Statin-Induced Myopathy: A Meta-Analysis of Randomized Controlled Trials." *Mayo Clinic Proceedings* 90, no. 1 (January 2015): 24–34.

Banach, M., C. Serban, S. Ursoniu, et al. "Statin Therapy and Plasma Coenzyme Q10 Concentrations–A Systematic Review and Meta-Analysis of Placebo-Controlled Trials." *Pharmacological Research* 99 (September 2015): 329–336.

Bookstaver, David A., Nancy A. Burkhalter, and Christos Hatzigeorgiou. "Effect of Coenzyme Q10 Supplementation on Statin-Induced Myalgias." *American Journal of Cardiology* 110, no. 4 (August 2012): 526–529.

Fotino, A. D., A. M. Thompson-Paul, and L. A. Bazzano. "Effect of Coenzyme Q10 Supplementation on Heart Failure: A Meta-Analysis." *American Journal of Clinical Nutrition* 97, no. 2 (February 2013): 268–275.

Gaul, Charly, Hans-Christoph Diener, Ulrich Danesch and on Behalf of the Migravent® Study Group. "Improvement of Migraine Symptoms with a Proprietary Supplement Containing Riboflavin, Magnesium and Q10: A Randomized, Double-Blind, Multicenter Trial." *The Journal of Headache and Pain* 16 (2015): 32–39.

Holloway, C. J., A. J. Murray, K. Mitchell, et al. "Oral Coenzyme Q10 Supplementation Does Not Prevent Cardiac Alternations during a High Altitude Trek to Everest Base Camp." *High Altitude Medicine & Biology* 15, no. 4 (December 2014): 459–467.

Kon, Michihiro, Kai Tanabe, Takayuki Akimoto, et al. "Reducing Exercise-Induced Muscular Injury in *Kendo* Athletes with Supplementation of Coenzyme Q10." *British Journal of Nutrition* 100 (2008): 903–909.

Lee, Bor-Jen, Chi-Hua Yen, Hui-Chen Hsu, et al. "A Significant Correlation between the Plasma Levels of Coenzyme Q10 and Vitamin B-6 and a Reduced Risk of Coronary Artery Disease." *Nutrition Research* 32 (2012): 751–756.

Lesser, G. J., D. Case, N. Stark, et al. "A Randomized, Double-Blind, Placebo-Controlled Study of Oral Coenzyme Q10 to Relieve Self-Reported Treatment-Related Fatigue in Newly Diagnosed Patients with Breast Cancer." *Journal of Supportive Oncology* 11, no. 1 (March 2013): 31–42.

Littlefield, N., R. L. Beckstrand, and K. E. Luthy. "Statins' Effect on Plasma Levels of Coenzyme Q10 and Improvement in Myopathy with Supplementation." *Journal of the American Association of Nurse Practitioners* 26, no. 2 (February 2014): 85–90.

Liu, Hsiao-Tien, Yi-Chia Huang, Shao-Bin Cheng, et al. "Effects of Coenzyme Q10 Supplementation on Antioxidant Capacity and Inflammation in Hepatocellular Carcinoma Patients After Surgery: A Randomized, Placebo-Controlled Trial." *Nutrition Journal* 15 (2016): 85–93.

Mizuno, K., M. Tanaka, S. Nozaki, et al. "Antifatigue Effects of Coenzyme Q10 during Physical Fatigue." *Nutrition* 24, no. 4 (April 2008): 293–299.

Mortensen, S. A., F. Rosenfeldt, A. Kumar, et al. "The Effect of Coenzyme Q10 on Morbidity and Mortality in Chronic Heart Failure: Results from Q-SYMBIO: A Randomized Double-Blind Trial." *JACC: Heart Failure* 2, no. 6 (December 2014): 641–649.

Young, J. M., C. M. Florkowski, S. L. Molyneux, et al. "A Randomized, Double-Blind, Placebo-Controlled Crossover Study of Coenzyme Q10 Therapy in Hypertensive Patients with the Metabolic Syndrome." *American Journal of Hypertension* 25, no. 2 (February 2012): 261–270.

Collagen

Collagen is the most important protein in the human body, and is a major component of connective tissues, ligaments, skin, and muscles. Collagen gives skin structure and strengthens bones. Between 1% and 19% of muscle tissue is composed of collagen. Collagen is necessary to maintain muscle strength and its proper functioning. Moreover, because bones are made of collagen, as collagen in the body deteriorates, bone mass diminishes.

Collagen helps maintain the integrity of cartilage, the rubber-like tissue that protects joints. When the body ages, it produces less collagen, which results in dry skin and wrinkles.

Collagen is found in the connective tissue of animals. Sources include chicken skin, pork skin, and fish scales. Foods that contain gelatin also have collagen. Gelatin is a protein substance derived from cooked collagen.

There are more than a dozen types of collagen, each composed of different peptides or amino acids. Most supplements contain a hydrolyzed type I collagen, which supports healthy skin. (Hydrolyzed implies that the amino acid chains have been broken down into smaller units that are easier to absorb.) Type II collagen is primarily found in cartilage and is useful for joint health, and type III collagen promotes skin health by improving elasticity.

Though humans naturally synthesize collagen, with increasing age, the production of collagen slows. Eating foods rich in collagen will probably not produce sufficient amounts of collagen to compensate for this loss.

HEALTH BENEFITS AND RISKS

Collagen supplementation may boost muscle mass, especially in people with sarcopenia (muscle loss caused by aging), and prevent bone loss. It may increase the strength of nails and help leaky gut syndrome. In addition, collagen supplementation may support brain health and aid weight loss.

Collagen supplements are generally safe for most people. However, some supplements are made from common food allergens such as fish, shellfish, and eggs. Higher doses of collagen may be associated with digestive discomfort such as gas and bloating. People with kidney disease should use collagen with caution and under the guidance of a medical provider.

HOW IT IS SOLD AND TAKEN

Collagen supplementation is most often sold as a powder, but is also available in capsules, tablets, and gummies. Dosage recommendations tend to range from

5 g per day to 30 g per day. It is best to consult a medical provider before initiating supplementation.

RESEARCH FINDINGS

When Taken with Other Vitamins and Bioactive Compounds, Collagen Supplementation Improves Skin Elasticity, Joints, and General Wellbeing, and, Consequently, Has Antiaging Properties

In a double-blind, randomized, placebo-controlled clinical trial published in 2018 in the journal *Nutrition Research*, researchers from Italy and the United Kingdom hypothesized that collagen supplementation that also contained vitamins and bioactive compounds would have several antiaging benefits. The initial cohort had 122 healthy male and female participants, who were divided into two groups of 61 between the ages of 21 and 70 years. Eighty percent of the supplement group and 70% of the placebo group were women. For 90 days, the participants consumed the supplement or a placebo. One hundred and twenty participants completed the entire trial. During the trial, the participants were told to follow their normal skin routines. There were no reported adverse effects. The researchers learned that the participants consuming the supplement had a significant improvement in skin elasticity, a reduction in skin photoaging, and an improvement in general wellbeing. Interestingly, they also observed a significant improvement in joint health, with reductions in joint discomfort and increases in joint mobility in a subgroup of participants between the ages of 51 and 70 years. The researchers commented that the participants in the supplement group wanted "to continue with the oral supplementation . . . after the end of the study."[1]

When Combined with Resistance Training, Collagen Supplementation May Be Useful for Elderly Men

In a randomized, double-blind, placebo-controlled trial published in 2015 in the *British Journal of Nutrition*, researchers from Germany wanted to learn if the combination of collagen supplementation and resistance training would be useful for elderly men dealing with the loss of muscle mass and muscle function. The initial cohort consisted of 60 males. For 12 weeks, they took either 15 g of collagen peptides per day or a placebo; both were given in a powder form and were dissolved by the participants in 250 mL water. During the trial, all participants participated in a 60-min resistance training program three times per week. Assessments were made at baseline and at the end of the trial. Fifty-three men, with a mean age of 72.2 years, completed the trial. The researchers found that collagen supplementation increased the benefits associated with resistance training. The participants who consumed collagen supplements while they participated in the resistance training program had higher increases in fat-free mass and muscle strength as well as higher reduction in fat mass. These improvements appeared to be more pronounced than the findings in previous studies. The researchers underscored the need for similar studies in other populations, "including sex and different age groups and should focus on the mode of action as well as on the required dosage."[2]

Collagen Supplementation May Help the Symptoms of Osteoarthritis

In a double-blind, placebo-controlled, randomized clinical trial published in 2015 in the *Journal of the Science of Food and Agriculture*, researchers from India and Japan wanted to learn if pork and bovine collagen supplements would help people dealing with the symptoms of osteoarthritis, such as joint pain and stiffness and reduced mobility. The cohort consisted of 30 men and women between the ages of 30 and 65 years; all participants had been diagnosed with knee osteoarthritis. For 13 weeks, 20 participants consumed 10 g of collagen supplements per day, and the other 10 consumed placebos. During the treatment period, the participants had seven clinical visits. The researchers learned that the participants in the collagen supplement group had significant improvement in their osteoarthritis symptoms. The researchers concluded "that collagen peptides are potential therapeutic agents as nutritional supplements for the management of osteoarthritis and maintenance of joint health."[3]

Collagen Supplementation Appears to Improve Nail Growth and Reduces the Symptoms of Brittle Nails

In an open-label, single-center trial published in 2017 in the *Journal of Cosmetic Dermatology*, researchers from Brazil and Germany investigated the ability of a specific brand of bioactive collagen peptides (VERISOL) to improve nail growth and reduce the symptoms of brittle nails, including nail peeling, edge irregularities, and nail roughness. The cohort consisted of 25 healthy women between the ages of 18 and 50 years, who consumed 2.5 g VERISOL once daily for 24 weeks. The trial was followed by a 4-week off-therapy period. All women had brittle nails. Assessments were conducted at baseline, after 12 and 24 weeks, and 4 weeks after completing the trial. In addition, the participants evaluated their satisfaction with the treatment. The researchers learned that the participants experienced "considerable clinical improvement" in their brittle nail symptoms. There was an increase in nail growth rate and a significant decrease in the frequency of broken nails. Most participants were satisfied with the treatment and believed that their nails were stronger. By the end of the 4-week washout period, 88% of the women had "clinical global improvement." According to the researchers, "perhaps the most telling result is the high participant satisfaction." They also noted that the participants had "previously tried other treatments without success."[4]

Collagen Supplementation May Support Heart Health

In an open-label, single-dose trial published in 2017 in the *Journal of Atherosclerosis and Thrombosis*, researchers from Japan tested the ability of collagen to support heart health in generally healthy participants. The initial cohort consisted of 16 men and 16 women who had never received treatments for cardiovascular disease or diabetes. For 6 months, they consumed 2.4 g per day of collagen dissolved in beverages or soup. Thirty participants completed the entire trial. Several indices were used to assess the effect of collagen supplementation on the development of atherosclerosis. These included levels of total cholesterol, low-density lipoprotein cholesterol (LDL or "bad" cholesterol), high-density lipoprotein cholesterol (HDL or "good" cholesterol), and triglycerides. The researchers found that the collagen supplement significantly increased the levels of HDL cholesterol and significantly reduced the LDL cholesterol/HDL cholesterol ratio in 12 participants with the most cardiovascular risk. Other tests, such as the cardio-ankle vascular index, which measured arterial stiffness, were also conducted. From these tests, the researchers concluded that collagen supplementation "resulted in significant improvements in several predictors of atherosclerosis," and supported "the prevention and treatment of atherosclerosis in healthy humans."[5]

Collagen Supplementation Has Beneficial Effects on the Skin

In a double-blind, placebo-controlled trial published in 2014 in the journal *Skin Pharmacology and Physiology*, researchers from Germany and Brazil examined the ability of collagen hydrolysate supplements to improve skin elasticity, skin moisture, transepidermal water loss, and skin roughness. The initial cohort consisted of 69 healthy females between the ages of 35 and 55 years; for 8 weeks, the participants consumed 2.5 g or 5 g of collagen hydrolysate each day or a placebo (maltodextrin). Each group had 23 participants. The products were dissolved in water or another cold liquid. Assessments were conducted at baseline, at 4 weeks, at the end of the trial, and at 4 weeks after the trial ended. The researchers learned that both collagen doses improved skin physiology. For example, after 4 weeks, the skin had a statistically significant increase in elasticity. After 8 weeks, some of the women had an increase in elasticity of up to 30%. Compared to younger women, women over 50 years of age had a more pronounced increase in skin elasticity. This positive effect was still evident 4 weeks after the trial ended. Hence, the researchers concluded that "skin elasticity is a very important marker for skin aging."[6]

In a double-blind, randomized, placebo-controlled clinical trial published in 2015 in the *Journal of Medical Nutrition & Nutraceuticals*, researchers from the United Kingdom investigated the use of collagen supplementation for facial wrinkles, skin elasticity, and hydration. The cohort consisted of 18 postmenopausal women. For 12 weeks, nine participants consumed a daily drink containing hydrolyzed collagen, hyaluronic acid, and other vitamins and nutrients. The participants in the other group consumed a placebo drink containing no active ingredients. Assessments were conducted at baseline, at 3 weeks, at 6 weeks, at 9 weeks, and at the end of the trial. All participants completed the trial, and no adverse effects were noted. The researchers learned that the supplement reduced wrinkles. In fact, the deeper the wrinkle, the greater the reduction in depth. The supplement also enhanced skin elasticity and significantly improved skin hydration. At 6 weeks, the water content of the dermis had increased by 14%. The researchers concluded that the daily intake of this supplement induced "a clinically measurable improvement in the depth of facial wrinkles, skin elasticity and hydration."[7]

In a prospective, controlled, open trial published in 2014 in the *Journal of Cosmetic and Laser Therapy*, researchers from South Korea randomized 32 healthy volunteers to consume either no supplement, 3 g collagen, 3 g collagen and 500 mg vitamin C, or 500 mg vitamin C every day for 12 weeks. Each group had eight participants. There were 24 women and eight men aged 30–48 years. The researchers determined that collagen supplementation appeared to improve skin hydration and elasticity; however, it seemed to have no effect on skin erythema (redness) and pigmentation. The addition of a low dose of vitamin C did not enhance the effects of collagen. The researchers concluded that "further double-blinded, large-scale studies including elderly subjects will . . . be necessary to establish general clinical recommendations."[8]

Collagen Supplementation Appears to Support Wound Healing and Skin Recovery

Some South Korean researchers in the previous trial (the trial just noted in the previous paragraph) joined other researchers to participate in a trial investigating the use of collagen supplement for wound healing and skin recovery following a fractional photothermolysis treatment. This pilot trial was published in 2014 in the journal *Clinical and Experimental Dermatology*. Eight healthy Korean women were randomly divided into two groups. All eight participants received a fractional photothermolysis treatment. The participants in the treatment group consumed 3 g per day of oral collagen peptide for 2 weeks before the procedure and 2 weeks after the procedure. The participants were assessed 2 weeks before the treatment and at days 1, 3, 7, and 14 after the treatment. All eight participants completed the trial and follow-up. The researchers found that the posttreatment erythema resolved faster among women consuming collagen; the supplement group had significantly greater improvement in erythema than the control group. In addition, the treatment group had better recovery of skin hydration and higher levels of skin elasticity. At their final visit, the participants were asked to assess their satisfaction with their results. Seventy-five percent of the participants in the supplement group were either satisfied or very satisfied compared to 50% of those in the control group. None of the participants reported supplement-related gastrointestinal problems. The researchers concluded that "collagen tripeptide treatment appears to be an effective and conservative therapy for cutaneous wound healing and skin recovery after fractional photothermolysis treatment."[9]

When Taken with Calcium and Vitamin D, Collagen May Be Useful for Postmenopausal Women with Osteopenia

In a randomized, double-blind, placebo-controlled trial published in 2015 in the *Journal of Medicinal Food*, researchers from Florida, California, and Oklahoma (USA) investigated the association between intake of collagen hydrolysate, calcium, and vitamin D and osteopenia in postmenopausal women. The initial cohort consisted of 39 women with a mean age of 55.7 years, who completed up to 6 months of the study. Twenty-two women with a mean age of 56.2 years completed up to 12 months of the study. The participants in the treatment group consumed daily doses of 5 g collagen, 500 mg calcium, and 200 IU vitamin D; the participants in the control group consumed daily doses of 500 mg calcium and 200 IU vitamin D. Bone density was assessed at baseline, at 6 months, and at 12 months. The researchers found that collagen altered the ratio of bone formation over bone resorption, thereby decreasing the rate of bone loss. The researchers concluded that collagen supplementation "may provide protection against excessive bone loss and turnover which supplementation with calcium and vitamin D alone could not prevent."[10]

Collagen Supplementation Seems to Improve Bone Mineral Density and Bone Markers in Postmenopausal Women

In a randomized, controlled, double-blind clinical trial published in 2018 in the journal *Nutrients*, researchers from Germany wanted to learn more about the use of collagen supplementation and bone formation and bone mineral density in postmenopausal women. The initial cohort consisted of 131 postmenopausal women with a reduced bone mineral density in the lower spine or the femoral neck. For 12 months, they consumed either 5 g per day of specific collagen peptides or a placebo (maltodextrin). All participants were told to dissolve the contents of one sachet into water and drink it before breakfast. The collagen and placebo were similar in appearance, flavor, and texture. Bone mineral density measurements of the lower lumbar spine and femoral neck were measured at baseline and at the end of the trial. The researchers learned that the women in the supplement group experienced significant increases in the bone mineral density of the spine and femoral neck; the women consuming placebos did not have these beneficial changes. Nevertheless, the researchers underscored the need for more collagen supplementation studies in humans.[11]

Collagen Supplementation May Be a Complementary Therapy for the Prevention and Treatment of Osteoporosis and Osteoarthritis

In a systematic review published in 2016 in the journal *Revista Brasileira de Geriatria e Gerontologia*, researchers from Brazil identified nine studies that addressed the use of collagen supplement to prevent and treat osteoporosis and osteoarthritis. Of these, five were research studies involving humans. The researchers learned that collagen hydrolysate was useful in the prevention and treatment of both osteoporosis and osteoarthritis. It appeared to increase bone mineral density while it had a protective effect on articular cartilage, primarily by reducing pain. Unfortunately, their research failed to find any consensus on a specific recommended dosage. However, a daily dosage equivalent to 12 g was seen to result in significant improvements in the symptoms of osteoarthritis and osteoporosis. Still, the researchers concluded that there is a need for more research "to determine the pathogenic factors involved in osteoporosis and osteoarthritis, its early diagnosis, and from which stage of life it would be recommended to start supplementation, as well as the suitable dosage, in order to achieve significant therapeutic potential."[12]

Collagen Supplementation Seems to Be Useful for Articular Pain

In a double-blind, randomized, multicenter trial published in 2012 in the journal *Complementary Therapies in Medicine*, researchers from Belgium and France wanted to assess the ability of collagen supplements to alleviate articular pain or pain at the lower or upper limbs or at the lumbar spine. The initial cohort consisted of 200 men and women who were at least 50 years old with articular pain over 30 mm on a 0–100 mm visual analog scale. With each participant, the researchers targeted and focused on the joint that was initially considered the most painful. For 6 months, the participants consumed a daily dose equivalent to 1200 mg collagen hydrolysate or an identical hard gel placebo. Clinical assessments were conducted at baseline, at 3 months, and at 6 months. Fifty-six participants—33 in the collagen group and 23 in the placebo group—withdrew from the trial. Still, while there was no significant difference between the groups at 3 months, at the end of the trial, the researchers found that the participants in the supplement group had more people who improved by at least 20% than those in the placebo group. The researchers emphasized the need for more well-designed studies.[13]

NOTES

1. Czajka, A., E. M. Kania, L. Genovese, et al. "Daily Oral Supplementation with Collagen Peptides Combined with Vitamins and Other Bioactive Compounds Improves Skin Elasticity and Has a Beneficial Effect on Joint and General Wellbeing." *Nutrition Research* 57 (September 2018): 97–108.

2. Zdzieblik, Denise, Steffen Oesser, Manfred W. Baumstark, et al. "Collagen Peptide Supplementation in Combination with Resistance Training Improves Body Composition and Increases Muscle Strength in Elderly Sarcopenic Men: A Randomised Controlled Trial." *British Journal of Nutrition* 114 (2015): 1237–1245.

3. Kumar, S., F. Sugihara, K. Suzuki, et al. "A Double-Blind, Placebo-Controlled, Randomised, Clinical Study on the Effectiveness of Collagen Peptide on Osteoarthritis." *Journal of the Science of Food and Agriculture* 95, no. 4 (March 2015): 702–707.

4. Hexsel, Doris, Vivian Zague, Michael Schunck, et al. "Oral Supplementation with Specific Bioactive Collagen Peptides Improves Nail Growth and Reduces Symptoms of Brittle Nails." *Journal of Cosmetic Dermatology* 16, no. 4 (December 2017): 520–526.

5. Tomosugi, Nachisa, Shoko Yamamoto, Masayoshi Takeuchi, et al. "Effect of Collagen Tripeptide on Atherosclerosis in Healthy Humans." *Journal of Atherosclerosis and Thrombosis* 24 (2017): 530–538.

6. Proksch, E., D. Segger, J. Degwert, et al. "Oral Supplementation of Specific Collagen Peptides Has Beneficial Effects on Human Skin Physiology: A Double-Blind, Placebo-Controlled Study." *Skin Pharmacology and Physiology* 27, no. 1 (2014): 47–55.

7. Borumand, Maryam and Sara Sibilla. "Effects of Nutritional Supplement Containing Collagen Peptides on Skin Elasticity, Hydration and Wrinkles." *Journal of Medical Nutrition & Nutraceuticals* 4, no. 1 (2015): 47–53.

8. Choi, S. Y., E. J. Ko, Y. H. Lee, et al. "Effects of Collagen Tripeptide Supplement on Skin Properties: A Prospective, Randomized, Controlled Study." *Journal of Cosmetic and Laser Therapy* 16, no. 3 (June 2014): 132–137.

9. Choi, S. Y., W. G. Kim, E. J. Ko, et al. "Effect of High Advanced-Collagen Tripeptide on Wound Healing and Skin Recovery after Fractional Photothermolysis Treatment." *Clinical and Experimental Dermatology* 39, no. 8 (December 2014): 874–880.

10. Elam, M. L., S. A. Johnson, S. Hooshmand, et al. "A Calcium-Collagen Chelate Dietary Supplement Attenuates Bone Loss in Postmenopausal Women with Osteopenia: A Randomized Controlled Trial." *Journal of Medicinal Food* 18, no. 3 (March 2015): 324–331.

11. König, Daniel, Steffen Oesser, Stephan Scharila, et al. "Specific Collagen Peptides Improve Bone Mineral Density and Bone Markers in Postmenopausal Women–A Randomized Controlled Study." *Nutrients* 10, no. 1 (2018): 97–107.

12. Porfírio, Elisângela and Gustavo Bernardes Fanaro. "Collagen Supplementation as a Complementary Therapy for the Prevention and Treatment of Osteoporosis and Osteoarthritis: A Systematic Review." *Revista Brasileira de Geriatria e Gerontologia* 19, no. 1 (January–February 2016): 153–164.

13. Bruyère, O., B. Zegels, L. Leonori, et al. "Effect of Collagen Hydrolysate in Articular Pain: A 6-Month Randomized, Double-Blind, Placebo-Controlled Study." *Complementary Therapies in Medicine* 20, no. 3 (June 2012): 124–130.

REFERENCES AND FURTHER READING

Borumand, Maryam, and Sara Sibilla. "Effects of Nutritional Supplement Containing Collagen Peptides on Skin Elasticity, Hydration and Wrinkles." *Journal of Medical Nutrition & Nutraceuticals* 4, no. 1 (2015): 47–53.

Bruyère, O., B. Zegels, L. Leonori, et al. "Effect of Collagen Hydrolysate in Articular Pain: A 6-Month Randomized, Double-Blind, Placebo-Controlled Study." *Complementary Therapies in Medicine* 20, no. 3 (June 2012): 124–130.

Choi, S. Y., W. G. Kim, E. J. Ko, et al. "Effect of High Advanced-Collagen Tripeptide on Wound Healing and Skin Recovery After Fractional Photothermolysis Treatment." *Clinical and Experimental Dermatology* 39 (2014): 874–880.

Choi, S. Y., E. J. Ko, B. G. Kim, et al. "Effects of Collagen Tripeptide Supplement on Skin Properties: A Prospective, Randomized, Controlled Study." *Journal of Cosmetic and Laser Therapy* 16, no. 3 (June 2014): 132–137.

Czajka, A., E. M. Kania, L. Genovese, et al. "Daily Oral Supplementation with Collagen Peptides Combined with Vitamins and Other Bioactive Compounds Improves Skin Elasticity and Has a Beneficial Effect on Joint and General Wellbeing." *Nutrition Research* 57 (September 2018): 97–108.

Elam, M. L., S. A. Johnson, S. Hooshmand, et al. "A Calcium-Collagen Chelate Dietary Supplement Attenuates Bone Loss in Postmenopausal Women with Osteopenia: A Randomized Controlled Trial." *Journal of Medicinal Food* 18, no. 3 (March 2015): 324–331.

Hexsel, D., V. Zague, M. *Schunck*, et al. "Oral Supplementation with Specific Bioactive Collagen Peptides Improves Nail Growth and Reduces Symptoms of Brittle Nails." *Journal of Cosmetic Dermatology* 16, no. 4 (December 2017): 520–526.

König, Daniel, Steffen Oesser, Stephan Scharla, et al. "Specific Collagen Peptides Improve Bone Mineral Density and Bone Markers in Postmenopausal Women–A Randomized Controlled Study." *Nutrients* 10 (2018): 97–107.

Kumar, S., F. Sugihara, K. Suzuki, et al. "A Double-Blind, Placebo-Controlled, Randomized, Clinical Study on the Effectiveness of Collagen Peptides on Osteoarthritis." *Journal of the Science of Food and Agriculture* 95, no. 4 (March 2015): 702–707.

Porfírio, Elisângela and Gustavo Bernardes Fanaro. "Collagen Supplementation as a Complementary Therapy for the Prevention and Treatment of Osteoporosis and Osteoarthritis: A Systematic Review." *Revista Brasileira de Geriatria e Gerontologia* 19, no. 1 (January–February 2016): 153–164.

Proksch, E., D. Segger, J. Degwert, et al. "Oral Supplementation of Specific Collagen Peptides Has Beneficial Effects on Human Skin Physiology: A Double-Blind, Placebo-Controlled Study." *Skin Pharmacology and Physiology* 27, no. 1 (2014): 47–55.

Tomosugi, Naohisa, Shoko Yamamoto, Masayoshi Takeuchi, et al. "Effect of Collagen Tripeptide on Atherosclerosis in Healthy Humans." *Journal of Atherosclerosis and Thrombosis* 24 (2017): 530–538.

Zdzieblik, Denise, Steffen Oesser, Manfred W. Baumstark, et al. "Collagen Peptide Supplementation in Combination with Resistance Training Improves Body Composition and Increases Muscle Strength in Elderly Sarcopenic Men: A Randomized Controlled Trial." *British Journal of Nutrition* 114 (2015): 1237–1245.

Cranberry

For centuries, cranberry, which is indigenous to North America and grown in bogs (wet muddy ground), has been considered both a food and a medicine. Also known as *Vaccinium macrocarpon*, Native Americans used cranberries to treat bladder and kidney diseases. The early settlers from England used cranberries for stomach problems, blood disorders, appetite loss, and scurvy. Today, the United States is the world's single largest producer of cranberries, with Wisconsin and Massachusetts being the two leading states.

Related to blueberry and bilberry, cranberry is an evergreen shrub with upright branches. In the months of June and July, it has blossoming pink flowers and red-black fruits. Fresh cranberries are harvested in the fall, particularly during the month of October.

Cranberry is very high in disease-fighting antioxidants. In fact, researchers have identified over two dozen antioxidant phytonutrients in cranberries, such as proanthocyanidins and anthocyanins. Consuming any form of cranberry raises the levels of these antioxidants in the blood. Antioxidants neutralize free radicals that damage DNA and contribute to diseases, such as heart disease, cancer, and diabetes. In addition, cranberry is an excellent source of vitamin C.

HEALTH BENEFITS AND RISKS

Cranberry is probably best known for preventing urinary tract infections from the bacteria *Escherichia coli*. While researchers initially thought that cranberry made urine sufficiently acidic to kill bacteria, it now appears that cranberry prevents bacteria from attaching to the walls of the urinary tract. At present, cranberry is not considered useful for treating urinary tract infections, it simply prevents them. These infections need to be treated with antibiotics. Cranberry may be helpful for cancer prevention, reducing high cholesterol levels, and treating viral and bacterial illnesses.

Cranberry contains significant amounts of salicylic acid, which is found in aspirin. Regular intake of cranberry increases the amount of salicylic acid in the body, which reduces swelling, prevents blood clots, and may have antitumor properties.

Cranberry juice is generally considered safe, however, it may be combined with sugar, which can be problematic for people with diabetes. Cranberry has high levels of oxalate, which may increase the risk of kidney stones in some people. People with a history of kidney stones should avoid cranberry extract products or drinking more than small amounts of juice. People on blood-thinning medications, such as warfarin, or those who regularly take aspirin should avoid cranberry as it may increase the risk of bleeding.

HOW IT IS SOLD AND TAKEN

Cranberry is sold in a juice and supplement, generally as a capsule, extract, powder, tablet, or softgel. It is considered safe for children to drink cranberry juice, but they should not take supplements, unless under the supervision of a medical provider. There are no standard doses for cranberry. For adults, some studies have used between 10 and 16 oz of cranberry juice cocktail per day. Other studies have used between 800 and 1600 mg of cranberry supplement per day. Before initiating supplementation, medical providers should be consulted.

On the other hand, it is safe for adults and children to consume fresh or dried cranberries. Fresh cranberries are normally available in the fall, especially around the Thanksgiving holiday in the United States. Dried cranberries are usually available throughout the year; however, they often contain sugar, which may be problematic.

RESEARCH FINDINGS

Cranberry Supplement May or May Not Help Prevent Urinary Tract Infections

In a trial published in 2015 in the journal *European Review for Medical and Pharmacological Sciences*, researchers from Italy evaluated the ability of cranberry supplementation to prevent recurrent urinary tract infections. The cohort consisted of 44 participants who were placed on a capsule containing cranberry extract or a placebo for 60 days. During the 2 months before the trial began, the participants in the cranberry group had a total of 75 urinary tract infections; throughout the trial, that number was 20—a reduction of 73.3%. The reduction was only 15.4% in the placebo group. The difference between the two groups was statistically significant. Seven of the 22 participants in the intervention group were symptom free during the trial; none of the participants in the placebo group were symptom free. Three participants in the cranberry group and eight in the placebo group required medical consultations for urinary tract infections. At the end of the trial, urine evaluation for blood or bacteria was negative in 20 of the 22 participants on cranberry and 11 of the 22 participants in the placebo group. The researchers concluded that "these preliminary results, obtained in a field practice setting, indicate the effectiveness and safety of a well-standardized cranberry extract in the prevention of R-UTI [recurrent lower-urinary tract infections].[1]

The lead researcher in the previous study directed another cranberry trial published in 2016 in the *European Review for Medical and Pharmacological Sciences*. The researchers investigated the use of a high-concentration cranberry extract for elderly men with prostatic hyperplasia (enlargement of the prostate caused by increase in the reproduction rate of its cells). The initial cohort consisted of 44 men over the age of 65 years, all of whom had benign prostatic hyperplasia. For 2 months, 23 men consumed a supplement with a high concentration of cranberry extract. The remaining 21 men did not consume this supplement. Evaluations were made regarding the clinical effectiveness of the supplement by determining the number of new urinary tract infections that the men experienced during the trial. The researchers found that, in the supplement group, the mean number of urinary tract infections significantly decreased. No significant differences were observed in the control group, and no adverse effects were seen in either group. The researchers concluded that "these results suggest that cranberry supplement could be an effective and safe approach, within a SM [standard management] program, for the prevention of recurrent UTIs in elderly men suffering from BPH [benign prostate hyperplasia] avoiding some antibiotic treatments."[2]

In a study published in 2009 in the *Scandinavian Journal of Urology and Nephrology*, researchers from Italy investigated the use of cranberry juice for children who experienced recurrent urinary tract infections. The cohort consisted of 85 girls between the ages of 3 and 14 years, with a mean age of 7.5 years. All participants had more than one urinary tract infection in the previous year. The participants were randomly placed in one of three groups. The participants in the first group, including 28 girls, received 50 mL of cranberry concentrate juice everyday for 6 months. The participants in the second group, including 27 girls, received 100 mL of *Lactobacillus* GG drink 5 days a month for 6 months. The remaining girls served as controls. Only four participants dropped out of the study. During the trial, the participants had 34 urinary tract infections. While the rate was 18.5% in the cranberry group, the rates were 42.3% in the *Lactobacillus* group and 48.1% in the control group. Compared to the *Lactobacillus* and placebo groups, the participants in the cranberry group had a significant reduction in urinary tract infections. There were no negative reactions other than a few reports about the taste of the cranberry juice. The researchers concluded that "considering that cranberry juice is a natural alternative and a widely and easily available product, it seems a very useful and self-administrable means of preventing UTIs [urinary tract infections] in children, reducing the use of antibiotics."[3]

In a double-blind, randomized, placebo-controlled efficacy trial published in 2016 in *JAMA*, researchers from New Haven, Connecticut (USA), wanted to learn if cranberry would help prevent "bacteriuria plus pyuria" in elderly women who were nursing home residents. The cohort consisted of 185 English-speaking women who were 65 years or older, "with or without bacteriuria plus pyuria" at baseline. In fact, 31.4% suffered from this condition at baseline. The women lived in 21 nursing homes located within 50 miles of New Haven. For 1 year, the women were placed on a cranberry supplement or a placebo. One hundred and forty-seven women completed the trial. Laboratory assessments were conducted every 2 months. The researchers found no significant differences in the levels of "bacteriuria plus pyuria" in these two groups of women. They concluded that "among older women residing in nursing homes, administration of cranberry capsules, compared with placebo, results in no significant difference in presence of bacteriuria plus pyuria over one year."[4]

In a prospective, randomized, double-blind trial published in 2011 in the journal *Clinical Infectious Diseases*, researchers based in Ann Arbor, Michigan (USA), assembled an initial cohort of 319 college women with an average age of 21 years. The women were seen at the University of Michigan Health Service Laboratory between August 2005 and October 2007 for symptoms of a urinary tract infection. The women were assigned to consume either 8 oz of a 27% low-calorie cranberry juice cocktail drink twice a day (n = 155) or 8 oz of a placebo juice twice a day (n = 164) for 6 months. The placebo juice was formulated to imitate the flavor and color of the cranberry juice. Laboratory testing was conducted at baseline, at 3 months, and at 6 months. Participants also completed questionnaires. Two hundred and thirty women finished the entire trial, with 116 women in the treatment group and 114 in the placebo group. Compliance assessment was based on self-reporting. Overall, the recurrence rate of urinary tract infections was 16.9% (19.3% in cranberry group and 14.6% in placebo group). Hence, the participants consuming the cranberry drink had higher rates of infection than those in the placebo group. Among this group of women, the cranberry drink appeared to offer no protection from urinary tract infections.[5]

In a study published in 2012 in *Cochrane Database of Systematic Reviews*, researchers from the United Kingdom conducted an overview of randomized and "quasi" randomized studies of the use of cranberry products to prevent urinary tract infections. They included 24 studies with a total of 4473 participants. Thirteen studies with 2380 participants evaluated only cranberry juice/concentrate; nine studies with 1032 participants evaluated only cranberry tablets and capsules; one study compared cranberry juice and tablets; and one study compared cranberry capsules and tablets. After analyzing their data, the researchers found that cranberry products did not significantly reduce the overall occurrence of symptomatic urinary tract infections. It also did not significantly reduce the incidence in women with recurrent urinary tract infections, older people, pregnant women, children with recurrent infections, people with neuropathic bladder or spinal injury, and cancer patients. In many studies, there was low compliance and high withdrawal and dropout rates. Thus, the researchers concluded that "although some of the small studies demonstrated a small benefit for women with recurrent UTIs, there were no statistically significant differences when the result of a much larger study were included."[6]

Cranberry Juice May Reduce Cardiometabolic Risk

In a double-blind, placebo-controlled, parallel-arm trial published in 2015 in *The Journal of Nutrition*, researchers from Maryland and Massachusetts (USA) examined the association between intake of cranberry juice and cardiometabolic risk or the risk of cardiovascular disease, diabetes, or stroke. The cohort consisted of 30 women and 26 men. For 8 weeks, the participants consumed either 8 oz of a low-calorie cranberry juice or 8 oz of similar tasting placebo twice a day. The researchers provided all the food; the diet was designed to prevent people from gaining or losing weight. The researchers measured levels of 22 indicators of cardiometabolic risk. At the end of the trial, five of these indicators were lower—triglycerides (8%), C-reactive protein (44%), diastolic blood pressure (3%), glucose (2%), and a health indicator known as homeostasis model assessment of insulin resistance (3%). The researchers concluded that the "consumption of LCCJ [low calorie cranberry juice] for eight weeks results in lowering of several factors associated with cardiometabolic risk in an adult population."[7]

Cranberry Supplementation May Provide Some Benefit for Athletes

In a double-blind study published in 2017 in the *Journal of the International Society of Sports Nutrition*, researchers from Poland and Turkey wanted to learn if cranberry supplementation would benefit rowers subjected to exhaustive exercise. The cohort consisted of 16 members of the Polish Rowing Team. Nine members were randomly assigned to consume cranberry supplementation and seven were randomly placed in a placebo group. For 6 weeks, during a training camp, they took either the highly concentrated cranberry supplements or a placebo. The athletes performed a controlled 2000-m test prior to supplementation and at the end of the training camp, after the supplementation ended. Blood samples were collected before the 2000-m test, 1 min after completing the test, and after a 24-h recovery period. The researchers learned that the athletes who consumed the supplements appeared to have higher levels of serum antioxidants. Thus, they concluded that the cranberry supplement "contributed to a significant strengthening of antioxidant potential in individuals exposed to strenuous physical exercise." However, the supplementation did not affect other analyzed parameters such as inflammation markers and indices of iron metabolism.[8]

Cranberry May or May Not Improve Arterial Stiffness in Overweight Men

In a controlled, double-blind, crossover trial published in 2013 in the journal *Nutrition Research*, researchers from Québec, Canada wanted to learn if cranberry would be useful for arterial stiffness in abdominally obese men. The cohort consisted of 35 men who were obese and sedentary; for 4 weeks, they were randomly assigned to drink 500 mL of low-calorie cranberry juice per day or 500 mL per day of a placebo juice. After a 4-week washout period, the participants were assigned to participate in the alternate protocol. Blood samples were collected, blood pressure readings were recorded, and food questionnaires were completed. The researchers found that the intake of cranberry juice did not appear to have any effect on arterial stiffness. Yet, when the participants were divided into those who had metabolic syndrome (n = 13) and those who did not (n = 22), the researchers observed a significant within-group decrease in resting arterial stiffness values in the participants drinking cranberry juice who had metabolic syndrome. The researchers commented that this finding "surely deserves to be further investigated with regards to its clinical and physiological relevance."[9]

Cranberry Appears to Reduce Inflammation

In a study published in 2015 in the journal *Nutrition Research*, researchers from Virginia and New Hampshire (USA) investigated the ability of cranberry juice cocktail to reduce inflammation. They used data drawn from the cross-sectional National Health and Examination Survey, which had 10,334 adult participants aged 19 years and older. Of these, 330 were consumers of cranberry juice cocktail, defined as anyone consuming this drink for two nonconsecutive 24-h dietary recalls. The researchers observed that there were "very few differences" in the sociodemographic characteristics of cranberry consumers and nonconsumers. However, the researchers did learn that consumers of the cranberry juice cocktail had significantly lower levels of the measure of inflammation known as C-reactive protein. Further, though the drink contains sugar, there was no evidence that "consumption was associated with higher weight or an increased likelihood for overweight or obesity." Hence, the researchers concluded that "intake of cranberry polyphenols may play a role in promoting anti-inflammatory markers."[10]

Cranberry May Be Useful for Men Diagnosed with Prostate Cancer

In a single-center, randomized, placebo-controlled intervention trial published in 2016 in the journal *Biomedical Papers of the Medical Faculty of the University Palacký, Olomouc, Czech Republic*, researchers from the Czech Republic wanted to learn if cranberry would be useful for men diagnosed with prostate cancer. Prior to their radical prostatectomy surgery, 64 men with prostate cancer were randomized to consume either cranberry or a placebo. The 32 men in the cranberry group consumed 1500 mg cranberry fruit powder each day for at least 21 days before surgery; the 32 men in the control group consumed a similar amount of the placebo. The researchers determined that the men on cranberry supplement had significant reductions in their prostate-specific antigen levels. In fact, on the day they arrived for surgery, the levels dropped by 22.5%. The researchers concluded that "these data suggest that further studies to evaluate cranberry consumption as a prophylactic against the biochemical recurrence of prostate cancer in patients after surgery is warranted."[11]

People Who Take Warfarin Should Not Consume Cranberry

In a report published in 2011 in the journal *Annals of Pharmacotherapy*, medical providers from Memphis, Tennessee (USA), described the case of a 46-year-old woman who was taking a weekly dose of 56 mg warfarin, an anticoagulant medication. During the previous 4 months, her average internalized normalized ratio (INR, a clotting measure) was 2.0, ranging 1.6–2.2. After drinking approximately 1.5 quarts of cranberry juice cocktail for 2 days, her INR increased to 4.6. After 14 days without drinking any cranberry juice cocktail, her INR reduced to 2.3. For the next 3 months, while taking warfarin at a dose of 56 mg per week, her average INR was 2.1, ranging 1.4–2.5. Then, she drank two quarts of cranberry juice cocktail daily for 3 or 4 days, and her INR levels increased to 6.5. Warfarin was discontinued for 3 days, and her INR level dropped to 1.86. Seven days after she resumed her warfarin medication, the INR was 3.2. Thus, the ingestion of cranberry juice cocktail was able to derail the INR levels of a patient who was "previously stable on warfarin."[12]

NOTES

1. Ledda, A., A. Bottari, R. Luzzi, et al. "Cranberry-Supplementation in the Prevention of Non-Severe Lower Urinary Tract Infections: A Pilot Study." *European Review for Medical and Pharmacological Sciences* 19 (2015): 77–80.

2. Ledda, A., G. Belcaro, M. Dugall, et al. "Supplementation with High Titer Cranberry Extract (Anthocran®) for the Prevention of Recurrent Urinary Tract Infections in Elderly Men Suffering from Moderate Prostatic Hyperplasia: A Pilot Study." *European Review for Medical and Pharmacological Sciences* 20 (2016): 5205–5209.

3. Ferrara, Pietro, Luciana Romaniello, Ottavio Vitelli, et al. "Cranberry Juice for the Prevention of Recurrent Urinary Tract Infections: A Randomized Controlled Trial in Children." *Scandinavian Journal of Urology and Nephrology* 43 (2009): 369–372.

4. Juthani-Mehta, M., P. H. Van Ness, L. Bianco, et al. "Effect of Cranberry Capsules on Bacteriuria Plus Pyuria Among Older Women in Nursing Homes: A Randomized Clinical Trial." *JAMA* 316, no. 18 (November 8, 2016): 1879–1887.

5. Barbosa-Cesnik, Cibele, Morton B. Brown, Miatta Buxton, et al. "Cranberry Juice Fails to Prevent Recurrent Urinary Tract Infection: Results from a Randomized Placebo-Controlled Trial." *Clinical Infectious Diseases* 52, no. 1 (January 1, 2011): 23–30.

6. Jepson, R. G., G. Williams, and J. C. Craig. "Cranberries for Preventing Urinary Tract Infections." *Cochrane Database of Systematic Reviews* 10 (October 17, 2012): CD001321.

7. Novotny, J. A., D. J. Baer, C. Khoo, et al. "Cranberry Juice Consumption Lowers Markers of Cardiometabolic Risk, Including Blood Pressure and Circulating C-Reactive Protein, Triglyceride, and Glucose Concentrations in Adults." *The Journal of Nutrition* 145, no. 6 (June 2015): 1185–1193.

8. Skarpańska-Steijnborn, A., P. Basta, J. Trzeciak, et al. "Effects of Cranberry (*Vaccinum macrocarpon*) Supplementation on Iron Status and Inflammatory Markers in Rowers." *Journal of the International Society of Sports Nutrition* 14 (February 28, 2017): 7.

9. Ruel, Guillaume, Annie Lapointe, Sonia Pomerleau, et al. "Evidence that Cranberry Juice May Improve Augmentation Index in Overweight Men." *Nutrition Research* 33, no. 1 (January 2013): 41–49.

10. Duffey, Kiyah J. and Lisa A. Sutherland. "Adult Consumers of Cranberry Juice Have Lower C-Reactive Protein Levels Compared with Nonconsumers." *Nutrition Research* 35, no. 2 (February 2015): 118–126.

11. Student, V., A. Vidlar, J. Bouchal, et al. "Cranberry Intervention in Patients with Prostate Cancer Prior to Radical Prostatectomy. Clinical, Pathological and Laboratory Findings." *Biomedical Papers of the Medical Faculty of the University Palacký, Olomouc, Czech Republic* 160, no. 4 (December 2016): 559–565.

12. Hamann, G. L., J. D. Campbell, and C. M. George. "Warfarin-Cranberry Juice Interaction." *Annals of Pharmacotherapy* 45, no. 3 (March 2011): e17.

REFERENCES AND FURTHER READING

Barbosa-Cesnik, Cibele, Morton B. Brown, Miatta Buxton, et al. "Cranberry Juice Fails to Prevent Recurrent Urinary Tract Infection: Results from a Randomized Placebo-Controlled Trial." *Clinical Infectious Diseases* 52, no. 1 (January 1, 2011): 23–30.

Duffey, Kiyah J., and Lisa A. Sutherland. "Adult Consumers of Cranberry Juice Cocktail Have Lower C-Reactive Protein Levels Compared with Nonconsumers." *Nutrition Research* 35, no. 2 (February 2015): 118–126.

Ferrara, Pietro, Luciana Romaniello, Ottavio Vittelli, et al. "Cranberry Juice for the Prevention of Recurrent Urinary Tract Infections: A Randomized Controlled Trial in Children." *Scandinavian Journal of Urology and Nephrology* 43, no. 5 (2009): 369–372.

Hamann, G. L., J. D. Campbell, and C. M. George. "Warfarin-Cranberry Juice Interaction." *Annals of Pharmacotherapy* 45, no. 3 (March 2011): e17.

Jepson, R. G., G. Williams, and J. C. Craig. "Cranberries for Preventing Urinary Tract Infections." *Cochrane Database of Systematic Reviews* 10 (October 17, 2012): CD001321.

Juthani-Mehta, M., P. H. Van Ness, L. Bianco, et al. "Effect of Cranberry Capsules on Bacteriuria Plus Pyuria Among Older Women in Nursing Homes: A Randomized Clinical Trial." *JAMA* 316, no. 18 (November 8, 2016): 1879–1887.

Ledda, A., G. Belcaro, M. Dugall, et al. "Supplementation with High Titer Cranberry Extract (Anthocran®) for the Prevention of Recurrent Urinary Tract Infections in Elderly Men Suffering from Moderate Prostatic Hyperplasia: A Pilot Study." *European Review for Medical and Pharmacological Sciences* 20 (2016): 5205–5209.

Ledda, A., A. Bottari, R. Luzzi, et al. "Cranberry Supplementation in the Prevention of Non-Severe Lower Urinary Tract Infections: A Pilot Study." *European Review for Medical and Pharmacological Sciences* 19 (2015): 77–80.

Novotny, J. A., D. J. Baer, C. Khoo, et al. "Cranberry Juice Consumption Lowers Markers of Cardiometabolic Risk, Including Blood Pressure and Circulating C-Reactive Protein, Triglyceride, and Glucose Concentrations in Adults." *The Journal of Nutrition* 145, no. 6 (June 2015): 1185–1193.

Ruel, Guillaume, Annie Lapointe, Sonia Pomerleau, et al. "Evidence That Cranberry Juice May Improve Augmentation Index in Overweight Men." *Nutrition Research* 33, no. 1 (January 2013): 41–49.

Skarpańska-Stejnborn, A., P. Basta, J. Trzeciak, et al. "Effects of Cranberry (*Vaccinum macrocarpon*) Supplementation on Iron Status and Inflammatory Markers in Rowers." *Journal of the International Society of Sports Nutrition* 13 (February 28, 2017): 7.

Student, V., A. Vidlar, J. Bouchal, et al. "Cranberry Intervention in Patients with Prostate Cancer Prior to Radical Prostatectomy. Clinical, Pathological and Laboratory Findings." *Biomedical Papers of the Medical Faculty of the University, Palacký, Olomouc, Czech Republic* 160, no. 4 (December 2016): 559–565.

Creatine

Creatine is a naturally occurring combination of three amino acids—L-arginine, glycine, and L-methionine—that is found in fish and meat. In the human body, it is primarily found in muscles, as well as in the brain. Everyday, humans require between 1 and 3 g of creatine. (Athletes may need more.) Approximately half of this is obtained from diet, and the rest is synthesized by the body in the pancreas, kidneys, and liver. The body transforms creatine into creatine phosphate or phosphocreatine and stores it in muscles, where it is used for energy.

Most often, creatine is needed to improve exercise performance and increase muscle mass. In the United States, the majority of sports nutrition supplements contain creatine. And many people dealing with a wide variety of chronic and debilitating illnesses consume creatine to obtain a degree of relief. Consequently, it is not uncommon for people with congestive heart failure, depression, diabetes, and a host of other medical problems to consume creatine. Though there may or may not be actual research to support the use of creatine, it is thought that some degree of relief may be obtained from the placebo effect.

HEALTH BENEFITS AND RISKS

Creatine is a popular supplement for bodybuilders and competitive athletes. Many believe that it enhances athletic performance and increases lean muscle mass, especially during high-intensity, short-duration sports. While others doubt these claims, and not all bodybuilders and athletes notice any difference on creatine supplementation. Thus, people who already have higher amounts of creatine in their muscles may not experience an energy boost from supplementation. Further, creatine may or may not improve performance in exercises that require sustained endurance, such as running. Some contend that creatine may reduce cramping and help athletes recover from injuries. Though the use of creatine is controversial, it is not banned by the National Collegiate Athletic Association or the International Olympic Committee.

While generally considered safe, there are a number of side effects associated with creatine including weight gain, water retention, muscle cramps, high blood pressure, stomach upset, diarrhea, dizziness, muscle strains and pulls, and liver dysfunction. When used in high doses, there may be more serious negative side effects, such as kidney damage. High doses may also cause the body to stop making creatine. People with kidney, heart, or liver disease and high blood pressure should not consume creatine. Pregnant or breastfeeding women should not consume creatine. The long-term safety of creatine supplement has not been proven.

HOW IT IS SOLD AND TAKEN

Though most creatine is sold as a powder mixed with a liquid such as water, milk, or juice, it is also available in capsules and tablets. Medical providers who recommend creatine often suggest adults begin with a loading or high dose, such as 5 g of creatine monohydrate four times a day for a total of 20 g per day for 2 to 5 days. Subsequently, they should consume 2 g per day. But, many recommend higher doses. Creatine should not be taken by children or teens unless under the close supervision of a medical provider.

RESEARCH FINDINGS

Creatine Supplementation May Be Useful for Knee Osteoarthritis

In a randomized, double-blind, placebo-controlled trial published in 2011 in the journal *Medicine & Science in Sports & Exercise,* researchers from Brazil wanted to determine if creatine supplementation would be an effective treatment for knee osteoarthritis, an illness associated with pain and stiffness in the knee joints. The cohort consisted of 24 women between the ages of 50 and 65 years who were diagnosed with knee osteoarthritis. For 12 weeks, the participants consumed either creatine supplementation or a placebo and participated in a resistance training program. All participants reported 100% compliance with the protocol. The researchers observed that there was evidence that creatine supplementation had a positive effect on the physical functioning of the women. In addition, the supplementation appeared to improve the lower limb lean mass and the quality of life. They concluded that creatine supplementation "along with a lower limb resistance training program led to significant improvements in physical function when compared with resistance training alone." Further, there were no negative side effects.[1]

Creatine May Improve Lower Limb Strength Performance

In a meta-analysis and systematic review published in 2015 in the journal *Sports Medicine,* researchers from Australia and France examined studies on the association between creatine supplementation and lower limb strength performance. The cohort consisted of 60 randomized controlled trials with 646 participants in the creatine supplementation groups and 651 in the control groups. The majority of the studies were double-blind. In more than 80% of the studies, the supplementation was associated with sports training. Participants were trained for endurance, strength, or both. On average, they were trained three times per week. The researchers learned that creatine supplementation improved lower limb strength performance, primarily at the site of the quadriceps. With creatine supplementation, the maximum weight lifted during squats and total weight lifted at leg press increased by approximately 8% and 3%, respectively. Responses to creatine supplementation did not differ between males and females or between physically active or inactive people. Moreover, results did not vary by age. Thus, the researchers concluded that "creatine supplementation is effective in lower limb strength performance for exercise with a duration of less than three minutes, independent of population characteristic, training protocols, and supplementary doses and duration."[2]

Creatine Supplementation Appears to Improve Upper Limb Strength Performance

In 2017, the same researchers from Australia and France published another meta-analysis and systematic review in *Sports Medicine*. The researchers reviewed trials on the association between creatine supplementation and upper limb strength performance. The analysis included 53 studies with 563 participants on creatine supplementation and 575 on controls. All the studies were double-blind, randomized, and placebo-controlled. Only 25% of the participants were women. Forty percent of the studies recruited recreationally trained participants; 28% recruited competitive athletes; and 21% were conducted on sedentary people. The remaining studies did not report the training status of the participants. The researchers learned that creatine supplementation improved upper limb strength performance, primarily at the site of the pectoral muscles. With creatine supplementation, performances in bench pressing increased by about 5.3%. According to the researchers, "creatine supplementation is effective in upper limb strength performance for exercise with a duration of less than 3 minutes, mainly at the site of the pectoral group of muscles." This occurred independent "of population characteristics, training protocols, and supplementary doses or duration."[3]

Creatine Supplementation May Have Some Limited Benefits for People with Fibromyalgia

In a randomized, double-blind, placebo-controlled, parallel-group trial published in 2013 in the journal *Arthritis Care & Research*, researchers based in Brazil wanted to determine if people dealing with fibromyalgia would benefit from creatine supplementation. (Fibromyalgia is a chronic syndrome characterized by generalized pain, muscle dysfunction, disability, fatigue, psychological distress, cognitive dysfunction, and sleep and mood disturbances.) Twenty-eight patients with fibromyalgia were randomly assigned to consume creatine monohydrate (n = 15) or a placebo (n = 13). The participants were evaluated at baseline and after 16 weeks when the trial ended. The researchers learned that creatine supplementation significantly increased muscle phosphoryl creatine content and lower and upper muscle function; however, it had only a minor impact on the symptoms of fibromyalgia. Yet, because no negative side effects were observed, the researchers concluded that creatine could improve muscle function in people dealing with fibromyalgia.[4]

Creatine Supplementation May or May Not Be Useful for Older Women

In a randomized, double-blind, placebo-controlled trial published in 2013 in the *European Journal of Applied Physiology*, researchers from Brazil wanted to determine if creatine supplementation would be useful for older women who practice resistance training routines. Eighteen healthy women, with an average age of 64.9 years, completed a 12-week supervised resistance training program that met three times per week. It was hoped that this program would enable them to obtain similar fitness levels. The training regimen was designed to work all the major muscle groups. Then, the women were randomly assigned to consume creatine supplementation or a placebo. The women in both groups completed a second 12-week supervised resistance training program that also met three days per week. At the end of the trial, which everyone completed, the women on creatine supplementation had greater increase in training volume, bench press, knee extension, and biceps curl performance than those in the placebo group. In addition, the supplement group gained significantly more fat-free mass and muscle mass and was more efficient in performing submaximal strength functional tests than the placebo group. The researchers concluded that their findings "indicate that long-term creatine supplementation combined with RT [resistance training] improves the ability to perform submaximal-strength functional tasks and promotes a greater increase in maximal strength, fat-free mass and muscle mass in older women."[5]

In a double-blind, randomized, parallel-group, placebo-controlled trial published in 2015 in the journal *Experimental Gerontology*, researchers from Brazil and Germany investigated the effects of a 1-year low-dose creatine supplementation on bone health, lean mass, and muscle function in older postmenopausal women. Conducted between November 2011 and November 2013, the trial included 109 women postmenopausal women with osteopenia. Fifty-six women were placed on creatine supplementation and 53 took a placebo. Testing was conducted at baseline and after a 1-year intervention. The researchers learned that there was no difference in bone mineral density between the two groups. Moreover, there were no significant changes in other factors such as body weight, muscle function, and body lean mass. The researchers concluded that "a one-year low-dose creatine supplementation (1 g/d), although free of adverse effects, did not affect bone health parameters, lean mass, and muscle function in older women."[6]

Creatine May Provide Benefits for Some People with Muscle Disorders

In an analysis published in 2013 in the *Cochrane Database of Systematic Reviews*, researchers from Germany evaluated 14 randomized controlled trials or quasi-randomized controlled trials with 364 participants that examined the use of creatine for people with hereditary and acquired muscle diseases. Of the six trials on muscular dystrophies, which included 192 participants, the creatine supplementation groups had significant increases in muscle strength. The pooled data of four trials that had 115 participants showed that people on creatine supplementation "felt better during creatine treatment." In one trial, the participants, who had idiopathic inflammatory myopathies, "showed a significant improvement in functional performance." In metabolic myopathies, three trials with 33 participants revealed no significant difference in muscle strength. Still, one trial found a significant deterioration of activities of daily living and an increase in muscle pain during high-dose creatine treatment for McArdle disease, an inherited rare condition in which the body is unable to break down glycogen.[7] (Symptoms of McArdle disease include muscle weakness, stiffness, cramps, and fatigue.)

Creatine May Be Somewhat Helpful for Young Competitive Swimmers

In a trial published in 2011 in the journal *Procedia Social and Behavioral Sciences*, a researcher from Iran investigated the ability of creatine supplementation to improve the performance of young competitive swimmers. The cohort consisted of 20 women between the ages of 17 and 26 years. Ten women were randomly assigned to consume 5 g of the creatine supplement four times per day, and ten were randomly assigned to take a placebo four times per day. All the athletes participated in a 6-day conditioning program that focused on swimming. Testing was conducted at baseline and at the end of the program. The researchers determined that the women consuming creatine had significant improvements in bench press, vertical jump, and 60-yard sprint running. In addition, the women consuming creatine had improvements in swimming, but were not statistically significant. The researcher concluded that "creatine supplementation in conjunction with a good conditioning program can improve athletic performance in female competitive swimmers."[8]

Vegetarians and Omnivores May Have Different Cognitive Responses to Creatine Supplementation

In a study published in 2011 in the *British Journal of Nutrition*, researchers from the United Kingdom wanted to learn more about the influence creatine supplementation has on the cognitive functioning of omnivores (meat eaters) and vegetarians. The researchers recruited 121 female undergraduate students with a mean age of 20.3 years. At baseline, none of the participants took creatine supplementation, and all reported good health. Fifty-one participants were omnivores, and 70 were vegetarians. The participants were randomly placed on creatine supplementation (n = 61) or placebo (n = 60). Cognitive testing was completed at baseline and after 5-day consumption of the supplements/placebos. The researchers determined that, before the supplementation began, the memory of omnivores and vegetarians was similar. After 4 days of consuming the supplement, the vegetarians had better memory. The researchers concluded that "it was found that vegetarians were more sensitive to supplementation with creatine." Creatine supplementation did not have any influence on verbal fluency and vigilance.[9]

Short-Term Creatine Supplementation Does Not Improve the Anaerobic Upper Body Power of Trained Wrestlers

In a double-blind, placebo-controlled, parallel-group trial published in 2015 in the *Journal of the International Society of Sports Nutrition*, researchers from Estonia tested the ability of creatine supplementation to improve the upper body strength of trained wrestlers, with a mean age of 25.6 years. Normally, the wrestlers' training consisted of 3 to 4 2-h sessions per week. Each session included a combination of calisthenics, technical and tactical drills, and training matches. During the trial, the wrestlers were assigned to either a creatine supplementation or a placebo group. Both groups participated in two simulated competition days with exactly 7 days in between. The first simulated competition day was completed without any prior dietary supplementation. The second simulated competition day was completed after a 5-day creatine monohydrate or placebo supplementation period. A number of different tests were conducted to evaluate the wrestlers. Although the researchers had hypothesized that creatine supplementation would increase upper body anaerobic power, it did not occur. Creatine supplementation appeared to have no impact on upper body anaerobic power. According to the researchers, "considering the great practical importance of upper body muscular performance not only for combat sports athletes but also for disabled people who use wheelchair in their everyday life, further studies in this area of interest are warranted."[10]

Creatine Supplementation Does Not Appear to Improve Cognition and Psychomotor Performance in Young Adults

In a trial published in 2008 in the journal *Physiology & Behavior*, researchers from Pennsylvania and Massachusetts (USA) tested the ability of creatine supplementation to improve the cognition and psychomotor performance of young adults. The cohort consisted of 22 nonvegetarian participants with an average age of 21 years, including 13 males and 9 females. Before the trial began, they all completed tests. For 6 weeks, they took creatine supplementation or a placebo, followed by more testing. Although the researchers had hypothesized that creatine supplementation would improve cognitive functioning and psychomotor performance, contrary to the results of previous studies that did not occur. The researchers were unable "to demonstrate any effect of the creatine supplement on cognitive processing or psychomotor performance."[11]

Creatine Supplementation with or without Strength Training Did Not Improve the Emotional Health or Cognitive Performance of Older Women

In a 24-week, parallel-group, double-blind, randomized, placebo-controlled trial published in 2013 in the online journal *PLoS ONE*, researchers from Brazil investigated the association between the intake of creatine supplementation and emotional and cognitive measures in older women. They wanted to determine if creatine supplementation could be used as a tool to improve the mental health of older women. The cohort consisted of 56 healthy older women aged 60–80 years. None of the participants had engaged in any regular physical activity for at least 1 year prior to the study. The researchers formed four groups of 14 women. The members of the first group took placebos; the second group took creatine supplementation; the third group took placebos and participated in strength training; and the fourth group took creatine supplementation and participated in strength training. The strength training was performed in a hospital gymnasium; the supervised 40-min sessions were completed twice each week. Comprehensive emotional and cognitive testing was conducted at baseline, after 12 weeks, and after 24 weeks of intervention. The researchers learned that creatine supplementation with or without strength training did not improve the emotional or cognitive health of the women. The researchers concluded that "further studies involving frailer older individuals undergoing strength training and ingesting creatine supplementation are necessary to test the efficacy of this intervention."[12]

NOTES

1. Neves, M., Jr., B. Gualano, H. Roschel, et al. "Beneficial Effect of Creatine Supplementation in Knee Osteoarthritis." *Medicine & Science in Sports & Exercise* 43, no. 8 (August 2011): 1538–1543.

2. Lanhers, Charlotte, Bruno Pereira, Geraldine Naughton, et al. "Creatine Supplementation and Lower Limb Strength Performance: A Systematic Review and Meta-Analysis." *Sports Medicine* 45, no. 9 (September 2015): 1285–1294.

3. Lanhers, Charlotte, Bruno Pereira, Geraldine Naughton, et al. "Creatine Supplementation and Upper Limb Strength Performance: A Systematic Review and Meta-Analysis." *Sports Medicine* 47, no. 1 (January 2017): 163–173.

4. Alves, C. R., B. M. Santiago, F. R. Lima, et al. "Creatine Supplementation in Fibromyalgia: A Randomized, Double-Blind Placebo-Controlled Trial." *Arthritis Care & Research* 65, no. 9 (September 2013): 1449–1459.

5. Aguiar, Andreo Fernando, Renata Selvatici Borges Januário, Raymundo Pires Junior, et al. "Long-Term Creatine Supplementation Improves Muscular Performance During Resistance Training in Older Women." *European Journal of Applied Physiology* 113 (2013): 987–996.

6. Lobo, Daniel Medeiros, Aline Cristina Tritto, Luana Rodrigues da Silva, et al. "Effect of Long-Term Low-Dose Dietary Creatine Supplementation in Older Women." *Experimental Gerontology* 70 (2015): 97–104.

7. Kley, Rudolf A., Mark A. Tarnopolsky, and Matthias Vorgerd. "Creatine for Treating Muscle Disorders." *Cochrane Database of Systematic Reviews* 6 (June 5, 2013): CD004760.

8. Azizi, Masoumeh. "The Effect of Short-Term Creatine Supplementation on Some of the Anaerobic Performance and Sprint Swimming Records of Female Competitive Swimmers." *Procedia Social and Behavioral Sciences* 15 (2011): 1626–1629.

9. Benton, D., and R. Donohoe. "The Influence of Creatine Supplementation on the Cognitive Functioning of Vegetarians and Omnivores." *British Journal of Nutrition* 105, no. 7 (April 2011): 1100–1105.

10. Aedma, M., S. Timpmann, E. Lätt, and V. Ööpik. "Short-Term Creatine Supplementation Has No Impact on Upper-Body Anaerobic Power in Trained Wrestlers." *Journal of the International Society of Sports Nutrition* 12 (December 9, 2015): 45–53.

11. Rawson, Eric S., Harris R. Lieberman, Talia M. Walsh, et al. "Creatine Supplementation Does Not Improve Cognitive Function in Young Adults." *Physiology & Behavior* 95 (2008): 130–134.

12. Alves, C. R., C. A. Merege Filho, F. B. Benatti, et al. "Creatine Supplementation Associated or Not with Strength Training upon Emotional and Cognitive Measures in Older Women: A Randomized Double-Blind Study." *PLoS ONE* 8, no. 10 (October 3, 2013): e76301.

REFERENCES AND FURTHER READING

Aedma, M., S. Timpmann, E. Lätt, and Ööpik. "Short-Term Creatine Supplementation Has No Impact on Upper-Body Anaerobic Power in Trained Wrestlers." *Journal of the International Society of Sports Nutrition* 12 (December 2015): 45–53.

Aguiar, Andreo Fernando, Renata Selvatici Borges Januário, Raymundo Pires Junior, et al. "Long-Term Creatine Supplementation Improves Muscular Performance during Resistance Training in Older Women." *European Journal of Applied Physiology* 113 (2013): 987–996.

Alves, C. R., C. A. Merege Filho, F. B. Benatti, et al. "Creatine Supplementation Associated or Not with Strength Training upon Emotional and Cognitive Measures in Older Women: A Randomized Double-Blind Study." *PLoS ONE* 8, no. 10 (October 3, 2013): e76301.

Alves, C. R., B. M. Santiago, F. R. Lima, et al. "Creatine Supplementation in Fibromyalgia: A Randomized, Double-Blind, Placebo-Controlled Trial." *Arthritis Care & Research* 65, no. 9 (September 2013): 1449–1459.

Azizi, Masoumeh. "The Effect of a Short-Term Creatine Supplementation on Some of the Anaerobic Performance and Sprint Swimming Records of Female Competitive Swimmers." *Procedia Social and Behavioral Sciences* 15 (2011): 1626–1629.

Benton, D., and R. Donohoe. "The Influence of Creatine Supplementation on the Cognitive Functioning of Vegetarians and Omnivores." *British Journal of Nutrition* 105, no. 7 (April 2011): 1100–1105.

Kley, Rudolf A., Mark A. Tarnopolsky, and Matthias Vorgerd. "Creatine for Treating Muscle Disorders." *Cochrane Database of Systematic Reviews* 6 (June 5, 2013): CD004760.

Lanhers, Charlotte, Bruno Pereira, Geraldine Naughton, et al. "Creatine Supplementation and Lower Limb Strength Performance: A Systematic Review and Meta-Analysis." *Sports Medicine* 45, no. 9 (September 2015): 1285–1294.

Lanhers, Charlotte, Bruno Pereira, Geraldine Naughton, et al. "Creatine Supplementation and Upper Limb Strength Performance: A Systematic Review and Meta-Analysis." *Sports Medicine* 47, no. 1 (January 2017): 163–173.

Lobo, Daniel Medeiros, Aline Cristina Tritto, Luana Rodrigues de Silva, et al. "Effects of Long-Term Low-Dose Dietary Creatine Supplementation in Older Women." *Experimental Gerontology* 70 (2015): 97–104.

Neves, M., Jr., B. Gualano, H. Roschel, et al. "Beneficial Effect of Creatine Supplementation in Knee Osteoarthritis." *Medicine & Science in Sports & Exercise* 43, no. 8 (August 2011): 1538–1543.

Rawson, Eric S., Harris R. Lieberman, Talia M. Walsh, et al. "Creatine Supplementation Does Not Improve Cognitive Function in Young Adults." *Physiology & Behavior* 95 (2008): 130–134.

Echinacea

Echinacea, one of the most popular supplements, is a Native American medicinal perennial plant that derives its name from the prickly scales in its conical seed head. The scales are believed to resemble the spines of an angry hedgehog—*echinos* is the Greek word for hedgehog. Fully grown, the plant is approximately 1–2 ft. tall and has large purple-to-pink flowers.

There is good evidence that people have been using echinacea for centuries to treat various illnesses, such as viruses, infections, wounds, scarlet fever, malaria, diphtheria, and syphilis. Echinacea was introduced to Western medicine in the 1890s; at that time, it was thought to be useful for skin problems, respiratory tract infections, and sinus infections.

Echinacea contains several chemicals believed to contribute to its therapeutic properties. These include flavonoids, polysaccharides, glycoproteins, alkamides, and volatile oils. While the upper part of the plant has high concentrations of polysaccharides, the roots have high concentrations of volatile oils.

Three species of echinacea are generally used for medicinal purposes: *Echinacea angustifolia, E. pallida,* and *E. purpurea.* Commercially available echinacea may contain one, two, or all three of these species.

HEALTH BENEFITS AND RISKS

Today, people frequently use echinacea to shorten the duration of symptoms associated with cold and flu viruses, such as sore throat, cough, and fever. Often, people consume echinacea as the first signs of illness emerge. Some maintain that it may prevent cold and flu. It is not uncommon for an herbalist to recommend echinacea to boost immunity and overall health. Some contend that echinacea reduces pain and inflammation, and may be recommended for urinary tract infections, vaginal infections, yeast infections, ear infections, athlete's foot, allergies, or used topically for hard-to-heal wounds.

People with certain medical problems may be advised to not consume echinacea including connective tissue disorders, autoimmune disorders, tuberculosis, leukemia, diabetes, multiple sclerosis, HIV/AIDS, and liver problems. Because echinacea may reduce the effectiveness of medications that suppress the immune system, people who have undergone organ transplants should avoid echinacea.

Though it is thought to be rare, some people may develop allergic reactions to echinacea. Those who have allergies or asthma are at an increased risk for an allergic reaction. People with allergies to plants in the daisy family should avoid echinacea. Mild side effects from echinacea supplementation include stomach upset, nausea, dizziness, and dry eyes.

HOW IT IS SOLD AND TAKEN

Echinacea is sold as an extract, tincture, tablets, capsules, teas, juices, and ointments. It may also be combined with other herbs, vitamins, and minerals.

Do not consume echinacea for more than 10 days. Echinacea should be taken with food or a large glass of water, and should not be taken on an empty stomach. Children should be given alcohol-free echinacea.

Dosing recommendations vary, and it is best to follow instructions on the label. Still, following are some suggested recommendations administered three times per day: 300 mg dry powdered extract, 0.25–1.25 mL liquid extract, 1–2 mL tincture, 2–3 mL expressed juice *E. purpurea*, and 0.5–1 g dried root or tea.

RESEARCH FINDINGS

Echinacea May or May Not Be Useful for Respiratory Infections

In a meta-analysis published in 2015 in the journal *Advances in Therapy*, researchers from Switzerland, Germany, and the United Kingdom examined the association between echinacea and respiratory illnesses. The analysis included six clinical studies with a total of 2458 participants. Studies varied in the type of echinacea preparation and the doses administered. The participants in all the studies consumed the supplement for up to 4 months. The researchers found that echinacea was significantly associated with a reduced risk of recurrent respiratory tract infections. Moreover, in people who are at an increased risk for infections, echinacea consumption reduced the risk of recurrent infections by 50%. Common complications of respiratory infections such as pneumonia, ear infections, tonsillitis, and pharyngitis occurred less often in those taking echinacea. The researchers concluded that echinacea "presents an effective option for the longer term management of recurrent RTIs [respiratory tract infections] and related complications."[1]

In a randomized, double-blind, placebo-controlled clinical trial published in 2012 in the journal *Evidence-Based Complementary and Alternative Medicine*, researchers from the United Kingdom and Germany investigated the safety and efficacy of *E. purpurea* extract in the prevention of common cold episodes over a 4-month period. The cohort consisted of 755 healthy participants who were 18 years old or older. The participants, who had at least two cold episodes each year, were placed on either echinacea (2400 mg of extract per day) or a placebo. The participants kept diaries of their cold-related issues and adverse events and were seen during monthly visits. Six hundred and seventy-three participants completed the trial. The researchers learned that echinacea and placebo had almost the same number of adverse effects. As a result, echinacea and placebo were equally safe. Moreover, echinacea inhibited virally confirmed colds and prevented viral infections. Echinacea was especially useful in the prevention of recurrent infections. The preventive effects were particularly apparent when participants were compliant and followed the protocol. The researchers concluded that "compliant prophylactic intake of *E. purpurea* over a 4-month period appeared to provide a positive risk to benefit ratio."[2]

In an article published in 2012 in the journal *Alternative Medicine Review*, researchers from Italy described two "explorative pilot investigations" that they conducted on the ability of echinacea (*E. angustifolia*) to prevent respiratory infections. One of the trials was conducted among adults with three different respiratory disorders—chronic bronchitis, respiratory insufficiency, or asthma. The second trial was conducted among healthy children. The first trial included 38 volunteers between the ages of 38 and 79 years, who were divided into three groups. The members of the first group received an influenza vaccine; the members of the second group consumed echinacea supplementation; the members of the third group had the vaccine and supplementation. The vaccine was administered between October 15 and November 15, 2008. The echinacea supplements were administered from October to December 2008. Assessments were based on symptoms.

Eight of the 14 participants in the vaccine group had respiratory symptoms; two of the 12 participants in the echinacea group had symptoms; and only one of the 12 participants in the vaccine and echinacea group had symptoms.

The second trial included 34 healthy pediatric volunteers between the ages of 9 and 15 years. They were all placed on echinacea or a multivitamin—Be Total Plus. Supplementation took place from October to December 2008. Similar to the adult group, the participants in the pediatric group were evaluated for respiratory symptoms. Two of the 14 volunteers in the echinacea group experienced respiratory symptoms, while six of the 20 volunteers in the multivitamin group had symptoms and another two had suspected symptoms. Overall, there was excellent tolerance of the products used. The researchers concluded that their preliminary results are "encouraging."[3]

In a randomized controlled trial published in 2010 in the journal *Annals of Internal Medicine*, researchers from Wisconsin (USA) assessed "the potential benefits of echinacea as a treatment of [the] common cold." The cohort consisted of 719 patients between the ages of 12 and 80 years, who had early cold symptoms. The patients, enrolled from January 2004 to August 2008, were assigned to one of four groups. The members of the first group took no pills; the second group took placebos; the third group took blinded echinacea pills; and the fourth group took open-label echinacea pills. Only six patients did not complete the trial. Sixty-four percent of the participants were female and 88% were white; the mean age of the participants was 33.7 years. The researchers determined that echinacea groups had shorter duration of illness and lower severity of illness; however, the results were not statistically significant. The researchers concluded that "this echinacea formulation did not make a large impact on the course of the common cold." On average, echinacea supplementation reduced the duration of the cold by half a day; and there was a 10% reduction in the severity of the colds. Finally, the researchers concluded that "unfortunately, echinacea is not the long sought cure for the common cold."[4]

In a 2014 article published in the journal *Cochrane Database of Systematic Reviews*, researchers based in Germany evaluated 24 double-blind trials with 4631 participants. As expected, different types of echinacea were used in the various trials. Ten of the trials were believed to have a low risk of bias, whereas eight were thought to have a high risk of bias. The risk of bias was unclear in six of the trials. Ten trials investigated the prevention of colds. In individual trials, there was no association between echinacea products and the prevention of the common cold. However, further analysis found that echinacea may slightly reduce the incidence of colds. The researchers concluded that "echinacea products have not here been shown to provide benefits for treating colds, although it is possible that there is a weak benefit from some echinacea products."[5]

Echinacea Appears to Be Useful for Acute Sore Throats

In a randomized, double-blind, controlled trial published in 2009 in the *European Journal of Medical Research*, researchers from Switzerland and Germany assessed the efficacy of a echinacea/sage spray and a chlorhexidine/lidocaine spray for the treatment of acute sore throats, a very common medical problem. (Chlorhexidine is a disinfectant and antiseptic. Lidocaine is a local anesthetic.) A total of 154 patients, who were 12 years old or older, from 11 general medical practices in Switzerland participated in the study. The participants were treated with either spray—up to 10 times a day—until they were symptom free for a maximum of 5 days. Each patient also received a placebo spray corresponding to the other spray treatment that was similar in appearance, taste, and smell. The participants recorded diary entries three times each day and noted symptoms of throat pain, difficulty in swallowing, salivation, erythema, and fever. One hundred and thirty-three participants were included in the final analysis. The researchers determined that during the treatment the two sprays had similar rates of efficacy. They concluded that "an echinacea/sage preparation is as efficacious and well tolerated as a chlorhexidine/lidocaine spray in the treatment of acute sore throats."[6]

According to One Study, Echinacea Is Safe to Use during Pregnancy

In a study published in 2016 in the *European Journal of Clinical Pharmacology*, researchers wanted to learn if it is safe to use echinacea supplementation during pregnancy. The researchers used data from the Norwegian Mother and Child Cohort Study (MoBa) that included 68,522 women and their children. Information from the women was obtained twice during pregnancy and 6 months after delivery. To retrieve pregnancy outcomes, they also used data from the Medical Birth Registry of Norway (MBRN). Among 68,522 women, 363 (0.5%) reported using echinacea while pregnant. No association was found between the use of echinacea and an increased risk for malformations or adverse pregnancy outcomes, such as preterm birth, low birth weight, or too small for gestational age. The researchers concluded that their findings are "reassuring and will assist women and their healthcare providers when discussing treatment options during pregnancy and the benefit-risk ratio of the echinacea."[7]

Echinacea Does Not Appear to Increase Aerobic Capacity

In trial published in 2014 in the journal *ISRN Nutrition*, researchers from Louisiana and Indiana (USA) wanted to determine if echinacea supplementation would improve aerobic capacity in "recreationally active college students" who were not competitive athletes. The cohort consisted of 13 healthy males who were provided with a 30-day supply of a concentrated dose of echinacea (*E. purpurea*) supplementation. The supplement also contained other vitamins, minerals, and herbs. The students were asked to adhere to their usual routine, and data on maximum aerobic capacity were collected throughout the trial. The researchers found that the echinacea supplement did not increase maximum aerobic capacity. This supplement was "not an effective intervention to increase aerobic capacity" in these students. The researchers suggested that further studies should be conducted in "populations where oxygen delivery limits functional capacity," such as people who are transitioning to higher altitudes.[8]

Echinacea Supplementation Combined with Osteopathic Manipulative Treatment Did Not Help Children with Recurrent Otitis Media

In a randomized placebo-controlled trial published in 2008 in the journal *BMC Complementary and Alternative Medicine*, researchers from Tucson, Arizona (USA), wanted to determine if children with recurrent middle ear inflammation would benefit from echinacea supplementation combined with osteopathic manipulative treatment. The initial cohort consisted of 90 children between the ages of 12 and 60 months, with a median age of 1.5 years. All children had recurrent otitis media, defined as three or more separate episodes within 6 months or at least four episodes in 1 year. The children were assigned to one of four protocols: placebo supplement and sham osteopathic manipulation, echinacea supplement plus sham osteopathic manipulative treatment, placebo plus osteopathic manipulative treatment, or echinacea supplement plus osteopathic manipulative treatment. Eighty-four children were followed for 3 or more months. Fifty-two percent had one or more episodes of acute otitis media. The highest rates of otitis media were among the children receiving echinacea alone. Thus, treatment with echinacea and/or osteopathic manipulation did not result in a statistically significant reduction in the incidence of otitis media in otitis-prone children. The researchers concluded that "the borderline increased risk associated with echinacea treatment make a protective effect of this form and dosage schedule of echinacea very unlikely, despite the sample size."[9]

NOTES

1. Schapowal, Andreas, Peter Klein, and Sebastian L. Johnstron. "Echinacea Reduces the Risk of Recurrent Respiratory Tract Infections and Complications: A Meta-Analysis of Randomized Controlled Trials." *Advances in Therapy* 32 (2015): 187–200.

2. Jawad, M., R. Schoop, A. Suter, et al. "Safety and Efficacy Profile of *Echinacea purpurea* to Prevent Common Cold Episodes: A Randomized, Double-Blind, Placebo-Controlled Trial." *Evidence-Based Complementary and Alternative Medicine* 2012 (2012): Article ID: 841315.

3. Di Pierro, Francesco, Giuliana Rapacioli, Tarcisio Ferrara, and Stefano Togni. "Use of Standardized Extract from *Echinacea angustifolia* (Polinacea®) for the Prevention of Respiratory Tract Infections." *Alternative Medicine Review* 17, no. 1 (2012): 36–41.

4. Barrett, B., R. Brown, D. Rakel, et al. "Echinacea for Treating the Common Cold: A Randomized Trial." *Annals of Internal Medicine* 153, no. 12 (December 21, 2010): 769–777.

5. Karsch-Völk, M., B. Barrett, D. Kiefer, et al. "Echinacea for Preventing and Treating the Common Cold." *Cochrane Database of Systematic Reviews* 2 (February 20, 2014): CD000530.

6. Schapowal, A., D. Berger, P. Klein, and A. Suter. "Echinacea/Sage or Chlorhexidine/Lidocaine for Treating Acute Sore Throats: A Randomized Double-Blind Trial." *European Journal of Medical Research* 14 (2009): 406–412.

7. Heitmann, K., G. C. Havnen, L. Holst, and H. Nordeng. "Pregnancy Outcomes after Prenatal Exposure to Echinacea: The Norwegian Mother and Child Care Cohort Study." *European Journal of Clinical Pharmacology* 72 (2016): 623–630.

8. Bellar, David, Kaitlyn M. Moody, Nicholas S. Richard, and Lawrence W. Judge. "Efficacy of a Botanical Supplement with Concentrated *Echinacea purpurea* for Increasing Aerobic Capacity." *ISRN Nutrition* 2014 (2014): Article ID: 149549.

9. Wahl, R. A., M. B. Aldous, K. A. Worden, and K. L. Grant. "*Echinacea purpurea* and Osteopathic Manipulative Treatment in Children with Recurrent Otitis Media: A Randomized Controlled Trial." *BMC Complementary and Alternative Medicine* 8 (October 2, 2008): 56–64.

REFERENCES AND FURTHER READING

Barrett, B., R. Brown, D. Rakel, et al. "Echinacea for Treating the Common Cold: A Randomized Trial." *Annals of Internal Medicine* 153, no. 12 (December 21, 2010): 769–777.

Bellar, David, Kaitlyn M. Moody, Nicholas S. Richard, and Lawrence W. Judge. "Efficacy of a Botanical Supplement with Concentrated *Echinacea purpurea* for Increasing Aerobic Capacity." *ISRN Nutrition* 2014 (2014): Article ID: 149549.

Di Pierro, Francesco, Giuliana Rapacioli, Tarcisio Ferrara, and Stefano Togni. "Use of Standardized Extract from *Echinacea angustifolia* (Polinacea®) for the Prevention of Respiratory Tract Infections." *Alternative Medicine Review* 17, no. 1 (2012): 36–41.

Heitmann, K., G. C. Havnen, L. Holst, and H. Nordeng. "Pregnancy Outcomes after Prenatal Exposure to Echinacea: The Norwegian Mother and Child Cohort Study." *European Journal of Clinical Pharmacology* 72 (2016): 623–630.

Jawad, M., R. Schoop, A. Suter, et al. "Safety and Efficacy Profile of *Echinacea purpurea* to Prevent Common Cold Episodes: A Randomized, Double-Blind, Placebo-Controlled Trial." *Evidence-Based Complementary and Alternative Medicine* 2012 (2012): Article ID: 841315.

Karsch-Völk, M., B. Barrett, D. Kiefer, et al. "Echinacea for Preventing and Treating the Common Cold." *Cochrane Database of Systematic Reviews* 2 (February 20, 2014): CD000530.

Ross, Stephanie Maxine. *"Echinacea purpurea*: A Proprietary Extract of *Echinacea purpurea* Is Shown to Be Safe and Effective in the Prevention of the Common Cold." *Holistic Nursing Practice* 30, no. 1 (January–February 2016): 54–57.

Schapowal, A., D. Berger, P. Klein, and A. Suter. "Echinacea/Sage or Cholorhexidine/ Lidocaine for Treating Acute Sore Throats: A Randomized Double-Blind Trial." *European Journal of Medical Research* 14 (2009): 406–412.

Schapowal, A., P. Klein, and S. L. Johnston. "Echinacea Reduces the Risk of Recurrent Respiratory Tract Infections and Complications: A Meta-Analysis of Randomized Controlled Trials." *Advances in Therapy* 32, no. 3 (March 2015): 187–200.

Wahl, R. A., M. B. Aldous, K. A. Worden, and K. L. Grant. *"Echinacea purpurea* and Osteopathic Manipulative Treatment in Children with Recurrent Otitis Media: A Randomized Controlled Trial." *BMC Complementary and Alternative Medicine* 8 (October 2, 2008): 56–64.

Evening Primrose Oil

Derived from the seeds of the evening primrose plant (*Oenothera biennis*), evening primrose oil is a very popular supplement containing rich amounts of omega-6 essential fatty acids, specifically gamma-linolenic acid (GLA) and linolenic acid. These are essential components of myelin, the protective coating around nerve fibers and the neuronal cell membrane. Evening primrose oil supplements are frequently standardized to 8% GLA and 72% linoleic acid.

Evening primrose oil has been used since ancient times, and was considered a treatment for skin disorders, such as eczema, psoriasis, and acne. Native Americans used evening primrose seeds, leaves, and roots for food. In addition, they made poultices from the whole plant to treat bruises. Moreover, they used leaves to heal wounds, gastrointestinal problems, and sore throats.

HEALTH BENEFITS AND RISKS

Evening primrose oil is thought to be useful for a wide variety of medical problems including skin disorders such as eczema, psoriasis, and acne, rheumatoid arthritis, osteoporosis, Raynaud's syndrome, multiple sclerosis, Sjögren's syndrome, chronic fatigue, diabetes-related nerve damage, gastrointestinal disorders, attention deficit hyperactivity disorder, and heart disease. Pregnant women use evening primrose oil to prevent high blood pressure, trigger labor, and shorten labor. However, some contend that it is unsafe to consume evening primrose oil during pregnancy. Nonpregnant women use evening primrose to address menopausal symptoms, such as hot flashes, premenstrual syndrome, endometriosis, and breast pain (mastalgia).

Because of its blood-thinning properties, people on blood-thinning medication, such as warfarin, or people with an upcoming surgical procedure should not use evening primrose oil. Generally, it is recommended that people stop consuming evening primrose oil 2 weeks before a surgery. People with seizure disorders should not consume evening primrose oil as it may increase the risk of seizures. Side effects associated with evening primrose oil include stomach upset, nausea, diarrhea, and headache. True allergic reactions to evening primrose oil are thought to be rare. Symptoms of an allergic reaction include inflammation of the hands and feet, rash, wheezing, and difficulty in breathing.

HOW IT IS SOLD AND TAKEN

Evening primrose oil is sold in capsules or as a liquid. Because it can easily become rancid, it should be stored in the refrigerator or purchased in a light-resistant container. Recommended doses vary widely. For most adults, two capsules per day at a dose of 500 mg is probably sufficient. However, capsules are often sold in doses of 1300 mg. In clinical trials, evening primrose oil has been administered at doses of 6–8 g per day in adults and 2–4 g per day in children. Evening primrose oil may also be used topically.

RESEARCH FINDINGS

Evening Primrose Oil May or May Not Help Atopic Dermatitis, Also Known as Eczema

In a trial published in 2013 in the journal *Annals of Dermatology*, researchers based in Seoul, Korea wanted to determine if evening primrose oil was an effective treatment for atopic dermatitis, a condition that makes skin red and itchy. The researchers recruited 40 children and adolescents (24 males and 16 females between the ages of 2 and 15 years) with atopic dermatitis and randomly divided them into two groups. The participants in the first group consumed 160 mg per day of evening primrose oil for 8 weeks, whereas the participants in the second group consumed 320 mg twice each day for 8 weeks. As expected, the serum fatty acid levels in the second group were higher than the first group, and they were statistically significant. The researchers observed that the participants in both groups experienced improvements in their atopic dermatitis symptoms, though the participants in the 320-mg group had more improvement than those in the 160-mg group. The researchers concluded that evening primrose oil "may be useful for treating AD [atopic dermatitis] patients in a dose-dependent manner."[1]

In a trial published in 2008 in the *Indian Journal of Dermatology, Venereology and Leprology*, researchers from India wanted to determine if evening primrose would be useful for people who have atopic dermatitis, which is chronic and relapsing. The initial cohort consisted of 65 patients who were randomly assigned to consume 500 mg of evening primrose oil capsules or a placebo that contained 300 mg of sunflower oil. All the participants were given the maximum allowable dosage for their age. The treatment continued for 5 months. Patients were told to visit the clinic for an evaluation every 4 weeks. The analysis was conducted on the first 25 patients from each group. The researchers learned that 96% of the participants consuming evening primrose oil had improvements in their condition, whereas only 32% of those on placebo improved. No significant adverse effects were reported. The researchers concluded that "evening primrose oil is a safe and effective medicine in [the] management of AD [atopic dermatitis]."[2]

In 2014, another trial on the use of evening primrose oil for atopic dermatitis was published in the journal *Advances in Therapy*. In this prospective, explorative, multicenter, open, noncontrolled trial, researchers from Switzerland recruited 23 patients with atopic dermatitis, with a mean age of 26.3 years. Six patients were under the age of 12 years, two were between the ages of 12 and 18 years, and 15 were older than 18 years. For 12 weeks, the patients consumed supplemental evening primrose oil. Fourteen patients were included in the analysis. By the time the trial ended, the researchers determined that the patients had an increase plasma

GLA and metabolite dihomo-gamma-linoleic acid, as well as significant improvement in their clinical symptoms. Patients saw healing as early as 4 weeks after beginning supplementation. Therefore, according to the researchers, patients could be evaluated after 4 weeks of supplementation and advised whether they should continue. They concluded that "remarkably, the significance of these preliminary results could be obtained despite the small sample size."[3]

In another analysis published in 2013 in the *Cochrane Database of Systematic Reviews*, researchers form Minnesota (USA) investigated studies on the ability of evening primrose oil and borage oil to relieve the symptoms associated with eczema. A total of 27 studies with 1596 participants from 12 countries met the inclusion criteria. Of these, 19 studies compared evening primrose oil supplementation to placebos. The researchers found some evidence that evening primrose oil was associated with mild or temporary improvements in eczema; however, compared to placebos, evening primrose oil did not have a statistically significant advantage. (Borage oil supplementation was also found to have little effect on eczema.) The researchers concluded that there is no reason for further studies on the effectiveness of evening primrose oil as a treatment for eczema.[4]

Evening Primrose Oil May Have Some Limited Benefits for People with Type 2 Diabetes

In a prospective, randomized, controlled, open-label trial published in 2017 in the *UK Journal of Pharmaceutical and Biosciences*, researchers from Iraq wanted to determine if evening primrose oil supplementation would benefit people with type 2 diabetes. They enrolled 26 overweight or obese participants (16 females and 10 males) who were newly diagnosed with type 2 diabetes; the participant's age ranged from 35 to 60 years. For 3 months, 13 participants were placed on metformin, a medication for type 2 diabetes, and 13 were placed on metformin and evening primrose oil supplementation. Fourteen healthy control participants were also enrolled in the study. The researches learned that the addition of evening primrose oil to metformin therapy reduced fasting serum glucose levels, but the results were not statistically significant. Further, after treatment, the participants in the first two groups had highly significant reductions in total cholesterol and low-density lipoprotein or "bad" cholesterol. The researchers concluded that "the addition of evening primrose oil to metformin in the current study did not show significant reduction in lipid profile compared to metformin treated patients at the same dose and duration."[5]

Topical Evening Primrose Oil May Be an Effective Treatment for Molluscum Contagiosum

In an open trial published in 2017 in the journal *Clinical and Experimental Dermatology*, researchers from Korea wanted to learn if topical evening primrose oil would be useful for molluscum contagiosum, a skin infection caused by a virus that produces benign raised lesions or bumps on the upper layers of the skin. From February 2014 to April 2016, they enrolled 41 children with a mean age of 6.3 years. The parents were instructed to apply evening primrose oil topically to all the lesions twice daily for 3 months. Twenty-four children (58.5%) completed the trial. The parents of the children who were lost to follow-up were telephoned and asked to assess the therapeutic response. Thus, the analysis included all the children. Twenty-two respondents had positive comments about the treatment. The remaining 19 experienced no change, or, in the case of two participants, the condition worsened. The researchers concluded that topical evening primrose oil "may be a noninvasive, alternative treatment option for children with MC considering the inconvenience of the current treatments."[6]

Evening Primrose Oil May or May Not Be Useful for Mastalgia

In a double-blind, randomized, placebo-controlled pilot trial published in 2010 in the journal *Alternative Medicine Review*, researchers from two locations in Minnesota (USA) wanted to learn if supplemental evening primrose oil and/or vitamin E were useful for mastalgia. The initial enrollment consisted of 85 women with premenstrual cyclical breast discomfort, with a mean age of 40.4 years. For 6 months, the participants were assigned to one of four groups: vitamin E (1200 mg per day), evening primrose oil (3000 mg per day), vitamin E (1200 mg per day) and evening primrose oil (3000 mg per day), or double placebo. Forty-one participants completed the trial. Although the dropout rate was high, it was consistent among the four groups. Compared to the women in the placebo group, the women in all three treatment groups experienced reductions in the severity of cyclical mastalgia. However, the reductions were not statistically significant. The researchers concluded that "it is reasonable in a clinical setting to offer premenopausal women with severe cyclical mastalgia a short-duration trial with either vitamin E at a daily dose of 1200 IU, EPO [evening primrose oil] at a daily dose of 3000 mg or the combination of vitamin E and EPO in these same dosages."[7]

In a trial published in 2017 in the *Journal of Education and Health Promotion*, researchers from Iran tested the ability of evening primrose oil, flaxseed, and vitamin E to reduce periodic breast pain. The initial cohort consisted of 90 patients between the ages of 18 and 45 years, who were referred to clinics for breast pain or residents living in the dormitories of a university. The cohort was divided into three groups. The members of the first group consumed powdered flaxseed; the members of the second group consumed two 1000 mg capsules of evening primrose oil, and the members of the third group consumed vitamin E. The trial continued for two menstrual cycles. By the end of the trial, four patients were eliminated. Cyclical breast pain was measured at the beginning and end of both intervention periods. While evening primrose oil reduced the duration of breast pain, the reduction was not significant. (Powdered flaxseed was the most effective supplement in the reduction of the duration of breast pain.)[8] Evening primrose oil should probably not be the supplement of choice for reducing the duration of breast pain.

Evening Primrose Oil Supplementation May Help People with Rheumatoid Arthritis

In a 3-month prospective, randomized controlled trial published in 2016 in the journal *Clinical Rheumatology*, researchers from Serbia wanted to learn if evening primrose would help people with rheumatoid arthritis. The cohort consisted of 60 postmenopausal patients with a mean age of 63.1 years; all the patients had rheumatoid arthritis. They were divided into three groups of 20 patients. The patients in the first group were controls; the patients in the second group consumed concentrated fish oil; and the patients in the third group consumed concentrated fish oil and 1300 mg of evening primrose oil. The researchers found no changes in oxidative stress parameters in the first group. However, in the second and third groups, there were improvements in antioxidant enzyme levels and decreases in oxidative stress. By increasing antioxidant enzyme levels, fish oil and evening primrose oil reduced inflammation and disease activity. The researchers concluded that their "findings indicate that intakes of fish oil and evening primrose oil may be of importance in mitigation of inflammation, disease activity, and oxidative stress biomarkers through increased activities of antioxidant enzymes."[9]

Evening Primrose Oil May Have Some Limited Usefulness for Menopausal Hot Flashes

In a 6-week, randomized, double-blind, placebo-controlled trial published in 2013 in the journal *Archives of Gynecology and Obstetrics*, researchers from Iran investigated the ability of evening primrose oil to reduce the severity of menopausal hot flashes. The cohort consisted of 56 women with menopausal hot flashes between the ages of 45 and 59 years, with a mean age of 51.9 years. During 2011 and 2012, the women were placed on either evening primrose oil or a placebo. Questionnaires were completed at baseline and at the end of the intervention. After 6 weeks, the frequency, severity, and duration of hot flashes remained statistically similar in the two groups. However, compared to the placebo group, only the severity of hot flashes was significantly reduced by evening primrose oil. The researchers commented that the small size of their sample and the "subjective perception" of the intensity of hot flashes may have influenced the results of their trial.[10]

Evening Primrose Oil May Help Cheilitis in People Taking Strong Acne Medication

In an article published in 2014 in the journal *Annals of Dermatology*, researchers from Seoul, Korea explained that isotretinoin, a strong medication used to treat acne, has numerous negative side effects, such as skin dryness, dry eyes, and cheilitis, cuts at the corner of the mouth. Because of these side effects, some patients discontinued the medication. Hence, they wanted to learn if evening primrose oil would be useful in preventing cheilitis. The cohort consisted of 40 Korean volunteers (23 women and 17 men) with moderate acne; the participants, age ranged from 18 to 31 years, were randomized to receive isotretinoin with or without evening primrose oil for 8 weeks. Those who were placed on evening primrose oil took six 450 mg capsules three times each day. By the end of the trial, the degree of acne was decreased significantly in both groups. Moreover, the proportion of patients presenting with xerotic cheilitis was significantly lower in the experimental group. The researchers noted that additional research is needed "before we can have a complete understanding of the role of EPO on xerotic cheilitis in acne patients being treated with oral isotretinoin."[11]

NOTES

1. Chung, B. Y., J. H. Kim, S. I. Cho, et al. "Dose-Dependent Effects of Evening Primrose Oil in Children and Adolescents with Atopic Dermatitis." *Annals of Dermatology* 25, no. 3 (2013): 285–291.

2. Senapati, S., S. Banerjee, and D. N. Gangopadhyay. "Evening Primrose Oil Is Effective in Atopic Dermatitis: A Randomized Placebo-Controlled Trial." *Indian Journal of Dermatology, Venereology and Leprology* 74, no. 5 (September–October 2008): 447–452.

3. Simon, Dagmar, Peter A. Eng, Siegfried Borelli, et al. "Gamma-Linolenic Acid Levels Correlate with Clinical Efficacy of Evening Primrose Oil in Patients with Atopic Dermatitis." *Advances in Therapy* 31, no. 2 (February 2014): 180–188.

4. Bamford, J. T., S. Ray, Musekiwa, et al. "Oral Evening Primrose Oil and Borage Oil for Eczema." *Cochrane Database of Systematic Reviews* 4 (April 30, 2013): CD004416.

5. Abdulridha, Menal Khalid, Mustafa Safaa Hussain, and Mahmood Shaker Khudhair. "Study Effect of Evening Primrose Oil Supplement on Type 2 Diabetes Mellitus–Associated Metabolic Parameters." *UK Journal of Pharmaceutical and Biosciences* 5, no. 2 (2017): 17–23.

6. Kwon, H. S., J. H. Lee, G. M. Kim, et al. "Topical Evening Primrose Oil as a Possible Therapeutic Alternative in Children with Molluscum Contagiosum." *Clinical and experimental Dermatology* 42, no. 8 (December 2017): 923–925.

7. Pruthi, S., D. L. Wahner-Roedler, C. J. Torkelson, et al. "Vitamin E an Evening Primrose Oil for Management of Cyclical Mastalgia: A Randomized Pilot Study." *Alternative Medicine Review* 15, no. 1 (April 2010): 59–67.

8. Jaafarnejad, F., E. Adibmoghaddam, S. A. Emaami, and A. Saki. "Compare the Effect of Flaxseed, Evening Primrose Oil and Vitamin E on Duration of Periodic Breast Pain." *Journal of Education and Health Promotion* 6 (October 4, 2017): 85.

9. Vasiljevic, D., M. Veselinovic, M. Jovanovic, et al. "Evaluation of the Effects of Different Supplementation on Oxidative Status in Patients with Rheumatoid Arthritis." *Clinical Rheumatology* 35, no. 8 (August 2016): 1909–1915.

10. Farzaneh, F., S. Fatehi, M. R. Sohrabi, and K. Alizadeh. "The Effect of Oral Evening Primrose Oil on Menopausal Hot Flashes: A Randomized Clinical Trial." *Archives of Gynecology and Obstetrics* 288, no. 5 (November 2013): 1075–1079.

11. Park, Kui Young, Eun Jung Ko, In Su Kim, et al. "The Effect of Evening Primrose Oil for the Prevention of Xerotic Cheilitis in Acne Patients Being Treated with Isotretinoin: A Pilot Study." *Annals of Dermatology* 26, no. 6 (2014): 706–712.

REFERENCES AND FURTHER READING

Abdulridha, Manal Khalid, Mustafa Safaa Hussain, and Mahmood Shaker Khudhair. "Study Effect of Evening Primrose Oil Supplement on Type 2 Diabetes Mellitus–Association Metabolic Parameters." *UK Journal of Pharmaceutical and Biosciences* 5, no. 2 (2017): 17–23.

Bamford, J. T., S. Ray, A. Musekiwa, et al. "Oral Evening Primrose Oil and Borage Oil for Eczema." *Cochrane Database of Systematic Reviews* 4 (April 30, 2013): CD004416.

Bayles, Bryan, and Richard Usatine. "Evening Primrose Oil." *American Family Physician* 80, no. 12 (December 15, 2009): 1405–1408.

Chung, B. Y., J. H. Kim, S. I. Cho, et al. "Dose-Dependent Effects of Evening Primrose Oil in Children and Adolescents with Atopic Dermatitis." *Annals of Dermatology* 25, no. 3 (2013): 285–291.

Farzaneh, F., S. Fatehi, M. R. Sohrabi, and K. Alizadeh. "The Effect of Oral Evening Primrose Oil on Menopausal Hot Flashes: A Randomized Clinical Trial." *Archives of Gynecology and Obstetrics* 288, no. 5 (November 2013): 1075–1079.

Jaafarnejad, F., E. Adibmoghaddam, S. A. Emami, and A. Saki. "Compare the Effect of Flaxseed, Evening Primrose Oil and Vitamin E on Duration of Periodic Breast Pain." *Journal of Education and Health Promotion* 6 (October 4, 2017): 85.

Kwon, H. S., J. H. Lee, G. M. Kim, et al. "Topical Evening Primrose Oil as a Possible Therapeutic Alternative in Children with Molluscum Contagiosum." *Clinical and Experimental Dermatology* 42, no. 8 (December 2017): 923–925.

Park, Kui Young, Eun Jung Ko, In Su Kim, et al. "The Effect of Evening Primrose Oil for the Prevention of Xerotic Cheilitis in Acne Patients Being Treated with Isotretinoin: A Pilot Study." *Annals of Dermatology* 26, no. 6 (2014): 706–712.

Pruthi, S., D. L. Wahner-Roedler, C. J. Torkelson, et al. "Vitamin E and Evening Primrose Oil for Management of Cyclical Mastalgia: A Randomized Pilot Study." *Alternative Medicine Review* 15, no. 1 (April 2010): 59–67.

Senapati, S., S. Banerjee, and D. A. Gangopadhyay. "Evening Primrose Oil Is Effective in Atopic Dermatitis: A Randomized Placebo-Controlled Trial." *Indian Journal of Dermatology, Venereology and Leprology* 74, no. 5 (September–October 2008): 447–452.

Simon, Dagmar, Peter A. Eng, Siegfried Borelli, et al. "Gamma-Linolenic Acid Levels Correlate with Clinical Efficacy of Evening Primrose Oil in Patients with Atopic Dermatitis." *Advances in Therapy* 31, no. 2 (February 2014): 180–188.

Vasiljevic, D., M. Veselinovic, M. Jovanovic, et al. "Evaluation of the Effects of Different Supplementation on Oxidative Status in Patients with Rheumatoid Arthritis." *Clinical Rheumatology* 35, no. 8 (August 2016): 1909–1915.

Fish Oil

Fish oil, derived from the tissues of oily fish, is a dietary source of omega-3 fatty acids. While the body is unable to make these fatty acids, it needs them for numerous functions. Fish oil contains large amounts of two types of omega-3 fatty acids—docosahexaenoic acid (DHA) and eicosapentaenoic acid (EPA). Dietary sources of DHA and EPA include fatty fish, such as trout, salmon, tuna, herring, anchovies, sardines, and mackerel, as well as shellfish, such as crab, oysters, and mussels.

Interest in fish oil began decades ago when reports emerged that Eskimos, who consume large amounts of cold water fish, had low rates of heart disease, despite a diet that is high in animal fat. In recent years, the low rate of heart disease among Eskimos has largely been discredited. Nevertheless, fish oil supplements remain hugely popular and, often, controversial.

HEALTH BENEFITS AND RISKS

Fish oil is believed to support cardiovascular health, prevent heart disease and lower high blood pressure, triglycerides, and total cholesterol. People with rheumatoid arthritis may take fish oil supplements to reduce pain, morning stiffness, and joint inflammation. Some consume fish oil for kidney problems and kidney complications arising due to diabetes. However, fish oil has been recommended for a host of other problems including multiple sclerosis, depression, mood disorders, attention deficit hyperactivity disorder (ADHD), migraine headaches, dry eyes, age-related macular degeneration, inflammatory bowel disease, breast pain, obesity, and asthma.

While generally considered safe, fish oil supplements may cause side effects including a fishy aftertaste, bad breath, indigestion, nausea, loose stools, and rashes. Taking high doses of fish oil may increase the risk of bleeding. People on medication for blood pressure should use fish oil with caution as blood pressure levels may drop significantly. Those who have fish allergies should not use fish oil. Allergic reactions to fish oil include difficulty in breathing and swelling of the face, lips, tongue, or throat.

HOW IT IS SOLD AND TAKEN

Fish oil is sold as liquids and capsules. It is best to take fish oil with food. Recommended doses vary widely, and it is important not to consume more than the recommended doses. A dose of 1000–1200 mg per day should be aimed for. It is important to ensure that the supplement contains good amounts of EPA and DHA.

RESEARCH FINDINGS

Fish Oil Supplementation May or May Not Support Cardiovascular Health

In a systematic review and meta-analysis published in 2013 in the *American Journal of Clinical Nutrition*, researchers from China examined the association between fish oil supplementation and heart rate variability (the variation in time between heartbeats). The analysis consisted of 15 randomized controlled trials, with 349 participants in the fish oil groups and 343 in the control groups. The duration of the investigations ranged from 6 to 24 weeks, and the dosages of fish oil ranged from 640 to 5900 mg per day. The researchers noted that the trials had a number of differences, such as the health status of the participants, doses and composition of fish oil supplements, conditions of heart rate variability measurements, and follow-up durations. Still, the researchers learned that heart rate variability was significantly improved with fish oil supplementation. They concluded that "short-term fish-oil supplementation may favorably influence the frequency domain of heart rate variability."[1]

In a systematic review and meta-analysis published in 2009 in the *International Journal of Cardiology*, researchers from Australia investigated the use of fish oil supplementation in people with elevated lipid levels (hyperlipidemia). The cohort consisted of 47 randomized trials with adults who had cardiovascular risk factors; the trials included data from a total of 16,511 participants. Most participants were males with a mean age of 49 years. The average trial treatment was 24 weeks. For each trial, the researchers calculated the mean difference between treatment and placebo groups for total cholesterol, high-density lipoprotein (HDL), low-density lipoprotein (LDL), and triglycerides. The researchers found that fish oil alone was effective in reducing triglyceride levels in participants with elevated triglyceride levels. Fish oil had no significant effect on total cholesterol, although there were minor effects on HDL and LDL. The researchers commented that high triglyceride levels "are independently associated with coronary heart disease, stroke, metabolic syndrome, obesity, type 2 diabetes, and pancreatitis."[2]

In a randomized double-blind trial published in 2017 in *Kardiogia Polska* (*Polish Heart Journal*), researchers from Poland wanted to learn if fish oil supplementation would benefit people who had recently experienced a heart attack (myocardial infarction). The cohort consisted of 30 patients with postinfarction heart failure. For 12 weeks, half of the group consumed a daily 846 mg fish oil supplement and the other consumed a daily corn oil placebo. Blood tests were administered at baseline and at the end of the trial; information on dietary intake was also collected during this time. Fourteen patients in each group completed the trial. One person died from an acute cardiovascular event, and another withdrew consent. Upon discharge from the hospital, all the former patients were provided only general information about the benefits of the Mediterranean diet, "without specific education by a dietician." The researchers hypothesized that the outcomes might have been different if the patients had not returned to their atherogenic diet, or a diet that promotes atheromas, inflamed plaques on the inside of arteries. The diet "nullified" any potential fish oil benefits. The researchers concluded that "apparently, supplementation of omega-3 fatty acids without simultaneous dietary education and nutrition control does not bring the expected effect."[3]

People with Rheumatoid Arthritis May Benefit from Omega-3 Fatty Acids, such as Fish Oil

In a systematic review and meta-analysis published in 2018 in the journal *Nutrition*, researchers evaluated the ability of omega-3 fatty acids, such as fish oil, to help those dealing with rheumatoid arthritis. The researchers included 20 randomized controlled trials with a total of 717 participants with rheumatoid arthritis in the intervention groups and 535 participants with rheumatoid arthritis in the control groups. Except for two studies that only had female participants, all the trials included men and women. The intervention periods ranged from 12 to 72 weeks, and the daily dose of omega-3 fatty acids ranged from 300 to 9600 mg. All the participants maintained their conventional drug treatment during the trials. Twenty-seven markers of rheumatoid arthritis severity and progression were evaluated. The researchers determined that omega-3 fatty acids significantly improved eight disease activity-related markers. Moreover, these findings confirmed the results found in previous meta-analyses.[4]

Fish Oil Appears to Be Useful for Depressive Disorders

In a systematic review and meta-analysis published in 2014 in the online journal *PLoS ONE*, researchers from Italy and Poland examined randomized controlled trials on the use of omega-3 fatty acids to cope with depressive disorders. The researchers included 47 trials on patients with major depressive disorder and those with depressive symptomology without a diagnosis of major depressive disorder. The trials lasted from 4 to 160 weeks, with a mean duration of about 16 weeks. Thirty-six studies used a mixed intervention of EPA and DHA; 14 had only EPA, and four had only DHA. The researchers learned that omega-3 fatty acids were useful for patients diagnosed with a major depressive disorder and those who experienced depressive symptoms. In addition, patients with bipolar disorder experienced benefits. Inconclusive results were observed in patients with other pathological conditions, such as schizophrenia and perinatal depression.[5]

Fish Oil Supplementation Does Not Support the Mental Well-Being of Older People

In a double-blind, placebo-controlled trial published in 2008 in the *American Journal of Clinical Nutrition*, researchers from the Netherlands investigated the effect of fish oil supplementation on the mental health of people who were at least

65 years old. The initial cohort consisted of 302 participants who lived independently, who were randomly assigned to consume a large dose of fish oil, a low dose of fish oil, or a placebo capsule for 26 weeks. The fish oil and placebo capsules were indistinguishable in appearance. Participants visited the research center at baseline, after 13 weeks, and 26 weeks. The final analysis included 299 participants; more than half were male. The supplementation was well-tolerated, and the main complaint was mild gastrointestinal discomfort. The researchers assessed changes in mental health. The researchers determined that the plasma concentrations of EPA and DHA increased by 238% in the high-dose fish supplementation and increased by 51% in the low-dose fish supplementation. Yet, the researchers observed that neither of the two doses had any mental health benefits. They concluded that "after 13 and 26 weeks of supplementation, there were no significant differential changes in the fish oil groups, compared with the placebo group for any of the measures of mental well-being."[6]

Fish Oil Supplementation May Increase Anxiety in Some People

In a case report published in 2015 in *Oxford Medical Case Reports*, medical providers from California (USA) described the case of a 55-year-old male who consulted his general practitioner for increased general anxiety and mild panic attacks, despite effective treatment for recurrent major depressive disorder, which included medication and fish oil supplementation. During the day, he experienced general nonspecific anxiety and a shortness of breath, and at night, he awakened with a shortness of breath and extreme anxiety. After several months of symptom onset, the man stopped taking his fish oil supplements, and his anxiety and insomnia ended. Several weeks later, he restarted the high-EPA fish oil supplements when his medical problems resumed. On finally stopping fish oil supplementation, both anxiety and insomnia did not return, and his depression remained in remission. Apparently, while fish oil benefitted the man for an extended period of time, at some point, it triggered problematic symptoms. The researchers hypothesized that the patient's "increasing age [may have] played a role in the change." Further, they concluded that "consumers and clinicians should be aware of potential idiosyncratic adverse events."[7]

Low Levels of Omega-3 Fatty Acids May Play a Role in Postpartum Depression

In a prospective study published in 2013 in the online journal *PLoS ONE*, researchers from Norway noted that postpartum depression is a common medical problem. In fact, between 10% and 15% of women are believed to experience postpartum depression, which may interfere with the early relationship between a mother and child. The study originated from a community-based examination of the consumption of seafood, mental health, and infant development in a municipality outside Bergen, Norway. Medical providers recruited pregnant women during their routine visits at the twenty-fourth week of gestation. The initial cohort consisted of 70 women. Of these, 69 provided blood samples for fatty acid analysis, 55 answered the online questionnaire, and 44 were screened for postpartum depression 3 months after their babies were born. The researchers learned that a lower level of serum omega-3 fatty acids was associated with higher levels of postpartum depressive symptoms. According to the researchers, lower levels of omega-3 fatty acids during pregnancy "could be a possible risk factor for postpartum depression."[8]

Fish Oil Does Not Appear to Be Useful for Reducing the Risks of Gestational Diabetes Mellitus, Pregnancy-Induced Hypertension, or Preeclampsia

In a meta-analysis published in 2015 in the journal *Medical Science Monitor*, researchers from China evaluated the association between intake of fish oil supplements during the second or third trimester of pregnancy and the risk of gestational diabetes mellitus, pregnancy-induced hypertension, or preeclampsia. The cohort consisted of 11 randomized controlled trials with more than 5000 participants. Four trials included women with high-risk pregnancies, while the other seven trials included women with low-risk pregnancies. Supplementation was initiated from the fourteenth to the thirty-three weeks of gestation. Fish oil doses ranged from 200 to 4950 mg per day. The researchers found no association between the intake of fish oil and the risk of the three medical problems; the results were consistent for both low-risk and high-risk pregnancies. Still, the researchers acknowledged that "gestational fish oil supplementation may have other potential benefits."[9]

When Combined with Vitamin E, Zinc, and Stinging Nettle, Fish Oil Benefits Those with Osteoarthritis of the Knee or Hip

In a randomized, double-blind, parallel-group clinical trial published in 2009 in the journal *Arthritis Research & Therapy*, researchers from France tested the ability of a supplement known as Phytalgic®, which contains fish oil, vitamin E, and stinging nettle, to help people with osteoarthritis of the knee or hip. The researchers wanted to determine if people on this supplement would be able to reduce their use of pain medication. The cohort consisted of 81 patients with osteoarthritis of the knee or hip who regularly used pain medication. They were placed on the supplement (14 men and 27 women, with a mean age of 56.8 years) or a placebo (12 men and 28 women, with a mean age of 57.5 years) for 3 months; the supplement and placebo were identical in appearance. Patients were told that they should keep a daily diary detailing their use of pain medication. Five patients did not complete the trial. The researchers learned that the patients consuming the supplement used less pain medication and better managed their osteoarthritis pain. Moreover, the ability of the supplement to reduce pain continued to improve over the course of the trial. In fact, the supplement enabled patients to reduce their pain medication by more than 50%. The researchers noted that "the effect of the present combination may be related to any one of the individual components, or more probably to the association of these compounds, since none of the compounds used alone seem to have demonstrated effects of the magnitude found here."[10]

Low-Dose Fish Oil Seems to Work Better Than High-Dose Fish Oil for Knee Osteoarthritis

In a randomized, double-blind, multicenter trial published in 2016 in the journal *Annals of Rheumatic Diseases*, researchers from South Australia and Australia wanted to learn if a higher dose of fish oil would be better for knee osteoarthritis than a lower dose. The initial cohort consisted of 202 patients over the age of 40 years, with knee osteoarthritis and regular knee pain. The patients were placed on either a high dose (4.5 g EPA+DHA per day) or low dose (0.45 g EPA+DHA per day) of fish oil. The low-dose fish oil also contained sunola oil, which was thought to be a placebo. Knee pain evaluations were conducted at baseline and at 3, 6, 12, and 24 months; magnetic resonance imaging was done at baseline and at 24 months to determine changes in cartilage volume. The researchers learned that the participants on the low-dose supplementation had less pain and better function than the high-dose group. The researchers noted that "the reasons for this unanticipated result remain unclear." Did sunola oil have some effect on the outcome? "It is still unknown." There were no differences in the structural outcomes of cartilage volumes. The researcher commented that "the unanticipated finding of better pain and function in the low-dose fish oil/sunola group requires further investigation."[11]

Fish Oil May Be Useful for the Symptoms Associated with Eye Strain

In a double-blind, randomized, parallel-group, placebo-controlled trial published in 2011 in the journal *Biomedical Research*, researchers from Japan tested the ability of a supplement containing fish oil, bilberry extract, and lutein to relieve the symptoms associated with asthenopia or eye strain. The cohort consisted of 20 participants aged 20 to 34 years. There were eight males and 12 females. For 4 weeks, the participants were placed on the supplement or a placebo. Before and after supplementation, the participants completed a questionnaire, which asked about their eye strain symptoms. The researchers found that the combination supplementation relieved numerous symptoms associated with eye strain, such as eye fatigue and eye redness. In addition, it appeared to improve "mental fatigue in humans."[12]

Fish Oil May Reduce Levels of Aggression in Healthy Adults

In a double-blind randomized trial published in 2018 in the journal *Psychiatry Research*, researchers from France, the Netherlands, and California and Ohio (USA) divided 194 French men and women, between the ages of 18 and 45 years, into two groups. The participants of one group consumed omega-3 supplements (total dose: 638 mg DHA and 772 mg EPA), and the other group consumed placebos—copra oil. Copra oil has no known behavioral effects. Self-reported aggressiveness was measured at baseline and after 6 weeks of treatment. The researchers learned that the omega-3 supplement significantly reduced levels of self-reported aggressiveness. The researchers concluded that their findings "suggested that omega-3 administration may reduce physical aggression in the general population."[13]

Fish Oil May Not Be Useful for Aggression in Children and Teens with Disruptive Behavior Disorders

In a prospective, randomized, placebo-controlled, crossover trial published in 2014 in the *Journal of Child and Adolescent Psychopharmacology*, researchers from Australia wanted to determine if fish oil would be useful for children and teens with disruptive behavior disorders. The cohort consisted of 21 children who ranged in age from 7 to 14 years; 81% of the participants were male. The participants consumed fish oil capsules (4000 mg per day) for 6 weeks followed by a placebo for 6 weeks. Alternatively, they consumed a placebo for 6 weeks followed by fish oil for 6 weeks. Serum concentrations of omega-3 and omega-6 fatty acids were measured at baseline, at 6 weeks, and at 12 weeks. As expected, fish oil treatments increased the levels of serum EPA and total omega-3 fatty acids. However, it did not lower aggression levels. As a secondary measure, fish oil appeared to increase aggression levels. Clinical evaluations were conducted every 2 weeks; research assessments were conducted at baseline, at 6 weeks, and at 12 weeks. The researchers concluded that "until evidence becomes available to support the use of fish oil or fatty acid supplementation for aggression and related behaviors, clinicians should be cautious about its use."[14]

Fish Oil May Have Some Benefits for Children with ADHD

In a systematic review and meta-analysis published in 2011 in the *Journal of the American Academy of Child and Adolescent Psychiatry*, researchers based in New Haven, Connecticut (USA), examined the association between omega-3 fatty acid supplementation and symptoms of ADHD. The researchers identified ten relevant trials that included 699 children. All the trials were randomized and placebo-controlled, and they ranged in duration from 4 weeks to 4 months. The researchers found that omega-3 fatty acid supplementation had a "small but significant benefit" on the symptoms of ADHD. Compared to the available pharmacological treatments, the results were "modest." Therefore, the researchers concluded that they would not recommend omega-3 fatty acids instead of traditional treatments for children with significant ADHD symptoms. They also concluded that "however, given evidence of modest efficacy of omega-3 supplementation and given its relatively benign side-effect profile, omega-3 fatty acid supplementation, particularly with higher doses of EPA, is a reasonable treatment strategy as augmentation to traditional pharmacotherapy or for those families reticent to use psychopharmacological agents."[15]

NOTES

1. Xin, W., W. Wei, and X. Y. Li. "Short-Term Effects of Fish-Oil Supplementation on Heart Rate Variability in Humans: A Meta-Analysis of Randomized Controlled Trials." *American Journal of Clinical Nutrition* 97, no. 5 (May 2013): 926–925.

2. Eslick, Guy D., Peter R. C. Howe, Caroline Smith, et al. "Benefits of Fish Oil Supplementation in Hyperlipidemia: A Systematic Review and Meta-Analysis." *International Journal of Cardiology* 136 (2009): 4–16.

3. Makarewicz-Wujec, M., G. Parol, A. Parzonko, and M. Kozlowska-Wojciechowska. "Supplementation with Omega-3 Acids after Myocardial Infarction and Modification of Inflammatory Markers in Light of the Patients' Diet: A Preliminary Study." *Kardiogia Polska (Polish Heart Journal)* 75, no. 7 (2017): 674–681.

4. Gioxari, A., A. C. Kaliora, F. Marantidou, and D. P. Panagiotakos. "Intake of ω-3 Polyunsaturated Fatty Acids in Patients with Rheumatoid Arthritis: A Systematic Review and Meta-Analysis." *Nutrition* 45 (January 2018): 114–124.

5. Grosso, Giuseppe, Andrzej Pajak, Stefano Marventano, et al. "Role of Omega-3 Fatty Acids in the Treatment of Depressive Disorders: A Comprehensive Meta-Analysis of Randomized Clinical Trials." *PLoS ONE* 9, no. 5 (May 2014): e96905.

6. van de Rest, O., J. M. Geleijnse, F. J. Kok, et al. "Effect of Fish-Oil Supplementation on Mental Well-Being in Older Subjects: A Randomized, Double-Blind, Placebo-Controlled Trial." *American Journal of Clinical Nutrition* 88, no. 3 (September 2008): 706–713.

7. Blanchard, Lauren B., and Gordon C. McCarter. "Insomnia and Exacerbation of Anxiety Associated with High-EPA Fish-Oil Supplements after Successful Treatment of Depression." *Oxford Medical Case Reports* 3 (2015): 244–245.

8. Markhus, Maria Wik, Siv Skotheim, Ingvild Eide Graff, et al. "Low Omega-3 Index in Pregnancy Is a Possible Biological Risk Factor for Postpartum Depression." *PLoS ONE* 8, no. 7 (2013): e67617.

9. Chen, B., X. Ji, L. Zhang, et al. "Fish Oil Supplementation Does Not Reduce Risks of Gestational Diabetes Mellitus, Pregnancy-Induced Hypertension, or Pre-Eclampsia: A Meta-Analysis of Randomized Controlled Trials." *Medical Science Monitor* 21 (August 9, 2015): 2322–2330.

10. Jacquet, Alain, Pierre-Olivier Girodet, Antoine Pariente, et al. "Phytalgic®, a Food Supplement, vs. Placebo in Patients with Osteoarthritis of the Knee or Hip: A Randomized Double-Blind Placebo-Controlled Clinical Trial." *Arthritis Research & Therapy* 11, no. 6 (2009): R192.

11. Hill, C. L., L. M. March, D. Aitken, et al. "Fish Oil in Knee Osteoarthritis: A Randomised Clinical Trial of Low Dose versus High Dose." *Annals of the Rheumatic Diseases* 75, no. 1 (January 2016): 23–29.

12. Kawabata, F., and T. Truji. "Effects of Dietary Supplementation with a Combination of Fish Oil, Bilberry Extract, and Lutein on Subjective Symptoms of Asthenopia in Humans." *Biomedical Research* 32, no. 6 (December 2011): 387–393.

13. Bègue, Laurent, Ap Zaalberg, Rébecca Shankland, et al. "Omega-3 Supplements Reduce Self-Reported Physical Aggression in Healthy Adults." *Psychiatry Research* 261 (2018): 307–311.

14. Dean, A. J., W. Bor, K. Adam, et al. "A Randomized, Controlled, Crossover Trial of Fish Oil Treatment for Impulsive Aggression in Children and Adolescents with

Disruptive Behavior Disorders." *Journal of Child and Adolescent Psychopharmacology* 24, no. 3 (April 2014): 140–148.

15. Bloch, M. H., and A. Qawasmi. "Omega-3 Fatty Acid Supplementation for the Treatment of Children with Attention-Deficit/Hyperactivity Disorder Symptomatology: Systematic Review and Meta-Analysis." *Journal of the American Academy of Child and Adolescent Psychiatry* 50, no. 10 (October 2011): 991–1000.

REFERENCES AND FURTHER READING

Bègue, Laurent, Ap Zaalberg, Rébecca Shankland, et al. "Omega-3 Supplements Reduce Self-Reported Physical Aggression in Healthy Adults." *Psychiatry Research* 261 (2018): 307–311.

Blanchard, Lauren B., and Gordon C. McCarter. "Insomnia and Exacerbation of Anxiety Associated with High-EPA Fish Oil Supplements after Successful Treatment of Depression." *Oxford Medical Case Reports* 3 (2015): 244–245.

Bloch, M. H., and A. Qawasmi. "Omega-3 Fatty Acid Supplementation for the Treatment of Children with Attention-Deficit/Hyperactivity Disorder Symptomatology: Systematic Review and Meta-Analysis." *Journal of the American Academy of Child and Adolescent Psychiatry* 50, no. 10 (October 2011): 881–1000.

Chen, B., X. Ji, L. Zhang, et al. "Fish Oil Supplementation Does Not Reduce Risks of Gestational Diabetes Mellitus, Pregnancy-Induced Hypertension, or Pre-Eclampsia: A Meta-Analysis of Randomized Controlled Trials." *Medical Science Monitor* 21 (August 9, 2015): 2322–2330.

Dean, A. J., W. Bor, K. Adam, et al. "A Randomized, Controlled, Crossover Trial of Fish Oil Treatment for Impulsive Aggression in Children and Adolescents with Disruptive Behavior Disorders." *Journal of Child and Adolescent Psychopharmacology* 24, no. 3 (April 2014): 140–148.

Eslick, Guy D., Peter R. C. Howe, Caroline Smith, et al. "Benefits of Fish Oil Supplementation in Hyperlipidemia: A Systematic Review and Meta-Analysis." *International Journal of Cardiology* 136 (2009): 4–16.

Gioxari, A., A. C. Kaliora, F. Marantidou, and D. P. Panagiotakos. "Intake of ω-3 Polyunsaturated Fatty Acids in Patients with Rheumatoid Arthritis: A Systematic Review and Meta-Analysis." *Nutrition* 45 (January 2018): 114–124.

Grosso, Giuseppe, Andrzej Pajak, Stefano Marventano, et al. "Role of Omega-3 Fatty Acids in the Treatment of Depressive Disorders: A Comprehensive Meta-Analysis of Randomized Clinical Trials." *PLoS ONE* 9, no. 5 (May 2014): e96905.

Hill, C. L., L. M. March, D. Aitken, et al. "Fish Oil in Knee Osteoarthritis: A Randomised Clinical Trial of Low Dose versus High Dose." *Annals of the Rheumatic Diseases* 75, no. 1 (January 2016): 23–29.

Jacquet, Alain, Pierre-Olivier Girodet, Antoine Pariente, et al. "Phytalgic®, a Food Supplement, vs. Placebo in Patients with Osteoarthritis of the Knee or Hip: A Randomised Double-Blind Placebo-Controlled Clinical Trial." *Arthritis Research & Therapy* 11, no. 6 (2009): R192.

Kawabata, F., and T. Tsuji. "Effects of Dietary Supplementation with a Combination of Fish Oil, Bilberry Extract, and Lutein on Subjective Symptoms of Asthenopia in Humans." *Biomedical Research* 32, no. 6 (December 2011): 387–393.

Makarewicz-Wujec, M., G. Parol, A. Parzonko, and M. Kozlowska. "Supplementation with Omega 3 Acids after Myocardial Infarction and Modification of Inflammatory

Markers in Light of the Patients' Diet: A Preliminary Study." *Kardiogia Polska (Polish Heart Journal)* 75, no. 7 (2017): 674–681.

Markhus, Maria Wik, Siv Skotheim, Ingvild Eide Graff, et al. "Low Omega-3 Index in Pregnancy Is a Possible Biological Risk Factor for Postpartum Depression." *PLoS ONE* 8, no. 7 (2013): e67617.

van de Rest, O., J. M. Geleojnse, F. J. Kok, et al. "Effect of Fish-Oil Supplementation on Mental Well-Being in Older Subjects: A Randomized, Double-Blind, Placebo-Controlled Trial." *American Journal of Clinical Nutrition* 88, no. 3 (September 2008): 706–713.

Xin, W., W. Wei, and X. Y. Li. "Short-Term Effects of Fish-Oil Supplementation on Heart Rate Variability in Humans: A Meta-Analysis of Randomized Controlled Trials." *American Journal of Clinical Nutrition* 97, no. 5 (May 2013): 926–935.

5-HTP

5-HTP, also known as 5-hydroxytryptophan, is a chemical that the body makes from tryptophan, an essential amino acid derived from food. After tryptophan is converted into 5-HTP, it is then changed into serotonin, a neurotransmitter that transmits signals between brain cells. As a result, 5-HTP supplementation raises serotonin levels in the brain. Because serotonin levels are associated with mood and behavior, 5-HTP supplementation is believed to improve sleep, mood, anxiety, appetite, and relieve pain.

While 5-HTP is not found in foods that most people consume, tryptophan is found in many foods including nuts, seeds, cheese, milk, potatoes, pumpkin, turnips, collard greens, seaweed, soya foods, red meat, chicken, turkey, fish, oats, beans, lentils, and eggs.

HEALTH BENEFITS AND RISKS

5-HTP is useful for several health problems. In addition to the previously noted health concerns, 5-HTP may be used to treat depression, fibromyalgia, insomnia, migraines and other headaches, premenstrual syndrome, premenstrual dysphonic disorder, attention deficit hyperactivity disorder, seizure disorder, Parkinson's disease, and obesity.

Further, 5-HTP may react with a number of different medications including those for depression, such as selective serotonin reuptake inhibitors, tricyclics, monoamine oxidase (MAO) inhibitors, and nefazodone. Combining 5-HTP with carbidopa, a medication for Parkinson's disease, may cause the skin to become hard, thick, and inflamed. Tramadol, which is used for pain relief, may result in unsafe serotonin levels. Even higher levels of serotonin may occur when 5-HTP is combined with dextromethorphan, which is found in Robitussin DM and other cough syrups. This condition is known as serotonin syndrome. Serotonin syndrome may also develop when Demerol, used for extreme pain, is taken with 5-HTP and when triptans, used for migraines, are combined with 5-HTP. Signs and symptoms of serotonin syndrome include agitation, restlessness, confusion, rapid heart rate, high blood pressure, dilated pupils, loss of muscle coordination, twitching muscles, muscle rigidity, heavy sweating, diarrhea, headache, shivering, and goose bumps. Signs and symptoms of severe serotonin syndrome include high fever, seizures, irregular heartbeat, and unconsciousness.

5-HTP should not be taken with other herbs or supplements that may cause drowsiness or sleepiness. If taken together, it may cause excessive sleepiness.

Supplements known to cause sleepiness include hops, kava, St. John's wort, skullcap, and valerian. Moreover, 5-HTP should not be taken with herbs or supplements that increase serotonin levels such as S-adenosylmethionine and St. John's wort.

The symptoms of serotonin syndrome include agitation, restlessness, confusion, rapid heart rate, high blood pressure, dilated pupils, loss of muscle coordination, twitching muscles, muscle rigidity, and heavy sweating. Very high doses of 5-HTP—ranging from 6 to 10 g per day—have been associated with severe stomach problems and muscle spasms. Moreover, some people known to have taken 5-HTP developed a condition known as eosinophilia–myalgia syndrome, which causes extreme muscle tenderness and blood abnormalities.

Because 5-HTP raises serotonin levels, it should be stopped at least 2 weeks before surgery. It may result in high levels of serotonin to accumulate in the brain. Very low doses may be safe in young children, but there is too little known about the use of 5-HTP to be sure. Therefore, it is best for children and pregnant and breastfeeding women to avoid 5-HTP.

To help prevent the myriad of related problems, it is best to check with a medical provider before initiating 5-HTP supplementation.

HOW IT IS SOLD AND TAKEN

5-HTP is produced commercially from the seeds of *Griffonia simplicifolia*, a West African plant. It is sold as tablets, time-release tablets, and capsules.

Dose recommendations vary widely. A typical dose may range between 100 and 400 mg, taken once daily or in divided doses. 5-HTP has been used safely in doses of up to 400 mg daily for up to 1 year. However, some medical providers recommend higher doses. 5-HTP should always be taken with a meal.

Ask a medical provider for dose recommendations.

RESEARCH FINDINGS

The Combination of 5-HTP and Prozac May Be a Useful Treatment for a First Depressive Episode

In a randomized, double-blind study published in 2013 in the *Asian Journal of Psychiatry*, researchers from India wanted to learn more about the antidepressive properties of 5-HTP and to compare with those of Prozac (fluoxetine). The initial cohort consisted of 70 patients, aged 20–50 years, who were diagnosed with their first episode of depression. The patients were divided into two groups. One group took Prozac, and the second group took 5-HTP. Over time, the doses were increased. All patients were assessed at baseline, at 2 weeks, at 4 weeks, and at 8 weeks. Sixty patients completed the entire study; there were 30 patients in each group. The researchers learned that, beginning with the second week, the participants in both groups experienced significant and nearly equal reduction in depressive symptoms. By 8 weeks, 22 patients in the 5-HTP group and 24 patients in the Prozac group demonstrated positive responses. The minimally effective dose to reduce depression was 150 mg per day. However, there were problems. Patients in both groups reported adverse effects such as nausea, anorexia, and headache. Nevertheless, the researchers concluded that 5-HTP worked essentially as well as Prozac for depression.[1]

5-HTP May Play a Role in the Alleviation of Alcohol Withdrawal Symptoms

In a study published in 2011 in the journal *Collegium Antropologicum*, researchers from Croatia and Slovenia tested the ability of a supplement containing 5-HTP, D-phenylalanine, and L-glutamine to help alleviate the symptoms of alcohol withdrawal such as anxiety, dysphoria, and restlessness. The cohort consisted of 20 hospitalized patients who were enrolled in a detoxification program for alcohol addiction. For 40 days, the patients were randomly treated with the supplementation or placebo; there were 10 patients in each group. Testing was administered at baseline and patients in both groups demonstrated high levels of psychiatric symptoms. Hospitalization and the beginning of abstinence were major sources of stress for the patients. By the fortieth day of hospitalization, there were statistically significant reductions in almost all symptoms. According to the researchers, "this may confirm our hypothesis that administration of such dietary supplements reduces symptoms of withdrawal from ethanol [alcohol for human consumption]."[2]

Adding 5-HTP to the Treatment Plan May Help Adults Who Have Not Responded Well to the More Common Prescription Treatments for Depression

In a pilot open-label study published in 2017 in the *Journal of Clinical Psychopharmacology*, researchers from Salt Lake City, Utah (USA), explained that many adult women with a major depressive disorder do not respond well to standard treatments, such as selective serotonin reuptake inhibitors and serotonin–norepinephrine reuptake inhibitors. This is a very serious concern, as major depressive disorder is a debilitating illness that is "associated with significant personal and social costs, diminished quality of life, and disability." The researchers aimed to investigate if addition of 5-HTP and creatine monohydrate to the standard treatment would improve the results. The initial cohort consisted of 15 women, with a mean age of 34 years, who were suffering from at least moderate depression and were on standard treatment for major depression. For 8 weeks, they were treated twice daily with 100 mg of 5-HTP and 5 g of creatine monohydrate. Twelve patients completed the trial. Overall, their depression levels were notably reduced. Moreover, they "demonstrated robust symptomatic improvement and good safety and tolerability." Of the 12 women, seven decided to continue supplementation, although they had to purchase their own supplements. However, only tentative conclusions may be obtained from such a small sample. The researchers concluded that, "Given the limitations of this small, open-label trial, future study in randomized, placebo-controlled trials is warranted."[3]

In a study published in 2016 in the journal *Trends in Pharmacological Sciences*, researchers from Durham, North Carolina (USA), commented that only one-third of patients respond adequately to the standard treatment for depression. According to the researchers, "Treatment-resistant depression (TRD) is a major unmet need." They also hypothesized that a slow-release form of 5-HTP might prevent some of the problems associated with regular 5-HTP supplementation. Further, they conducted an extensive review of the relevant literature to determine if there were supportive studies. They learned that slow-release 5-HTP would "substantially enhance the pharmacological action and transform 5-HTP into a clinically viable drug." It is possible that slow-release 5-HTP could become "an important new treatment" for treatment-resistant depression.[4]

5-HTP May Be Useful for Allergic Inflammation of the Lungs

In a study published in 2012 in the *American Journal of Physiology—Lung Cellular and Molecular Physiology*, researchers from Chicago, Illinois (USA), investigated the ability of 5-HTP to reduce allergic inflammation in the lungs. The researchers administered 5-HTP to mice and then exposed them to allergens, such as house dust and mite extract. After comparing mice on 5-HTP with control mice, the researchers determined that the mice that were given supplemental 5-HTP had 70%–90% less allergic lung inflammation. According to the researchers, "5-HTP reduced lung inflammation in two models of allergy/asthma."[5] Why is this important? Over the past decades, industrialized countries have witnessed dramatic increase in asthma and allergic illnesses. In fact, approximately half of all school children worldwide are sensitive to at least one allergen.

In Rats, Perinatal Treatment with 5-HTP Appears to Reduce One Type of Anxiety

In a study published in 2012 in the journal *Behavioural Brain Research*, researchers from Croatia tested the ability of 5-HTP to reduce anxiety and cognitive rigidity. The researchers treated Wistar rats with 5-HTP from gestational day 12 to postnatal day 21. (Other rats were treated with a nonselective MAO inhibitor tranylcypromine or served as controls.) Once they reached adulthood, the rats participated in several tests for anxiety-like behavior and cognitive flexibility. The researchers found that the rats treated with 5-HTP experienced reductions in only one type of anxiety-like behavior and increased exploratory activity. The researchers underscored the need for more studies "to elucidate the mechanisms underlying the observed behavior."[6]

5-HTP Does Not Appear to Be Useful for Menopausal Hot Flashes

In a study published in 2010 in the journal *Maturitas*, a researcher from Detroit, Michigan (USA), noted that hot flashes are a common symptom of menopause and are experienced by millions of women throughout the world. Would 5-HTP supplementation help these women? The study cohort consisted of 24 postmenopausal women who reported at least six hot flashes per day. The women were randomly assigned to take 5-HTP or placebo. A miniature, electronic, hot flash recorder was used to measure actual hot flashes. The trial continued for 4 weeks. The researcher failed to find a significant difference in hot flashes between the two groups. However, he acknowledged that his findings were "clearly limited" by the small sample size. In addition, there is a possibility that a higher dose of 5-HTP might yield different results.[7]

People Taking 5-HTP May Require More Time to Complete Certain Tasks

In a study published in 2013 in the journal *Human Psychopharmacology*, researchers from North Carolina (USA) wanted to learn if 5-HTP would have any influence on executive function testing. (An executive function test includes evaluating processes such as planning and logical thinking.) The study cohort consisted of 66 undergraduate students between the ages of 18 and 22 years. Each student was given either 5-HTP capsules or placebos; 34 received 5-HTP capsules and 32 had placebos. The participants were instructed to take the capsules at specific times before the testing began. The researchers determined that the students who took 5-HTP required significantly longer periods of time to complete the test. But, participants in both groups made approximately the same number of errors. As a result, 5-HTP does not appear to affect accuracy.[8]

5-HTP May Play a Role in the Treatment of Heroin Addiction

In a 6-day trial published in 2012 in the *Journal of Huazhong University of Sciences and Technology* [Medical Sciences], researchers from China wanted to determine if a supplement containing 5-HTP, tyrosine, lecithin, and L-glutamine would be useful for the syndromes and mental symptoms associated with detoxification from heroin. The cohort consisted of 83 detoxifying heroin addicts from a treatment center in Wuhan, China. Forty-one patients in the treatment group received the supplement, and 42 patients in the control group took placebo. The patients were not told if they were on the supplement or placebo. The researchers monitored sleep status and withdrawal symptoms, as well as mood status, both pre- and post-intervention group. Interestingly, the researchers observed that the participants in the intervention group had improvements in insomnia and withdrawal symptoms; they had greater reductions in tension-anxiety, depression-dejection, anger-hostility, fatigue-inertia, total mood disturbance; and a greater increase in their vigor and activity. The researchers concluded that "the neurotransmitter-precursor-supplement intervention is effective in alleviating the withdrawal and mood symptoms and it may become a supplementary method for patients' recovery from heroin addiction."[9]

NOTES

1. Jangid, Purushottam, Prerna Malik, Priti Singh, et al. "Comparative Study of Efficacy of L-5-Hydroxytryptophan and Fluoxetine in Patients Presenting with First Depressive Episode." *Asian Journal of Psychiatry* 6, no. 1 (February 2013): 29–34.

2. Jukić, Tomislav, Bojan Roje, Darja Boben-Bardutzky, et al. "The Use of a Food Supplementation with D-Phenylalanine, L-Glutamine, and L-5-Hydroxytriptophan in the Alleviation of Alcohol Withdrawal Symptoms." *Collegium Antropologicum* 35, no. 4 (December 2011): 1225–1230.

3. Kious, Brent, Hana Sabic, Young-Hoon Sung, et al. "An Open-Label Pilot Study of Combined Augmentation with Creatine Monohydrate and 5-Hydroxytryptophan for Selective Serotonin Reuptake Inhibitor- or Serotonin-Norepinephrine Reuptake Inhibitor-Resistant Depression in Adult Women." *Journal of Clinical Psychopharmacology* 37, no. 5 (October 2017): 578–583.

4. Jacobsen, J. P. R., A. D. Krystal, K. R. R. Krishnan, and M. G. Caron. "Adjunctive 5-Hydroxytryptophan Slow-Release for Treatment-Resistant Depression: Clinical and Preclinical Rationale." *Trends in Pharmacological Science* 37, no. 11 (November 2016): 933–944.

5. Abdala-Valencia, Hiam, Sergeis Berdnikovs, Christine A. McCary, et al. "Inhibition of Allergic Inflammation by Supplementation with 5-Hydroxytryptophan." *American Journal of Physiology –Lung Cellular and Molecular Physiology* 303, no. 8 (October 15, 2012): L642–L660.

6. Blazevic, Sofia, Lejla Colic, Luka Culig, and Dubravka Hranilovic. "Anxiety-Like Behavior and Cognitive Flexibility in Adult Rats Perinatally Exposed to Increased Serotonin Concentrations." *Behavioural Brain Research* 230, no. 1 (2012): 175–181.

7. Freedman, Robert R. "Treatment of Menopausal Hot Flashes with 5-Hydroxytryptophan." *Maturitas* 65 (2010): 383–385.

8. Gendle, Mathew H., Erica L. Young, and Alexandra C. Romano. "Effects of Oral 5-Hydroxytryptophan on a Standardized Planning Task: Insight into Possible Dopamine/Serotonin Interactions in the Forebrain." *Human Psychopharmacology* 28 (2013): 270–273.

9. Chen, D., Y. Liu, W. He, et al. "Neurotransmitter-Precursor-Supplement Intervention for Detoxified Heroin Addicts." *Journal of Huazhong University of Sciences and Technology* [Medical Sciences] 32, no. 3 (June 2012): 422–427.

REFERENCES AND FURTHER READING

Abdala-Valencia, Hiam, Sergeis Berdnikovs, Christine A. McCary, et al. "Inhibition of Allergic Inflammation by Supplementation with 5-Hydroxytryptophan." *American Journal of Physiology—Lung Cellular and Molecular Physiology* 303, no. 8 (October 15, 2012): L642–L660.

Blazevic, Sofia, Lejla Colic, Luke Culig, and Dubravka Hranilovic. "Anxiety-Like Behavior and Cognitive Flexibility in Adults Rats Perinatally Exposed to Increased Serotonin Concentrations." *Behavioural Brain Research* 230, no. 1 (2012): 175–181.

Chen, D., Y. Liu, W. He, et al. "Neurotransmitter-Precursor-Supplement Intervention for Detoxified Heroin Addicts." *Journal of Huazhong University of Sciences and Technology* [Medical Sciences] 32, no. 3 (June 2012): 422–427.

Freedman, Robert R. "Treatment of Menopausal Hot Flashes with 5-Hydroxytryptophan." *Maturitas* 65 (2010): 383–385.

Gendle, Mathew H., Erica L. Young, and Alexandra C. Romano. "Effects of Oral 5-Hydroxytryptophan on a Standardized Planning Task: Insight into Possible Dopamine/Serotonin Interactions in the Forebrain." *Human Psychopharmacology* 28 (2013): 270–273.

Jacobsen, J. P. R., A. D. Krystal, K. R. R. Krishnan, and M. G. Caron. "Adjunctive 5-Hydroxytryptophan Slow-Release for Treatment-Resistant Depression: Clinical and Preclinical Rationale." *Trends in Pharmacological Sciences* 37, no. 11 (November 2016): 933–944.

Jangid, Purushottam, Prerna Malik, Priti Singh, et al. "Comparative Study of Efficacy of L-5-Hydroxytryptophan and Fluoxetine in Patients Presenting with First Depressive Episode." *Asian Journal of Psychiatry* 6, no. 1 (February 2013): 29–34.

Jukić, Tomislav, Bojan Rojc, Darja Boben-Bardutzky, et al. "The Use of a Food Supplementation with D-Phenylalanine, L-Glutamine, and L-5-Hydroxytriptophan in the Alleviation of Alcohol Withdrawal Symptoms." *Collegium Antropologicum* 35, no. 4 (December 2011): 1225–1230.

Kious, Brent M., Hana Sabic, Young-Hoon Sung, et al. "An Open-Label Pilot Study of Combined Augmentation with Creatine Monohydrate and 5-Hydroxytryptophan for Selective Serotonin Reuptake Inhibitor—or Serotonin-Norepinephrine Reuptake Inhibitor-Resistant Depression in Adult Women." *Journal of Clinical Psychopharmacology* 37, no. 5 (October 2017): 578–583.

Mayo Clinic. www.mayoclinic.org.

Flaxseed Oil

Derived from flaxseed (*Linum usitatissimum*, which means very useful), flaxseed oil is a rich source of the essential fatty acid alpha-linolenic acid, a heart healthy omega-3 fatty acid. In addition to omega-3, flaxseed oil has omega-6 and omega-9 fatty acids. These essential fatty acids, which the body is unable to make, must be obtained through diet or supplementation. Flaxseed oil is naturally high in antioxidants, such as tocopherols and beta-carotene.

Flaxseed oil, also known as linseed oil, has been used since ancient times, and has been cultivated since the beginning of civilization.

Good-quality flaxseed oil is made from fresh-pressed seeds. It is processed at low temperatures without light, extreme heat, or oxygen, and has a nutty and slightly sweet flavor. Whether in liquid or capsule form, to reduce oxidation, flaxseed oil should be stored in an opaque or black bottle.

HEALTH BENEFITS AND RISKS

People consume flaxseed oil to support cardiovascular health, lower cholesterol and blood sugar levels, and treat constipation and inflammatory conditions, such as arthritis. They may also consume flaxseed oil for menopausal symptoms, such as hot flashes, and to improve bone health and balance hormones. Generally, it is safe for children to consume flaxseed oil for a short period of time.

Large doses of flaxseed oil, for example 30 g or more per day, may cause stomach upset, nausea, loose stools, and diarrhea. People may be allergic to flaxseed oil. Until more is known about the risks of flaxseed oil during pregnancy and breastfeeding, it should probably be avoided. People with bleeding disorders or on medication to slow blood clotting should avoid flaxseed oil as it may trigger severe bleeding. Those with diabetes must use flaxseed oil with caution. It may also interfere with certain medications, such as metformin. Flaxseed oil may alter the efficacy of oral contraceptives and hormone replacement therapy. Before beginning a flaxseed oil regime, women on these medications should have a discussion with a medical provider. It is probably best to consume flaxseed oil or fish oil—not both at the same time as their properties and side effects are similar. Flaxseed oil may interfere with medications for high blood pressure. Because flaxseed oil may increase bleeding during surgery, it should be discontinued 2 weeks before a scheduled surgical procedure.

HOW IT IS SOLD AND TAKEN

Flaxseed oil is sold as a liquid and as capsules. Recommended doses of flaxseed oil vary. It is best to follow the instructions on the bottle and start with the lowest dose, such as one teaspoon or one low-dose capsule. Some people recommend taking up to about one tablespoon per day or more. Flaxseed oil is somewhat fragile and readily breaks down when exposed to light, heat, or air. It may also easily become rancid. Flaxseed oil should be stored in the refrigerator. Flaxseed oil should never be heated or used for cooking. It may be used as a salad dressing or added to sauces, smoothies, yogurt, and protein shakes.

RESEARCH FINDINGS

Flaxseed Oil Appears to Have Anti-Inflammatory and Cardiovascular Support Properties in People with Chronic Renal Failure

In a randomized, double-blind, placebo-controlled, multicenter trial published in 2012 in the journal *Nutrition Research*, researchers from Brazil investigated the effects of flaxseed oil supplementation on patients with chronic renal failure undergoing hemodialysis. These patients have an increased risk for a number of medical problems including inflammation. The initial cohort consisted of 160 patients who received care at one of three different dialysis units in south Brazil, with a mean age of 59.3 years. For 120 days, they took either flaxseed oil or a placebo (mineral oil). The two different capsules were visually identical. At baseline, inflammation was observed in 89 patients (61%). One hundred and fourteen patients completed the trial. The group consuming flaxseed oil experienced a significant reduction in C-reactive protein, a measure of inflammation. The C-reactive protein levels of the members of the mineral oil group "remained stable." The flaxseed group also had lower levels of total cholesterol and low-density lipoprotein (LDL) cholesterol and higher levels of high-density lipoprotein (HDL) cholesterol. The researchers then compared patients who were inflamed and not inflamed at baseline. Among the noninflamed patients, neither intervention produced a significant decrease in C-reactive protein levels. On the other hand, a statistically significant decrease in C-reactive protein levels was noted in inflamed patients who consumed flaxseed oil. The researchers commented that "studies with a larger number of patients and over a longer duration are necessary to corroborate these findings."[1]

Benefits of Flaxseed Oil May Not Be as Apparent in Healthy Young Adults

In a crossover trial published in 2013 in the journal *Metabolism: Clinical and Experimental*, researchers from Greece tested the anti-inflammatory and antioxidant properties of flaxseed oil in healthy young adults. The cohort consisted of 37 healthy, normal weight, male and female young adults between the ages of 18 and

35 years. For 6 weeks, the participants were randomly placed on either flaxseed oil or olive oil supplementation. After the first intervention and a 6-week washout period, they were placed on an alternate intervention. The oils were provided in sealed dark bottles. Still, the participants were familiar with the flavor of olive oil, and were able to determine which oil they were taking. Various laboratory tests were administered at the beginning and end of the protocols. The researchers found that the dietary interventions did not trigger any significant changes in inflammatory markers or lipid profiles. According to the researchers, "daily consumption of FO [flaxseed oil] did not confer any benefit in inflammatory or biochemical markers in normal weight young adults, who traditionally use olive oil as the main edible oil."[2]

Flaxseed Supplementation May Reduce Skin Sensitivity and Improve Skin Barrier Function and Condition

In a randomized, double-blind trial published in 2011 in the journal *Skin Pharmacology and Physiology*, researchers from Germany and France investigated the ability of flaxseed oil supplementation to improve the skin of healthy females with skin sensitivity. Skin sensitivity is a very common problem in western society. The cohort consisted of 26 women between the ages of 18 and 65 years. For 12 weeks, they consumed either flaxseed oil or safflower oil supplementation. Skin parameters were evaluated at baseline, after 6 weeks, and after 12 weeks. Blood samples were drawn at the same time. The researchers determined that the women on flaxseed supplementation had a statistically significant decrease in skin sensitivity, transepidermal water loss, skin roughness, and scaling, as well as a statistically significant increase in smoothness. Supplementation with safflower oil only resulted in significant improvement in skin roughness and hydration, "however, these effects were less pronounced." The researchers concluded that the "daily intake of flaxseed oil modulates skin condition."[3]

Flaxseed Supplementation Seems to Support the HDL Levels in Older People

In a prospective, double-blind, placebo-controlled clinical trial published in 2015 in the journal *Clinical Interventions in Aging*, researchers from Brazil wanted to determine if flaxseed oil, which they called linseed oil, would help control lipid levels in older men and women. The cohort consisted of 110 men and women who were at least 60 years old. For 90 days, they consumed either 3 g per day of flaxseed oil or a placebo, which consisted of gelatin powder encapsulated in opaque capsules. The participants in both groups received nutritional guidelines. Food intake was assessed in two 24-h recalls at baseline and after the intervention, and blood samples were collected every month. The researchers learned that the intake of flaxseed oil resulted in significant reductions in the concentrations of total cholesterol, LDL cholesterol, and triglycerides, as well as increases in the concentrations of HDL cholesterol. Interestingly, the placebo group also had significant reductions in total cholesterol, LDL cholesterol, and triglycerides, but no changes in HDL. The researchers concluded that flaxseed oil "showed notable effects by increasing the HDL cholesterol concentration."[4]

Flaxseed Oil Appears to Lower Levels of Small Dense LDL

In a randomized, double-blind, crossover trial published in 2015 in *Nutrition Journal,* researchers based in Japan evaluated the association between flaxseed supplementation and levels of small dense LDL. (Small dense LDLs are smaller and denser than typical LDLs.) The cohort consisted of 15 Japanese men. For two consecutive 12-week periods, they consumed either 10 g of flaxseed oil or 10 g of corn oil each day with dinner. The two parts of the trial were separated by an 8-week washout period. Blood samples were collected at baseline, at 4 weeks, and at 12 weeks. Researchers interviewed the participants every 2 weeks. The researchers learned that the intake of flaxseed oil significantly and "markedly" reduced the levels of serum small dense LDL. This was particularly pronounced in participants with higher triglyceride levels.[5]

Flaxseed Oil Has Wound Healing Properties

In a study published in 2016 in the *Journal of Surgical Research*, researchers from Tunisia tested the ability of three different oils—flaxseed (which they termed linseed oil), prickly pear, and pumpkin—to heal second-degree burns on rats, with tissue damage, edema, and crusting. Thirty rats with laser-induced burns were divided into five groups. The rats in the first group were treated with a saline solution; the rats in the second group were treated with a standard drug "CYTOL BASIC" cream; and those in the third, fourth, and fifth group were treated with one of the three oils. The response to treatments was assessed by macroscopic, histologic, and biochemical parameters. The researchers discovered that after 7 days of treatment, the burns in all three oil groups demonstrated "a significant decrease in the healing time." The researchers noted that some medicinal plants have wound healing properties.[6]

In another wound-related study, published in 2017 in the *African Journal of Traditional, Complementary and Alternative Medicine*, researchers from Algeria tested crude flaxseed oil (which they also termed linseed oil), Vaseline gel, and Cicatryl-Bio, a wound ointment, on burn wounds in rabbits. The cohort consisted of eight healthy adult male New Zealand rabbits of the same flock, the same age, and about the same weight. After administering the burns, the wounds were treated with a topical application or left to heal "naturally" without any treatment. The wounds were inspected daily. By the end of the study, it was evident that flaxseed oil had the best overall healing properties, with no adverse effects. The researchers noted that their findings "confirmed that linseed oil compounds have bioactive properties that render it effective in promoting wound healing activity compared with well known commercial drugs."[7]

Flaxseed Oil Supplementation May Have Some Benefits for People with Metabolic Syndrome

In a randomized, controlled, interventional trial published in 2018 in the *Journal of Clinical Lipidology*, researchers from Iran examined the ability of flaxseed oil supplementation to help with signs associated with metabolic syndrome, such as elevated levels of serum glucose and high blood pressure. The cohort consisted of 60 volunteers between the ages of 30 and 60 years who were diagnosed with metabolic syndrome in Shiraz, Iran. Half of the volunteers were placed on flaxseed supplement, and the other half were placed on sunflower seed oil. All the participants ate an identical diet in terms of macronutrient composition, except for the type of oil they consumed. Testing was conducted at baseline and at the end of 7 weeks. While the results showed no significant difference between the two groups regarding blood lipid levels and fasting blood sugar, significant reductions in total cholesterol, LDL, and triglyceride levels were initially seen in both the flaxseed oil and sunflower seed oil groups. However, by the end of the study, these reductions were no longer statistically significant. In addition, the participants in the flaxseed group had significant reductions in systolic and diastolic blood pressure. The members of both groups had significant decreases in weight, however, waist circumference decreased significantly only in the flaxseed oil group. The researchers concluded that flaxseed oil may address some of the medical problems associated with metabolic syndrome.[8]

Flaxseed Oil Seems to Be Useful for Constipation, at Least in People Undergoing Hemodialysis

In a 4-week, double-blind, randomized controlled trial published in 2015 in the *Journal of Renal Nutrition*, researchers from Brazil compared the use of flaxseed oil, olive oil, and mineral oil for treating constipation in people undergoing hemodialysis. Constipation is a common complaint among people undergoing hemodialysis for profound renal disease. Varying symptoms included incomplete evacuation, lumpy or hard stools, anorectal obstruction, straining on evacuation, fewer than three evacuations per week, and manual maneuvers to facilitate evacuation. The cohort consisted of 50 patients (29% males) from a single dialysis unit who had constipation for at least 3 months; the participants were assigned to take daily doses of one of the oils. The initial dosage was 4 mL/day, however, individual adjustments were made during follow-up appointments. In the flaxseed oil group, 82% of the participants required an adjustment; the average final dose was 6.9 mL/day. The researchers learned that the daily use of either flaxseed or olive oil was as effective as mineral oil for the treatment of constipation in this population. They concluded that "the beneficial effects, the absence of significant adverse events, and the applicability of this intervention make the replacement of mineral oil by olive oil or flaxseed oil an alternative for the treatment of constipation in HD [hemodialysis] patients."[9]

Topical Flaxseed Oil May Be Useful for Knee Osteoarthritis

In a double-blind, randomized, placebo-controlled clinical trial published in 2018 in the journal *Complementary Therapies in Clinical Practice*, researchers from Iran wanted to determine if topical flaxseed oil, which they termed linseed oil, would be useful for knee osteoarthritis, a common form of arthritis in the elderly. The inclusion criteria for the trial were men and women between the ages of 40 and 70 years, with a body mass index of less than 35; all participants had knee osteoarthritis with a pain level of at least 4 on a 10-point scale. The initial cohort had 82 participants. Patients in the flaxseed group rubbed 20 drops of the oil on their knees every 8 h for 6 weeks. Patients in the placebo group followed the same procedure with liquid paraffin. All participants were permitted to use a pain and inflammation medication known as diclofenac up to three times per day. Thirty-five participants in the flaxseed group and 34 participants in the placebo group completed the trial. The researchers learned that flaxseed oil was significantly better than placebo in reducing the pain and symptoms of knee osteoarthritis. The members of the flaxseed group experienced improvements in "the activities of daily living, sport and recreation, and knee-related quality of life."[10]

Flaxseed Oil May Support Bone Health

In a study published in 2009 in the *International Journal of Food Safety, Nutrition and Public Health*, researchers from Cairo, Egypt wanted to determine if flaxseed oil would benefit bone mineral density and reduce markers associated with osteoporosis, a condition characterized by low bone mass, with increased risk of fractures. The researchers began with 70 female albino rats; they left them alone (control and sham) or treated them to fit the requirement of several different groups—control; sham; diabetic; diabetic fed flaxseed oil; ovarectomized; ovarectomized and diabetic; and ovarectomized, diabetic, and fed flaxseed oil. After 2 months, the researchers collected urine and blood samples from the rats and measured serum insulin-like growth factor 1 and the bone-creating protein osteocalcin. These compounds were present at higher levels in ovarectomized rats and ovarectomized rats with diabetes. However, in the non-ovariectomized rats without diabetes, these levels were low. The concentration of these compounds was raised when flaxseed oil was added to the rats' diets. The researchers also learned that the levels of deoxypyridinoline in the urine were raised in the diabetic group. Normally, deoxypyridinoline is present in healthy bones. When it is found in urine, it is a specific marker for bone resorption associated with osteoporosis. After the rats were given flaxseed oil, the levels of this marker reduced.

What do these findings mean? Diabetes increased the risk of declining bone health more than the ovariectomy surgery, which induced menopause. Further, diabetes in postmenopausal women appeared to be a greater risk factor for osteoporosis than the decline in sex hormones associated with menopause. Yet, supplementation with flaxseed oil reduced markers associated with osteoporosis, and may help menopausal women with diabetes reduce their risk for osteoporosis. The researchers concluded that diabetes is an incredibly significant risk factor for osteoporosis, and this risk may be attenuated by flaxseed oil supplementation.[11]

NOTES

1. Lemos, J. R., M. G. Alencastro, A. V. Konrath, et al. "Flaxseed Oil Supplementation Decreases C-Reactive Protein Levels in Chronic Hemodialysis Patients." *Nutrition Research* 32, no. 12 (December 2012): 921–927.

2. Kontogianni, M. D., A. Vlassopoulos, A. Gatzieva, et al. "Flaxseed Oil Does Not Affect Inflammatory Markers and Lipid Profile Compared to Olive Oil, in Young, Healthy, Normal Weight Adults." *Metabolism: Clinical and Experimental* 62, no. 5 (May 2013): 686–693.

3. Neukam, K., S. De Spirt, W. Stahl, et al. "Supplementation of Flaxseed Oil Diminishes Skin Sensitivity and Improves Skin Barrier Function and Condition." *Skin Pharmacology and Physiology* 24, no. 2 (2011): 67–74.

4. Avelino, A. P., G. M. Oliveira, C. C. Ferreira, et al. "Additive Effect of Linseed Oil Supplementation on the Lipid Profiles of Older Adults." *Clinical Interventions in Aging* 10 (October 22, 2015): 1679–1685.

5. Kawakami, Yuka, Hisami Yamanaka-Okumura, Yuko Naniwa-Kuroki, et al. "Flaxseed Oil Intake Reduces Serum Small Dense Low-Density Lipoprotein Concentrations in Japanese Men: A Randomized, Double Blind, Crossover Study." *Nutrition Journal* 14 (2015): 39.

6. Bardaa, S., N. Chabchoub, M. Jridi, et al. "The Effect of Natural Extracts on Laser Burn Wound Healing." *Journal of Surgical Research* 201, no. 2 (April 2016): 464–472.

7. Beroual, Katiba, Amir Agabou, Mohamed-Cherif Abdeldjelil, et al. "Evaluation of Crude Flaxseed (*Linum usitatissimum L.*) Oil in Burn Wound Healing in New Zealand Rabbits." *African Journal of Traditional, Complementary and Alternative Medicine* 14, no. 3 (2017): 280–286.

8. Akrami, A., F. Nikaein, S. Babajafari, et al. "Comparison of the Effects of Flaxseed Oil and Sunflower Oil Consumption on Serum Glucose, Lipid Profile, Blood Pressure, and Lipid Peroxidation in Patients with Metabolic Syndrome." *Journal of Clinical Lipidology* 12, no. 1 (January–February 2018): 70–77.

9. Ramos, C. I., A. F. Andrade de Lima, D. G. Grilli, and L. Cuppari. "The Short-Term Effects of Olive Oil and Flaxseed Oil for the Treatment of Constipation in Hemodialysis Patients." *Journal of Renal Nutrition* 25, no. 1 (January 2015): 50–56.

10. Mosavat, S. H., N. Masoudi, H. Hajimehdipoor, et al. "Efficacy of Topical *Linum usitatissimum* L. (Flaxseed) Oil in Knee Osteoarthritis: A Double-Blind, Randomized, Placebo-Controlled Clinical Trial." *Complementary Therapies in Clinical Practice* 31 (May 2018): 302–307.

11. Elwassef, M., M. Anwar, M. Harvi, et al. "Impact of Feeding Flaxseed Oil on Delaying the Development of Osteoporosis in Ovarectomized Diabetic Rats." *International Journal of Food Safety, Nutrition and Public Health* 2, no. 2 (2009): 189–201.

REFERENCES AND FURTHER READING

Akrami, A., F. Nikaein, S. Babajafari, et al. "Comparison of the Effects of Flaxseed Oil and Sunflower Seed Oil Consumption on Serum Glucose, Lipid Profile, Blood Pressure, and Lipid Peroxidation in Patients with Metabolic Syndrome." *Journal of Clinical Lipidology* 12, no. 1 (January–February 2018): 70–77.

Avelino, A. P., G. M. Oliveira, C. C. Ferreira, et al. "Additive Effect of Linseed Oil Supplementation on the Lipid Profiles of Older Adults." *Clinical Interventions in Aging* 10 (October 22, 2015): 1679–1685.

Bardaa, S., N. Chabchoub, M. Jridi, et al. "The Effect of Natural Extracts on Laser Burn Wound Healing." *Journal of Surgical Research* 201, no. 2 (April 2016): 464–472.

Beroual, Katiba, Amir Agabou, Mohammed-Cherif Abdeldjelil, et al. "Evaluation of Crude Flaxseed (*Linum usitatissimum L.*) Oil in Burn Wound Healing in New Zealand Rabbits." *African Journal of Traditional, Complementary and Alternative Medicine* 14, no. 3 (2017): 280–286.

Elwassef, M., M. Anwar, M. Harvi, et al. "Impact of Feeding Flaxseed Oil on Delaying the Development of Osteoporosis in Ovariectomised Diabetic Rats." *International Journal of Food Safety, Nutrition and Public Health* 2, no. 2 (2009): 189–201.

Kawakami, Yuka, Hisami Yamanaka-Okumura, Yuko Naniwa-Kuroki, et al. "Flaxseed Oil Intake Reduces Serum Small Dense Low-Density Lipoprotein Concentrations in Japanese Men: A Randomized, Double Blind, Crossover Study." *Nutrition Journal* 14 (2015): 39.

Kontogianni, M. D., A. Vlassopoulos, A. Gatzievae, et al. "Flaxseed Oil Does Not Affect Inflammatory Markers and Lipid Profile Compared to Olive Oil, in Young, Healthy, Normal Weight Adults." *Metabolism: Clinical and Experimental* 62, no. 5 (May 2013): 686–693.

Lemos, J. R., M. G. Alencastro, A. V. Konrath, et al. "Flaxseed Oil Supplementation Decreases C-Reactive Protein Levels in Chronic Hemodialysis Patients." *Nutrition Research* 32, no. 12 (December 2012): 921–927.

Mosavat, S. H., N. Masoudi, H. Hajimehdipoor, et al. "Efficacy of Topical *Linum usitatissimum L.* (Flaxseed) Oil in Knee Osteoarthritis: A Double-Blind, Randomized, Placebo-Controlled Clinical Trial." *Complementary Therapies in Clinical Practice* 31 (May 2018): 302–307.

Neukam, K., S. De Spirt, W. Stahl, et al. "Supplementation of Flaxseed Oil Diminishes Skin Sensitivity and Improves Skin Barrier Function and Condition." *Skin Pharmacology and Physiology* 24, no. 2 (2011): 67–74.

Ramos, C, I., A. F. Andrade de Lima, D. G. Grilli, and L. Cuppari. "The Short-Term Effects of Olive Oil and Flaxseed Oil for the Treatment of Constipation in Hemodialysis Patients." *Journal of Renal Nutrition* 25, no. 1 (January 2015): 50–56.

Ginger

Ginger, also known as *Zingiber officinale*, is a tropical plant with flowers and a fragrant underground stem, known as a rhizome. Texts from ancient cultures and languages, such as ancient Chinese, Greek, Roman, Sanskrit, and Arab mention the use of ginger for health-related problems. Dried ginger has been used in Asian medicine for thousands of years to treat gastrointestinal problems, such as diarrhea and nausea. Though indigenous to China and India, ginger is cultivated throughout the world. Ginger is a member of the *Zingiberaceae* family, which also includes cardamom and turmeric.

Scientific analyses have found that ginger contains hundreds of compounds and metabolites, which may support health and wellbeing. Of these, the most researched are gingerols and shogaols.

HEALTH BENEFITS AND RISKS

Most people recognize ginger for its antinausea properties. Medical providers may recommend ginger for nausea associated with surgical procedures or that related to chemotherapy treatment, pregnancy, or motion. Ginger supplementation is also thought to be useful for inflammation, rheumatoid arthritis, osteoarthritis, and menstrual pain.

Some people may experience mild side effects from ginger such as abdominal discomfort, heartburn, diarrhea, and gas. Because ginger may increase the flow of bile, people with gallstone disease should check with their medical provider before initiating ginger supplementation. Ginger and diabetes medications lower blood sugar levels. When taken together, levels of blood sugar may become too low. Furthermore, ginger supplementation may interact with anticoagulants or blood-thinning medications. Taking ginger with medications that slow blood clotting may increase the risk of bruising and bleeding.

HOW IT IS SOLD AND TAKEN

Ginger is sold in several forms such as tablets, fresh, dried, capsules, teas, juices, extracts, lozenges, and liquid extracts. Dosing recommendations for ginger supplements vary widely and tend to range from 500 to 2500 mg per day, or higher, in divided doses. It is probably best to discuss ginger supplementation with a medical provider and to follow the instructions on the label.

RESEARCH FINDINGS

Ginger Supplementation May or May Not Be Useful for Surgery-Related Nausea and Vomiting

In a randomized, double-blind, single-dose, parallel clinical trial published in 2018 in the *Journal of Traditional and Complementary Medicine*, researchers from Iran compared the postsurgical antinausea and antivomiting properties of ginger supplementation to ondansetron, a standard antinausea and vomiting medication. The cohort consisted of 100 patients with cholelithiasis (gallstones in their gallbladders); all patients had undergone laparoscopic surgical removal of their gallbladders (a procedure known as a laparoscopic cholecystectomy) from March 2013 to February 2014. Seventy-one percent of the patients were females; the patients had a mean age of 43.97 years. Fifty patients in group A received 500 mg of oral ginger 1 h before surgery, and 50 patients in group B received 4 mg of intravenous ondansetron before the surgery ended. Assessments were made at baseline and at 4, 8, 16, and 24 h after surgery. The researchers found that the incidence of nausea in the ginger group was significantly lower than the ondansetron group. On the other hand, there was no difference in the rate of vomiting between the two groups. The researchers concluded that ginger was a good substitute for ondansetron, commenting that "because ginger is an herbal, easily available, low price medication which is associated with low risk . . . [it] can be substituted for a chemical, scarce and expensive drug such as ondansetron."[1]

In a double-blind, placebo-controlled, randomized clinical trial published in 2017 in the journal *Electronic Physician*, researchers from Iran investigated the ability of presurgical administration of oral ginger to prevent the nausea and vomiting associated with cataract surgery performed under general anesthesia. The cohort consisted of 122 participants who underwent cataract surgery in 2015; the participants were placed in one of three groups. The average age of the participants in three groups ranged from 66.9 to 72 years. Before the surgery, the members of the first group consumed a single 1 g capsule of ginger; the members of the second group took two separate doses (the night and morning before the surgery) of 500 mg ginger; and the members of the third group took a placebo. For 6 h after surgery, nausea levels were assessed and incidences of vomiting were recorded. The researchers learned that the participants who took the two capsules had significantly less nausea and vomiting than those in the other two groups. The researchers noted that "ginger will be more effective if used regularly and in separate doses."[2]

In a double-blind, randomized clinical trial published in 2016 in the journal *Anesthesiology and Pain Medicine*, researchers from Iran evaluated the ability of ginger supplementation to reduce nausea and vomiting in women who underwent a cesarean section under spinal anesthesia. The cohort consisted of 92 pregnant women who delivered their babies via cesarean section under spinal anesthesia. One hour before the surgery, the women in the intervention group consumed 25 drops of ginger extract in 30 cc of water; the women in the control group had only 30 cc of water. The researchers learned that nausea and vomiting during and after the surgery was significantly lower in the intervention group than that in the control group. In addition, the rate of nausea decreased in both groups after 2 and 4 h of surgery, but, there was no significant difference between the groups. The frequency of vomiting decreased in both groups 2 h after the surgery, and again, there was no significant difference between the groups. Four hours after the surgery, there was no vomiting among the participants in either group. The researchers commented that "ginger is effective for the prevention of nausea and vomiting after cesarean section under spinal anesthesia, and no side effects related to this dose of ginger were observed."[3]

In a meta-analysis published in 2018 in the journal *Phytomedicine*, researchers from Hungary analyzed ten randomized, placebo-controlled trials that examined the use of ginger supplementation to prevent postoperative nausea and vomiting. In total, 918 patients were included in these trials. Trials that studied homeopathic preparations of ginger and/or combinations of ginger with other treatments were excluded. The included trials were conducted in six different countries—Thailand, the United Kingdom, Iran, Germany, India, and Australia. Doses of ginger ranged from 100 to 2000 mg. The researchers learned that ginger supplementation may reduce the incidence of postoperative nausea and vomiting. However, even at higher doses, the results were not statistically significant. Still, the researchers concluded that ginger is "safe and well tolerated," and since it may lower the incidence of postoperative nausea and vomiting, it may "reduce antiemetic drug demand."[4]

Ginger Supplementation May Benefit Pregnant Women with Nausea and Vomiting

In a systematic review and meta-analysis published in 2014 in *Nutrition Journal*, researchers from South Africa noted that nausea and vomiting are common medical problems associated with pregnancy. Therefore, the researchers wanted to learn if ginger supplementation would be a useful treatment. The researchers found 12 randomized controlled trials with 1278 pregnant women that met their criteria. The trials were published between 1991 and 2011. No restrictions were placed on the age of the women or their stage of pregnancy. Eleven trials had a parallel-group design and one trial had a crossover design. The trials ranged in size from 26 to 291 participants. Only two trials had more than 150 participants. The researchers learned that ginger supplementation was more effective than placebos in relieving the intensity of nausea; yet, it did not have a significant impact on vomiting episodes, even though there was a trend toward improvement. It did not increase the rates of spontaneous abortions or side effects, such as heartburn or drowsiness. The researchers commented that, "it is probably safe to assume that ginger has potential as a possible anti-emetic drug-alternative during pregnancy." In addition, a subgroup analysis found that doses of less than 1500 mg per day provided better nausea relief.[5]

In a meta-analysis published in 2014 in the *Journal of the American Board of Family Medicine*, researchers from Canada investigated the use of ginger for nausea and vomiting during early pregnancy. Six randomized, placebo-controlled trials met their criteria. Of the 508 participants in these studies, 256 were randomly assigned to consume a ginger supplement and 252 were randomly assigned to consume a placebo. Total sample sizes ranged from 23 to 235, and interventions continued for 4 days to 3 weeks. Ginger doses and methods of administration also varied. Reports of improvements in nausea and vomiting came from participants on ginger as well as on placebos. In fact, 180 of the 256 participants on ginger supplementation and 126 of the 252 participants taking placebos reported symptom improvements. Still, when ginger was used at a dose of about 1 g per day for at least 4 days, it offered better improvement than placebos. The researchers concluded that medical professionals "should be cognizant of the value of ginger as they contemplate pharmacological options for suitable patients with NVEP [nausea and vomiting in early pregnancy]."[6]

Ginger Supplementation May or May Not Be Useful for Chemotherapy-Related Nausea and Vomiting

In a randomized, double-blind, multicenter clinical trial, researchers from several locations in the United States but based in Rochester, New York (USA), noted that over 70% of patients on chemotherapy experience nausea. Therefore, they wanted to learn more about the ability of ginger supplementation to ease this common medical problem. The researchers initially placed 744 cancer patients in one of the four statistically similar groups—placebo, 0.5 g ginger per day, 1.0 g ginger per day, or 1.5 g ginger per day. All patients had experienced nausea with chemotherapy treatments. In addition to their regular chemotherapy-related medications, the participants took the ginger or placebo supplements during three rounds of chemotherapy, beginning 3 days before each treatment. A total of 576 patients were included in the final analyses. More than 90% were females who had a mean age of 53 years. The most common cancer types were breast, gastrointestinal, and lung. During the trial, the patients were asked to keep 4-day records of their use of antiemetic medications after their chemotherapy treatments. The researchers learned that ginger supplementation reduced the severity of acute nausea in the patients. The researchers concluded that "ginger had demonstrated a beneficial effect on acute nausea from chemotherapy."[7]

In a prospective, randomized trial published in 2016 in the *Asian Pacific Journal of Cancer Prevention*, researchers based in Iran tested the ability of ginger supplementation to help relieve nausea and vomiting among women suffering from breast cancer who were being treated with chemotherapy. The cohort consisted of 150 female breast cancer patients who received three cycles of doxorubicin-based chemotherapy; their mean age was 48.56 years. With each cycle, for 3 days, they consumed 500 mg ginger powder twice a day or a placebo; the ginger and placebo capsules had the same shape and color. The participants were asked to record the severity of their nausea and vomiting incidences. One hundred and nineteen participants completed all the requirements of the trial. After the first chemotherapy, the mean nausea in the ginger and placebo had no statistical difference. After the second chemotherapy, the nausea score was slightly higher in the ginger group. After the third chemotherapy, the mean nausea severity in the placebo group was less than the ginger group. During all three chemotherapy treatments, ginger reduced vomiting severity, but none of the differences were significant. The researchers commented that "further and larger studies are needed to draw conclusions."[8]

Ginger May Have Some Utility for People with Osteoarthritis

In a systematic review and meta-analysis published in 2015 in the journal *Osteoarthritis and Cartilage*, researchers from Denmark, Los Angeles, California (USA), and the United Kingdom investigated the efficacy and safety of using ginger supplementation for people with osteoarthritis. Their cohort consisted of five randomized controlled trials with 593 patients. The average age of the patients ranged from 47 to 66 years, and the percentage of women included in the trials ranged from 26% to 80%. The daily dose of ginger ranged from 500 to 1000 mg per day. The actual ginger products varied from trial to trial, and the duration of the trials ranged from 3 to 12 weeks. The researchers learned that ginger supplementation reduced osteoarthritis pain and disability, without any serious adverse effects. The researchers concluded that ginger supplementation "may be considered as part of the treatment of OA [osteoarthritis]."[9]

Ginger Supplementation May Have Some Benefits for People with Type 2 Diabetes

In a randomized, double-blind, placebo-controlled trial published in 2018 in the *Journal of Nutrition and Food Security*, researchers from Iran examined the use of ginger supplementation in people with type 2 diabetes. Eighty-eight participants were randomly divided into a group that consumed 3 g per day of ginger supplement or a group that consumed a placebo. The baseline characteristics of the participants did not differ significantly between the two groups. Assessments were periodically conducted throughout the 8-week trial. A 24-h dietary recall questionnaire was used at the beginning and end of the trial. Eighty-one participants were included in the final analyses, including 50 females and 31 males. The mean age of the participants in the ginger group was 49.83 years, and the mean age of the participants in the placebo group was 51.05 years. By the end of the trial, the researchers determined that ginger supplementation had a significant positive effect on diastolic blood pressure, systolic blood pressure, pulse pressure, and mean arterial pressure. No significant changes were observed in the placebo group. None of the participants reported any adverse effects. The researchers suggested that future trials should continue for longer periods of time. According to the researchers, the "consumption of this supplement is appropriate."[10]

Ginger Supplementation May Help Lower Blood Pressure

In a systematic review and meta-analysis published in 2019 in the journal *Phytotherapy Research*, researchers from Iran and the United Kingdom examined the usefulness of ginger supplementation for lowering blood pressure. The cohort consisted of six randomized clinical trials with 345 participants aged 22 to

54 years; 175 of the participants were in the supplement groups and 170 were in the control groups. The doses of ginger ranged from 0.5 to 3 g per day, and the duration of interventions ranged from 7 to 12 weeks. The researchers learned that ginger supplementation had clear blood pressure lowering properties. Pooled data analyses found that ginger supplementation has the potential to reduce blood pressure. This was more likely to occur when a higher dose of ginger supplementation was used for a shorter intervention period in people 50 years old or younger. Still, the researchers commented that "further studies are warranted before definitive conclusions may be reached."[11]

Ginger May Have Some Benefits for People with Nonalcoholic Fatty Liver Disease

In a randomized, double-blind, placebo-controlled clinical trial published in 2016 in the journal *Hepatitis Monthly*, researchers from Iran wanted to learn if people with nonalcoholic fatty liver disease would benefit from ginger supplementation. The initial cohort consisted of 50 participants with nonalcoholic fatty liver disease. For 12 weeks, they consumed either 2 g of ginger per day, in divided doses, or a placebo; there were 25 participants in each group. Participants were advised to follow a modified diet and physical activity plan. To assess food intake, all participants were asked to complete a 3-day food record at the beginning and end of the trial. Various other assessments were also conducted at baseline and when the trial ended. Twenty-three participants in the ginger group and 21 in the placebo group completed the trial. The researchers found that the participants consuming ginger had significant improvements in several factors associated with nonalcoholic fatty liver disease, such as the lowering of alanine aminotransferase (ALT) and gamma-glutamyl transferase (GGT) liver enzymes. The researchers concluded that "twelve weeks of two grams of ginger supplementation showed beneficial effects on some NAFLD [nonalcoholic fatty liver disease] characteristics."[12]

Ginger Supplementation May or May Not Have Weight Lowering Properties

In a systematic review published in 2018 in the journal *Phytotherapy Research*, researchers from Iran examined the antiobesity and weight lowering properties of ginger supplementation. Their review included six in vitro studies, 17 animal studies, and four human studies. The risk of bias for the included studies was low. The researchers determined that most experimental animal studies supported the weight lowering properties of ginger supplementation in obese animal models. On the other hand, the few clinical studies that the researchers evaluated showed either no changes or slight changes in the size, shape, and composition in obese participants. Interestingly, the researchers noted that most animal studies used high doses of ginger extract or its bioactive compounds instead of ginger powder. Finally, they concluded that "more randomized controlled trials are needed to make a definitive conclusion."[13]

Ginger Supplementation May Be Useful for Primary Dysmenorrhea, Pain Associated with Menstruation

In a randomized controlled clinical trial published in 2012 in the journal *BMC Complementary & Alternative Medicine*, researchers from Iran examined the use of ginger supplementation for the pain associated with primary dysmenorrhea. The cohort initially consisted of 120 university students who had moderate or severe primary dysmenorrhea. The severity of their symptoms was determined by a verbal multidimensional scoring system. During two different protocols, the women were randomly assigned to one of the two groups. Half of the women consumed 500 mg capsules of ginger root power three times each day, and the other half consumed the same number of placebos. In the first protocol, ginger and placebo were given 2 days before the onset of menstruation and continued through the first 3 days of the period. In the second protocol, ginger and placebo were given only during the first 3 days of the menstrual cycle. Pain severity was assessed before and after the interventions. One hundred and five students completed the trial. Compared to the placebos, both protocols significantly reduced pain levels. The researchers commented that "the effects of ginger are large enough to be clinically significant and to alleviate primary dysmenorrhea."[14]

When Combined with Artichoke Supplementation, Ginger Supplementation May Be Useful for Functional Dyspepsia

In a prospective, multicenter, double-blind, randomized, placebo-controlled trial, researchers from Italy wanted to learn if ginger and artichoke leaf extract supplementation would help people with functional dyspepsia or pain or discomfort in the upper middle part of the stomach, nausea, and bloating. The cohort consisted of 126 male and female participants with functional dyspepsia. For 4 weeks, 65 participants consumed two capsules per day containing 20 mg of ginger and 100 mg of artichoke or placebos. After 14 days of treatment, only the supplement group showed a significant improvement in symptoms. This improvement was maintained until the end of the trial. For example, the participants on the combination supplement had reductions in the severity of epigastric pain, epigastric fullness, bloating, nausea, and early satiety. The reductions in epigastric pain and nausea appeared to be statistically significant. The researchers concluded that "the association between ginger and artichoke leaf extracts appears efficacious in the treatment of functional dyspepsia and could represent a promising and safe treatment strategy for this frequent disease, even though additional studies are needed to confirm these results."[15]

Ginger Supplementation May or May Not Be Useful for Irritable Bowel Syndrome

In a randomized, double-blind, placebo-controlled, pilot trial published in 2014 in the journal *Complementary Therapies in Medicine*, researchers from North Carolina (USA) noted that ginger supplementation is frequently used for irritable bowel syndrome. Therefore, they wanted to determine if this supplementation actually improved symptoms, such as constipation, diarrhea, and bloating. The cohort consisted of 45 patients, who were all at least 18 years old, with a physician diagnosis of irritable bowel syndrome. For 28 days, 15 participants were assigned to one of three groups—placebo, 1 g ginger per day, or 2 g ginger per day. By the end of the trial, the participants in the placebo and 1-g ginger group had significant reductions in symptoms. The efficacy of ginger decreased in the higher dose. There was a 26% decrease in symptoms with the 1-g dose versus a 12% decrease in symptoms with a 2-g dose. Moreover, the placebo response was better than can normally be expected. The researchers concluded that "the current study does not find evidence for the use of ginger in treating IBS [irritable bowel syndrome] but future larger trials are needed before any definitive conclusions can be drawn."[16]

NOTES

1. Soltttani, E., A. Janqjoo, M. Afzal Aqhaei, and A. Dalili. "Effect of Preoperative Administration of Ginger (*Zingiber officinale* Roscoe) on Postoperative Nausea and Vomiting after Laparoscopic Cholecystectomy." *Journal of Traditional and Complementary Medicine* 8, no. 3 (July 2018): 387–390.

2. Seidi, Jamel, Shahrokh Ebnerasooli, Sirous Shahsawari, and Simin Nzarian. "The Influence of Oral Ginger before Operation on Nausea and Vomiting after Cataract Surgery under General Anesthesia: A Double-Blind Placebo-Controlled Randomized Clinical Trial." *Electronic Physician* 9, no. 1 (January 2017): 3508–3514.

3. Zeraati, Hossein, Javad Shahinfar, Shiva Imani Hesari, et al. "The Effect of Ginger Extract on the Incidence and Severity of Nausea and Vomiting after Cesarean Section under Spinal Anesthesia." *Anesthesiology and Pain Medicine* 6, no. 5 (October 2016): e38943.

4. Tóth, Barbara, Tamás Lantos, Péter Hegyi, et al. "Ginger (*Zingiber officinale*): An Alternative for the Prevention of Postoperative Nausea and Vomiting. A Meta-Analysis." *Phytomedicine* 50 (November 15, 2018): 8–18.

5. Viljoen, Estelle, Janicke Visser, Nelene Koen, and Alfred Musekiwa. "A Systematic Review and Meta-Analysis of the Effect and Safety of Ginger in the Treatment of Pregnancy-Associated Nausea and Vomiting." *Nutrition Journal* 13 (2014): 20.

6. Thomson, Maggie, Renee Corbin, and Lawrence Leung. "Effects of Ginger for Nausea and Vomiting in Early Pregnancy: A Meta-Analysis." *Journal of the American Board of Family Medicine* 27, no. 1 (2014): 115–122.

7. Ryan, Julie L., Charles E. Heckler, Joseph A. Roscoe, et al. "Ginger (*Zingiber officinale*) Reduces Acute Chemotherapy-Induced Nausea: A URCC CCOP Study of 576 Patients." *Supportive Care in Cancer* 20, no. 7 (July 2012): 1479–1489.

8. Ansari, Mansour, Pezhman Porouhan, Mohammad Mohammadianpanah, et al. "Efficacy of Ginger in Control of Chemotherapy Induced Nausea and Vomiting in Breast Cancer Patients Receiving Doxorubicin-Based Chemotherapy." 17, no. 8 (2016): 3877–3880.

9. Bartels, E. M., V. N. Folmer, H. Bliddal, et al. "Efficacy and Safety of Ginger in Osteoarthritis Patients: A Meta-Analysis of Randomized Placebo-Controlled Trials." *Osteoarthritis and Cartilage* 23, no. 1 (January 2015): 13–21.

10. Talaei, Behrouz, Hassan Mozaffari-Khosravi, and Shohreh Bahreini. "The Effect of Ginger Powder Supplementation on Blood Pressure of Patients with Type 2 Diabetes: A Double-Blind Randomized Clinical Controlled Trial." *Journal of Nutrition and Food Security* 3, no. 2 (2018): 70–78.

11. Hasani, Hossein, Arman Arab, Amir Hadi, et al. "Does Ginger Supplementation Lower Blood Pressure? A Systematic Review and Meta-Analysis of Clinical Trials." *Phytotherapy Research* 33, no. 6 (June 2019): 1639–1647.

12. Rahimlou, Mehran, Zahra Yari, Azita Hekmatdoost, et al. "Ginger Supplementation in Nonalcoholic Fatty Liver Disease: A Randomized, Double-Blind, Placebo-Controlled Pilot Study." *Hepatitis Monthly* 16, no. 1 (January 2016): e34897.

13. Ebrahimzadeh Attari, Vahideh, Aida Malek Mahdavi, Zeinab Javadivala, et al. "A Systematic Review of the Anti-Obesity and Weight Lowering Effect of Ginger (*Zingiber officinale* Roscoe) and Its Mechanisms of Action." *Phytotherapy Research* 32, no. 4 (April 2018): 577–585.

14. Rahnama, Parvin, Ali Montazeri, Hassan Falluh Huseini, et al. "Effect of *Zingiber officinale* R. Rhizomes (Ginger) on Pain Relief in Primary Dysmenorrhea: A Placebo Randomized Trial." *BMC Complementary & Alternative Medicine* 12 (2012): 92.

15. Giacosa, Attilio, Davide Guido, Mario Grassi, et al. "The Effect of Ginger (*Zingiber officinnalis*) and Artichoke (*Cynara cardunculus*) Extract Supplementation on Functional Dyspepsia: A Randomized, Double-Blind, and Placebo-Controlled Clinical Trial." *Evidence-Based Complementary and Alternative Medicine* 2015 (2015): Article ID: 915087.

16. van Tilburg, Miranda A. L., Olafur S. Palsson, Yehuda Ringel, and William E. Whitehead. "Is Ginger Effective for the Treatment of Irritable Bowel Syndrome? A Double Blind Randomized Controlled Pilot Trial." *Complementary Therapies in Medicine* 22 (2014): 17–20.

REFERENCES AND FURTHER READING

Annsari, Mansour, Pezhman Porouhan, Mohammad Mohammadianpanah, et al. "Efficacy of Ginger in Control of Chemotherapy-Induced Nausea and Vomiting in Breast Cancer Patients Receiving Doxorubicin-Based Chemotherapy." *Asian Pacific Journal of Cancer Prevention* 17, no. 8 (2016): 3877–3880.

Bartels, E. M., V. N. Folmer, H. Bliddal, et al. "Efficacy and Safety of Ginger in Osteoarthritis Patients: A Meta-Analysis of Randomized Placebo-Controlled Trials." *Osteoarthritis and Cartilage* 23, no. 1 (January 2015): 13–21.

Ebrahimzadeh Attari, V., A. Malek Mahdavi, Z. Javadivala, et al. "A Systematic Review of the Anti-Obesity and Weight Lowering Effect of Ginger (*Zingiber officinale* Roscoe) and Its Mechanisms of Action." *Phytotherapy Research* 32, no. 4 (April 2018): 577–585.

Giacosa, Attilio, Davide Guido, Mario Grassi, et al. "The Effect of Ginger (*Zingiber officinalis*) and Artichoke (*Cynara Cardunculus*) Extract Supplementation on Functional Dyspepsia: A Randomized, Double-Blind, and Placebo-Controlled Clinical Trial." *Evidence-Based Complementary and Alternative Medicine* 2015 (2015): Article ID: 915087.

Hasani, Hossein, Arman Arab, Amir Hadi, et al. "Does Ginger Supplementation Lower Blood Pressure? A Systematic Review and Meta-Analysis of Clinical Trials." *Phytotherapy Research* 33, no. 6 (June 2019): 1639–1647.

Rahimlou, Mehran, Zahra Yari, Azita Hekmatdoost, et al. "Ginger Supplementation in Nonalcoholic Fatty Liver Disease: A Randomized, Double-Blind, Placebo-Controlled Pilot Study." *Hepatitis Monthly* 16, no. 1 (January 2016): e34897.

Rahnama, Parvin, Ali Montazeri, Hassan Fallah Huseini, et al. "Effect of *Zingiber officinale* R. Rhizomes (Ginger) on Pain Relief in Primary Dysmenorrhea: A Placebo Randomized Trial." *BMC Complementary & Alternative Medicine* 12 (2012): 92.

Ryan, Julie L., Charles E. Heckler, Joseph A. Roscoe, et al. "Ginger (*Zingiber officinale*) Reduces Acute Chemotherapy-Induced Nausea: A URCC CCOP Study of 576 Patients." *Supportive Care in Cancer* 20, no. 7 (July 2012): 1479–1489.

Seidi, Jamal, Shahrokh Ebnerasooli, Sirous Shahsawari, and Simin Nzarian. "The Influence of Oral Ginger before Operation on Nausea and Vomiting after Cataract Surgery under General Anesthesia: A Double-Blind Placebo-Controlled Randomized Clinical Trial." *Electronic Physician* 9, no. 1 (January 2017): 3508–3514.

Soltani, E., A. Jangjoo, M. Afzal Aghaei, and A. Dalili. "Effects of Preoperative Administration of Ginger (*Zingiber officinale* Roscoe) on Postoperative Nausea and Vomiting After Laparoscopic Cholecystectomy." *Journal of Traditional and Complementary Medicine* 8, no. 3 (July 2018): 387–390.

Talaei, Behrouz, Hassan Mozaffari-Khosravi, and Shohred Bahreini. "The Effect of Ginger Powder Supplementation on Blood Pressure of Patients with Type 2 Diabetes: A Double-Blind Randomized Clinical Controlled Trial." *Journal of Nutrition and Food Security* 3, no. 2 (2018): 70–78.

Thomson, Maggie, Renee Corbin, and Lawrence Leung. "Effect of Ginger for Nausea and Vomiting in Early Pregnancy: A Meta-Analysis." *Journal of the American Board of Family Medicine* 27, no. 1 (2014): 115–122.

Tóth, Barbara, Tamás Lantos, Péter Hegyi, et al. "Ginger (*Zingiber officinale*): An Alternative for the Prevention of Postoperative Nausea and Vomiting. A Meta-Analysis." *Phytomedicine* 50 (November 15, 2018): 8–18.

van Tilburg, Miranda A. L., Olafur S. Palsson, Yehuda Ringel, and William E. Whitehead. "Is Ginger Effective for the Treatment of Irritable Bowel Syndrome? A Double Blind Randomized Controlled Pilot Trial." *Complementary Therapies in Medicine* 22 (2014): 17–20.

Viljoen, Estelle, Janicke Visser, Nelene Koen, and Alfred Musekiwa. "A Systematic Review and Meta-Analysis of the Effect and Safety of Ginger in the Treatment of Pregnancy-Associated Nausea and Vomiting." *Nutrition Journal* 13 (2014): 20.

Zeraati, Hossein, Javad Shahinfar, Shiva Imani Hesari, et al. "The Effect of Ginger Extract on the Incidence and Severity of Nausea and Vomiting After Cesarean Section under Spinal Anesthesia." *Anesthesiology and Pain Medicine* 6, no. 5 (October 2016): e38943.

Ginkgo Biloba

Ginkgo biloba, also known as gingko, is a very popular supplement believed to be useful for a wide variety of medical concerns. Gingko biloba contains high levels of flavonoids, antioxidants that provide protection against oxidative cell damage from free radicals, and terpenoids, which help improve circulation by dilating blood vessels and reduce the stickiness of platelets.

Ginkgo biloba extract is prepared from the dried green leaves of the maidenhair tree, one of the oldest species of trees in the world. These trees may grow to more than 130 ft. tall, and some are more than a thousand years old. Although the trees are native to China, Japan, and Korea, they have been grown in Europe since around 1730 and in the United States since around 1784.

Ginkgo biloba was first used for its medicinal properties in ancient China when it was thought to support cognition and alleviate the symptoms of asthma. Other traditional uses include bladder irritation, intestinal worms, bedwetting, and gonorrhea. Of course, in most of these instances, these uses are not supported by scientific studies.

HEALTH BENEFITS AND RISKS

Ginkgo biloba is said to heal blood disorders and improve cardiovascular function and blood flow. In addition, it is believed to enhance memory, cognitive function, and eye health. Some contend that people with dementia may benefit from ginkgo biloba supplementation. When used in moderate amounts, ginkgo biloba appears to be safe for healthy adults.

While ginkgo biloba may relieve anxiety, people on the prescription medication Xanax should not use the supplement as it may reduce the effectiveness of this drug. When combined with ibuprofen, ginkgo biloba may increase the risk of bleeding. People taking selective serotonin reuptake inhibitors should not consume ginkgo, which may reduce the usefulness of the medications. This is also true for those on certain statin medications, such as simvastatin (Zocor). People allergic to poison ivy and other plants with alkylphenols must also avoid this supplement. As there is some concern that ginkgo biloba may increase the risk of seizures, people who have ever had a seizure should not use ginkgo. It is important to stop taking this supplement at least 2 weeks before surgery. Potential side effects of ginkgo biloba include nausea, vomiting, heart palpitations, dizziness, constipation, diarrhea, allergic skin reactions, and headaches.

HOW IT IS SOLD AND TAKEN

Ginkgo biloba is sold in capsules, tablets, liquid extracts, and dried leaves for teas. Recommended doses vary widely. Studies show that adults generally use between 120 and 240 mg per day in divided doses. It may be 4 to 6 weeks of supplementation before any changes are observed. Pregnant and breastfeeding women, people with epilepsy, and those on blood-thinning medications should not use gingko biloba. Very little is known about the safety of gingko biloba in children. Before administering gingko biloba to a child, connect with a knowledgeable healthcare provider. People who are diabetic should not use the supplement without checking with a medical provider; people who are diabetic who take ginseng must be carefully monitored. Never eat raw or roasted ginkgo seeds as they may be poisonous.

RESEARCH FINDINGS

Ginkgo Biloba May Help People with Type 2 Diabetes Who Are Not Responding Well to the Medication Metformin

In a randomized, double-blind, placebo-controlled trial published in 2018 in the journal *Drug Design, Development and Theory*, researchers from Iraq and Malaysia evaluated the ability of ginkgo biloba to help people with type 2 diabetes who are not responding well to metformin, a common medication for this illness. Metformin alone was unable to control their glycemic status. The researchers recruited 60 patients with type 2 diabetes who were on metformin aged 25 to 65 years. For 90 days, they were placed on ginkgo biloba extract (120 mg/day) or a starch placebo. Each group initially had 30 patients. Twenty-seven patients from the treatment group and 20 patients from the placebo group completed the entire trial and were included in the final analysis. Assessments of type 2 diabetes factors, including hemoglobin A1C (HA1C), fasting glucose, insulin, waist circumference, and visceral adiposity index were made at baseline and at the end of the trial. The researchers determined that ginkgo biloba significantly reduced HA1c, fasting glucose, insulin, and waist circumference. Moreover, it reduced body mass index after 90 days. The researchers commented that their findings confirm "the beneficial role" of ginkgo biloba supplementation for people with type 2 diabetes.[1]

Ginkgo Biloba May Help People Who Suffered an Ischemic Stroke

In a multicenter, prospective, randomized, open-label, blinded, controlled clinical trial published in 2017 in the journal *Stroke and Vascular Neurology*, researchers from several locations in China investigated the ability of ginkgo biloba to help people who have suffered an ischemic stroke. The cohort consisted of 348 people who had experienced an ischemic stroke within the past week. They were enrolled between October 2012 and June 2014. The patients were assigned to one of two groups: 179 patients in the first group consumed 450 mg per day of ginkgo biloba extract and 100 mg aspirin per day; and the 169 patients in the control group consumed only aspirin. The interventions continued for 6 months after the stroke onset. At various points, the researchers conducted neurological and cognitive assessments. Eighteen patients were lost to follow-up. The researchers learned that the combination of ginkgo biloba and aspirin relieved cognitive and neurological deficits without increasing the incidence of vascular events. They concluded that those patients "manifested better memory function, executive functions, neurological function and daily life." Moreover, they did not have a higher incidence of adverse effects.[2]

Ginkgo Biloba May Have Some Benefits for People with Angina Pectoris

In a systematic review published in 2015 in the *Chinese Journal of Integrative Medicine*, researchers from China wanted to learn if ginkgo biloba would be useful for angina pectoris, or the short-lasting squeezing pains in the chest that radiate beyond the area. The researchers located 23 randomly controlled trials that included 2529 male and female patients of varying ages and ethnic origins. The average age of the participants ranged from 38 to 81 years, with mostly male participants. The average sample size was 110 patients. The ginkgo biloba supplements were taken alone or in combination with routine western medicine. There were also control groups and the use of placebos and Chinese patent medicine. All treatments continued for at least 1 month. Six trials reported adverse effects, however, no side effects were severe. The researchers determined that compared to the angina relief obtained from the supplement alone, the combination of the supplement and western medicine was more effective. The researchers commented that "ginkgo biloba extract may have beneficial effects on patients with angina pectoris, although the low quality of existing trials makes it difficult to draw a satisfactory conclusion."[3]

Ginkgo Biloba May or May Not Be Useful for Age-Related Macular Degeneration

In an analysis published in 2013 in the *Cochrane Database of Systematic Reviews*, a researcher from London, United Kingdom evaluated the ability of ginkgo biloba to limit the progression of age-related macular degeneration, a medical problem in which people lose central vision. Unfortunately, the researcher was only able to locate two randomized trials that included a total of 119 participants. In one trial, conducted in France, 20 participants were placed on either the ginkgo biloba extract known as EGb761 at a dose of 80 mg twice daily or a placebo. In the other trial, conducted in Germany, 99 participants were placed on two different doses of ginkgo biloba extract EGb761, at 240 mg per day or 60 mg per day. Both trials were conducted for 6 months. The researcher found some positive effects of ginkgo biloba on vision, however, the findings did not offer any definitive conclusions. According to the researchers, "future trials should be larger and longer."[4]

Ginkgo Biloba May Not Be Useful for Primary Hypertension

In a systematic review published in 2014 in the journal *Phytomedicine*, researchers from China, Canada, and Massachusetts (USA) wanted to learn if ginkgo biloba would be useful for people dealing with primary hypertension. The researchers identified a total of nine randomly controlled trials with 1012 people with hypertension (high blood pressure). The amounts of supplements varied, and the duration of treatments ranged from 8 weeks to 6 months. Interventions in all the trials included ginkgo biloba and antihypertensive medications. Controls included the use of only the antihypertensive drugs. However, the trials had a high risk of bias and a flawed study design. In addition, the quality of the methodology tended to be poor. Still, six of the trials found that ginkgo biloba was potentially useful for blood pressure reduction. The researchers concluded that there was "no convincing evidence to support the routine use" of ginkgo biloba for primary hypertension."[5]

Ginkgo Biloba May Help Children with Attention Deficit Hyperactivity Disorder (ADHD)

In a randomized, double-blind, placebo-controlled clinical trial published in 2015 in the journal *Complementary Therapies in Clinical Practice*, researchers from Iran evaluated the efficacy of using ginkgo biloba as a complementary therapy for ADHD. The research was conducted between September and December 2014; the researchers initially included 66 children between the ages of 6 and 12 years. All children were taking the prescription medication methylphenidate (such as Ritalin®) used to treat ADHD. For 6 weeks, half of the children were placed on 80–120 mg per day of ginkgo biloba and half were placed on a placebo. Six children dropped out after starting the trial. Interestingly, the children in both groups reported side effects such as nausea, headache, and diarrhea. Still, the children taking the supplement had significant improvements in their ADHD symptoms. The researchers concluded that ginkgo biloba "is an effective complementary treatment for ADHD."[6]

Ginkgo Biloba Appears to Have Antianxiety Properties

In a trial published in 2007 in the *Journal of Psychiatric Research*, researchers from Germany investigated the antianxiety properties of ginkgo biloba extract EGb761. The initial cohort consisted of 109 participants with generalized anxiety disorder or adjustment disorder with anxious mood. For 4 weeks, they were randomized to consume a daily dose of 480 mg EGb761, 240 mg EGb761, or a placebo. Using a standard rating scale for anxiety, anxiety assessments were quantified. The researchers learned that the subjects in both treatment groups had significantly better results than those in the placebo group. In all the outcome measures, the higher-dose group had more improvement than the lower-dose group. These findings were corroborated by the self-ratings of the participants. The researchers concluded that their extract had "a specific anxiolytic effect that was dose-dependent and significantly exceeded the placebo effect commonly seen in trials of psychoactive drugs."[7]

Ginkgo Biloba May Not Be Useful in Preventing Later-in-Life Dementia

In a systematic review and meta-analysis published in 2015 in the *Journal of the Medical Association of Thailand*, researchers from Thailand examined the ability of ginkgo biloba to lower the risk of later-in-life dementia. The cohort consisted of two trials with a total of 5889 participants, with mean ages in the mid-to-late 70s. Both trials compared ginkgo biloba extract to placebo in a multicenter, double-blind, parallel, and randomized controlled trial. The trials continued for 5 and 6 years using the same 240 mg/day treatment dose. Both trials had a low risk of bias. The researchers learned that the participants in the intervention and placebo groups had similar rates of dementia. While the supplement appeared to be safe for elders, it did not prevent the onset of this debilitating illness. The researchers concluded that "there is no convincing evidence from this review that demonstrated Ginkgo biloba in late-life can prevent the development of dementia."[8]

Ginkgo Biloba May Be Useful as a Treatment for Cognitive Impairment and Dementia

In a systematic review and meta-analysis published in 2015 in the *Journal of Alzheimer's Disease*, researchers from China and San Francisco, California (USA), analyzed the use of ginkgo biloba extract EGb761 for the treatment of cognitive impairment and dementia. The cohort consisted of nine randomized, double-blind, parallel-group, placebo-controlled trials with a total of 2561 patients; the trials lasted 22–26 weeks. Only two of the studies were conducted in the United States. The researchers found that the supplement stabilized or slowed the decline in cognition, function, behavior, and global change of patients with cognitive impairment or dementia. The clinical benefits were primarily seen in patients taking the 240 mg per day dose; the most notable improvements were seen in patients with neuropsychiatric symptoms. The researchers concluded that the "safety and tolerability" of the supplement was "excellent."[9]

In another systematic review and meta-analysis published in 2016 in the journal *Current Topics in Medicinal Chemistry*, researchers from China evaluated the ability of ginkgo biloba to treat mild cognitive impairment and Alzheimer's disease. The cohort consisted of 21 randomized, clinical trials with 2608 patients; nine trials addressed mild cognitive impairment and 12 trials included patients suffering from Alzheimer's disease. The duration of treatments ranged from 2 to 52 weeks, and the doses ranged from 60 to 450 mg per day. Eight of the trials were in English, while 13 were in Chinese. The researchers noted that the methodology quality of the trials was "moderate to poor." They learned that ginkgo biloba "had potential benefits in improving cognitive function, activities of daily living, and global critical assessment" for people with mild cognitive impairment and Alzheimer's disease. Still, the researchers cautioned that they were unable to offer "confirmative conclusions." The sample size was too small, the findings were sometimes inconsistent, and the methodological procedures were too often below expectations.[10]

Ginkgo Biloba Does Not Appear to Be Useful for Intermittent Claudication

In an analysis published in 2013 in the *Cochrane Database of Systematic Reviews*, researchers based in the Netherlands wanted to learn if ginkgo biloba would be useful for intermittent claudication, or pain in the legs caused by too little blood flow. The researchers located 14 relevant randomized trials with 739 participants. Eleven of the trials, with 477 participants, compared ginkgo biloba with a placebo and assessed the absolute claudication distance or the distance walked before the onset of claudication pain. The researchers found that the supplement did not appear to have any significant impact on intermittent claudication. They concluded that "overall, there is no evidence that Ginkgo biloba has a clinically significant benefit for patients with peripheral arterial disease."[11]

NOTES

1. Aziz, T. A., S. A. Hussain, T. O. Mahwi, et al. "The Efficacy and Safety of *Ginkgo biloba* Extract as an Adjuvant in Type 2 Diabetes Mellitus Patients Ineffectively Managed with Metformin: A Double-Blind, Randomized, Placebo-Controlled Trial." *Drug Design, Development and Therapy* 12 (April 5, 2018): 735–742.

2. Li, S., X. Zhang, Q. Fang, et al. "Ginkgo Biloba Extract Improved Cognition and Neurological Functions of Acute Ischaemic Stroke: A Randomised Controlled Trial." *Stroke and Vascular Neurology* 2, no. 4 (December 2017): 189–197.

3. Sun, T., X. Wang, and H. Xu. "Ginkgo Biloba Extract for Angina Pectoris: A Systematic Review." *Chinese Journal of Integrative Medicine* 21, no. 7 (July 2015): 542–550.

4. Evans, J. K. "Ginkgo Biloba Extract for Age-Related Macular Degeneration." *Cochrane Database of Systematic Reviews* 1 (January 31, 2013): CD001775.

5. Xiong, X. J., W. Liu, X. C. Yang, et al. "Ginkgo Biloba Extract for Essential Hypertension: A Systematic Review." *Phytomedicine* 21, no. 10 (September 15, 2014): 1131–1136.

6. Shakibaei, F., M. Radmanesh, E. Salari, and B. Mahakil. "Ginkgo Biloba in the Treatment of Attention-Deficit/Hyperactivity Disorder in Children and Adolescents. A Randomized, Placebo-Controlled, Trial." *Complementary Therapies in Clinical Practice* 21, no. 2 (May 2015): 61–67.

7. Woelk, H., K. H. Arnoldt, M. Kieser, and R. Hoerr. "Ginkgo Biloba Special Extract EGb 761 in Generalized Anxiety Disorder and Adjustment Disorder with Anxious Mood: A Randomized, Double-Blind, Placebo-Controlled Trial." *Journal of Psychiatric Research* 41 (2007): 472–480.

8. Charemboon, T., and K. Jaisin. "Ginkgo Biloba for Prevention of Dementia: A Systematic Review and Meta-Analysis." *Journal of the Medical Association of Thailand* 98, no. 5 (May 2015): 508–513.

9. Tan, M. S., J. T. Yu, C. C. Tan, et al. "Efficacy and Adverse Effects of Ginkgo Biloba for Cognitive Impairment and Dementia: A Systematic Review and Meta-Analysis." *Journal of Alzheimer's Disease* 43, no. 2 (2015): 589–603.

10. Yang, G., Y. Wang, J. Sun, et al. "Ginkgo Biloba for Mild Cognitive Impairment and Alzheimer's Disease: A Systematic Review and Meta-Analysis of Randomized Controlled Trials." *Current Topics in Medicinal Chemistry* 16, no. 5 (2016): 520–528.

11. Nicolaï, S. P., L. M. Kruidenier, B. L. Bendermacher, et al. "Ginkgo Biloba for Intermittent Claudication." *Cochrane Database of Systematic Reviews* 6 (June 6, 2013): CD006888.

REFERENCES AND FURTHER READING

Aziz, T. A., S. A. Hussain, T. O. Mahwi, et al. "The Efficacy and Safety of *Ginkgo Biloba* Extract as an Adjuvant in Type 2 Diabetes Mellitus Patients Ineffectively Managed with Metformin: A Double-Blind, Randomized, Placebo-Controlled Trial." *Drug Design, Development and Therapy* 12 (April 5, 2018): 735–742.

Charemboon, T., and K. Jaisin. "Ginkgo Biloba for Prevention of Dementia: A Systematic Review and Meta-Analysis." *Journal of the Medical Association of Thailand* 98, no. 5 (May 2015): 508–513.

Evans, J. R. "Ginkgo Biloba Extract for Age-Related Macular Degeneration." *Cochrane Database of Systematic Reviews* 1 (January 31, 2013): CD001775.

Li, S., X. Zhang, Q. Fang, et al. "Ginkgo Biloba Extract Improved Cognition and Neurological Functions of Acute Ischaemic Stroke: A Randomised Controlled Trial." *Stroke and Vascular Neurology* 2, no. 4 (December 18, 2017): 189–197.

Nicolaï, S. P., L. M. Kruidenier, B. L. Bendermacher, et al. "Ginkgo Biloba for Intermittent Claudication." *Cochrane Database of Systematic Reviews* 6 (June 6, 2013): CD006888.

Shakibaei, F., M. Radmanesh, E. Salari, and B. Mahaki. "Ginkgo Biloba in the Treatment of Attention-Deficit/Hyperactivity Disorder in Children and Adolescents: A Randomized, Placebo-Controlled Trial." *Complementary Therapies in Clinical Practice* 21, no. 2 (May 2015): 61–67.

Sun, T., X. Wang, and H. Xu. "Ginkgo Biloba Extract for Angina Pectoris: A Systematic Review." *Chinese Journal of Integrative Medicine* 21, no. 7 (July 2015): 542–550.

Tan, M. S., J. T. Yu, C. C. Tan, et al. "Efficacy and Adverse Effects of Ginkgo Biloba for Cognitive Impairment and Dementia: A Systematic Review and Meta-Analysis." *Journal of Alzheimer's Disease* 34, no. 2 (2015) 589–603.

Woelk, H., K. H. Arnoldt, M. Kieser, and R. Hoerr. "Ginkgo Biloba Special Extract EGb 761 in Generalized Anxiety Disorder and Adjustment Disorder with Anxious Mood: A Randomized, Double-Blind, Placebo-Controlled Trial." *Journal of Psychiatric Research* 41 (2007): 472–480.

Xiong, X. J., W. Liu, X. C. Yang, et al. "Ginkgo Biloba Extract for Essential Hypertension: A Systematic Review." *Phytomedicine* 21, no. 10 (September 15, 2014): 1131–1136.

Yang, G., Y. Wang, J. Sun, et al. "Ginkgo Biloba for Mild Cognitive Impairment and Alzheimer's Disease: A Systematic Review and Meta-Analysis of Randomized Controlled Trials." *Current Topics in Medicinal Chemistry* 16, no. 5 (2016): 520–528.

Ginseng

Ginseng is a herbaceous plant belonging to the genus *Panax*; panax means all healing, panacea, or, in Greek, "cure-all." Its use may be traced to ancient times, especially in China and Korea. Initially, ginseng was reserved only for royalty.

The root is considered the most important medicinal part of the plant. Typically, the root is dried, white ginseng, or is steamed, red ginseng. It may also be extracted as a concentrate. The leaves and berries are also used. Ginsenosides found in ginseng are thought to be responsible for the clinical effects of the herb; more than 20 ginsenosides have been identified to date.

Chinese ginseng (*Panax ginseng*) and American ginseng (*Panax quinquefolius*) are the two types of ginseng most commonly used. Chinese ginseng has been used in traditional Chinese medicine for thousands of years. American ginseng was first used by Native Americans.

HEALTH BENEFITS AND RISKS

Believed to have healing properties, ginseng is thought to reduce inflammation, fatigue, and menopausal symptoms; improve immunity, mood, and athletic performance; lower blood sugar levels; reduce stress; kill cancer cells; improve memory; lower the risk of obesity; lower blood pressure; and prevent heart disease. People use ginseng to treat nerve pain, respiratory tract infections, fever, attention deficit hyperactivity disorder, bleeding disorders, memory loss, and rheumatoid arthritis. In addition, ginseng is considered an antioxidant, antidiabetic, antimicrobial, and protector of the nervous system. Some even contend that ginseng is good for sexual dysfunction in men. In summary, people seem to use ginseng for wide-ranging, seemingly endless number of reasons.

Side effects associated with ginseng tend to be minor including gastric upset, insomnia, constipation, changes in blood sugar and blood pressure, irritability, blurred vision, skin reactions, edema, diarrhea, bleeding, dizziness, dry mouth, decreased heart rates, and headache. Women who use ginseng regularly may experience swollen breasts and vaginal bleeding. Higher doses of ginseng should be avoided. Until more relevant research becomes available, children, pregnant and breastfeeding women should avoid ginseng.

Ginseng may alter the effects of medication for blood pressure, diabetes, and heart problems. People on these medications should check with their medical provider before consuming ginseng. Likewise, ginseng may increase the risk of bleeding among those on blood thinners, intensify the effects of caffeine and other stimulants, and cancel out the painkilling effects of morphine. Ginseng should not be mixed with a class of antidepressants known as monoamine oxidase inhibitors as it can cause manic episodes and tremors.

To avoid the side effects of ginseng, it may be advisable to consume the supplement for relatively short periods of time. Periodic breaks from ginseng seem to be a good idea.

HOW IT IS SOLD AND TAKEN

As anticipated, the hugely popular ginseng is sold in various forms including capsules, tea, and liquid extract, as well as fresh, root slices, and combined in a complex supplement.

Ginseng products may vary markedly in their quality and medicinal properties. Check the label for ingredients, and try to purchase ginseng from a reliable company. Because ginseng tends to be costly, some manufacturers may market a poorer quality product for a lower price.

Dose recommendations vary widely. It is important to read the instructions on the label. Doses of 100 to 3000 mg per day have been used safely for up to 12 weeks.

RESEARCH FINDINGS

Ginseng May Be Useful for Fatigue Related to Chronic Illness

In a systematic review published in 2018 in the *Journal of Alternative and Complementary Medicine*, researchers from Arizona and Oregon (USA) noted that millions of people with chronic illness suffer from fatigue. Many people with fatigue report using ginseng and other herbal preparations. Therefore, the researchers wanted to evaluate the efficacy and safety of ginseng. The cohort included ten trials, with four using American ginseng and six using Asian ginseng. The trials varied considerably in doses and study durations. For example, in the American ginseng trials, sample sizes ranged from 56 to 364. Three studies included mostly white women, whereas one study had mostly male participants. Meanwhile, in the Asian ginseng studies, daily doses ranged from 80 to 2000 mg of ginseng, and study durations ranged from 4 weeks to 3 months. Most trials were double-blind, randomized, and controlled. In general, compared to the placebo groups, the intervention groups found that ginseng improved fatigue. The researchers concluded that "both American and Asian ginseng may be viable treatments for fatigue in people with chronic illness because of the low risk associated with its use, coupled with modest evidence for efficacy."[1]

Ginseng May Be Useful for People Experiencing Cancer-Related Fatigue

In a multisite, double-blind, randomized trial published in 2013 in the *Journal of the National Cancer Institute*, researchers from Minnesota, Kansas, Washington,

South Carolina, Michigan, and North Dakota (USA) wanted to learn if ginseng supplementation would be useful for the fatigue often experienced by cancer patients. The researchers enrolled 364 participants from 40 institutions, most of which were community cancer centers. All participants had experienced cancer-related fatigue for at least 1 month. The participants could still be receiving treatment, or they could have completed their current course of treatment. For 8 weeks, they were placed on either 2000 mg of American ginseng per day or a placebo. The participants were evaluated after 4 weeks and again after 8 weeks. Seventy-eight percent of the participants completed the entire trial. At baseline, there were no statistically significant differences in fatigue measures between the two groups. After 4 and 8 weeks, the participants undergoing cancer treatment and consuming ginseng had statistically significant improvements in fatigue levels. The researchers concluded that cancer patients may wish to try ginseng for fatigue, "taking into consideration that there are no other pharmacologic agents known to be effective."[2]

In a prospective, open-label study published in 2015 in the journal *Integrative Cancer Therapies*, researchers from Houston, Texas (USA), recruited 30 patients undergoing outpatient chemotherapy at a cancer center who were experiencing cancer-related fatigue. The patients were instructed to take a daily high dose (800 mg) of Asian ginseng for 29 days. Assessments were conducted at baseline, at 15 days, and at the end of the trial. Of the 30 patients enrolled, 24 were evaluated. Their mean age was 58 years and half of the participants were female. No severe adverse effects were reported. Of the 24 patients evaluated, 21 reported improvements in fatigue. The researchers concluded that Asian ginseng is safe and improves cancer-related fatigue "as well as overall quality of life, appetite, and sleep at night."[3]

Ginseng May Not Be as Useful for Fatigue in Patients with Advanced Cancer

In a randomized, double-blind, placebo-controlled trial published in 2017 in the *Journal of the National Comprehensive Cancer Network*, researchers from Houston, Texas (USA), and South Korea wanted to determine if ginseng would alleviate fatigue in people with advanced cancer. The initial cohort consisted of 127 patients. For 28 days, they consumed 400 mg of Chinese ginseng twice each day or a matching placebo. The researchers analyzed the results of 112 patients (56 in the intervention group and 56 in the placebo group). Although they had hypothesized that the patients in the supplementation group would experience reductions in fatigue, the researchers found no significant differences between the two groups. Interestingly, the patients in both groups improved. No benefits were obtained from the ginseng. As a result of these findings, the researchers concluded that "they could not recommend Chinese ginseng to relieve fatigue in patients with advanced cancer."[4]

Ginseng Improves Exercise Performance

In a randomized, double-blind, placebo-controlled clinical trial published in 2018 in the *Journal of Ginseng Research*, researchers from South Korea wanted to learn more about the ability of ginsenoside complex (UG0712) to act as an ergo-genic agent, a substance that enhances physical performance. The cohort included 117 people who tended to live sedentary lives; they were divided into one of three groups. For 12 weeks, the members of one group consumed low-dose ginsenoside supplementation (100 mg per day); the members of a second group consumed high-dose ginsenoside supplementation (500 mg per day); and the members of a third group consumed a placebo. Each of the groups included 39 participants. The supplementations were identical in color, shape, and taste. All of the participants took part in a supervised 12-week aerobic and resistance exercise training course at a sports center located in a university hospital. The exercise intervention con-sisted of programmed exercise for 60 min three times per week. Eighty-one par-ticipants completed all aspects of the trial and were included in the final analysis. Of these, 30 were in the high-dose group, 27 in the low-dose group, and 24 in the placebo group. The researchers learned that the participants on high-dose supplementation had better increases in maximal oxygen consumption. The researchers concluded that their findings "showed that high doses of ginseng sup-plementation could enhance aerobic capacity during exercise training." Moreover, because most comparable studies have been done on athletes, "the improvement of aerobic capacity by ginseng for sedentary people is more representative of the general population."[5]

Ginseng Appears to Improve Fasting Blood Glucose in People with and without Diabetes

In a systematic review and meta-analysis published in 2014 in the online jour-nal *PLoS ONE*, researchers from several locations in Canada noted that there is widespread use of ginseng among people with diabetes. Yet, there is little evi-dence supporting its antihyperglycemic properties. Therefore, they decided to investigate the use of ginseng among people with and without diabetes. They included only randomly controlled trials that lasted 30 days or longer. Nine trials had 339 participants with diabetes, and 7 trials had 431 participants without diabe-tes. The median age of the participants was 51 years. All but one of the trials were conducted in outpatient settings, and most trials included interventions that lasted for less than 12 weeks. Half of the trials were conducted in Asia, with the others conducted in North America or Europe. Eleven of the trials were found to be of high quality. The researchers learned that ginseng supplementation modestly, but significantly, lowered fasting blood glucose in people with or without diabetes. The researchers underscored the need for "larger and longer randomized con-trolled trials using standardized ginseng preparations."[6]

American Ginseng May Improve Arterial Stiffness in People with Type 2 Diabetes Who Have High Blood Pressure

In a double-blind, placebo-controlled, parallel design trial published in 2013 in the *Journal of Ethnopharmacology*, researchers from Croatia wanted to learn if people with type 2 diabetes and high blood pressure would benefit from American ginseng supplementation. The cohort consisted of 64 people with well-controlled type 2 diabetes and essential hypertension; for 12 weeks, 30 participants were assigned to a daily intake of 3 g of American ginseng, and 34 participants consumed placebos. Throughout the intervention, the participants were seen at the clinic every 6 weeks. Vascular assessments were performed at baseline and after 12 weeks. The researchers learned that the ginseng significantly lowered the levels of arterial stiffness (thickening and stiffening of arterial walls) and systolic blood pressure. No observable changes were seen in diastolic blood pressure. The researchers noted that there is a need for "further investigation" of this association.[7]

Ginseng Appears to Have No Cardiovascular Benefit for People with Metabolic Syndrome

In a randomized, double-blind, placebo-controlled, single-center trial published in 2012 in the *Korean Journal of Family Medicine*, researchers from South Korea investigated the association between Korean red ginseng and metabolic parameters, inflammatory markers, and arterial stiffness in participants suffering from metabolic syndrome. The researchers recruited 60 participants with metabolic syndrome who were over the age of 20 years. For 12 weeks, they took either 4.5 g per day of Korean red ginseng or a placebo. During the trial, the researchers assessed several different medical issues. Forty-eight participants completed the trial. The researchers concluded that Korean red ginseng supplementation did not significantly affect any of the metabolic syndrome factors that they tested. They noted that "these findings warrant subsequent longer-term prospective clinical investigations with a larger population."[8]

Ginseng Does Not Appear to Help Most Menopausal Symptoms

In a systematic review published in 2016 in the journal *Medicine*, researchers from South Korea and the United Kingdom evaluated the ability of ginseng to help alleviate menopausal symptoms. The researchers located ten randomly controlled trials that met their criteria, eight of which were from Korea. In these trials, the doses of ginseng ranged from 200 to 3000 mg per day, and the treatments continued for 2 to 16 weeks. The researchers determined that there was some evidence that ginseng was useful for sexual function and arousal in menopausal women. However, the findings failed to show any indication that ginseng was effective for vasomotor symptoms, hormones, biomarkers, and endometrial thickness. They concluded that "the level of evidence for these findings was low because of unclear risk of bias."[9]

Korean Red Ginseng Did Not Improve Insulin Sensitivity in Healthy But Overweight or Obese People

In a double-blind, placebo-controlled, randomized trial published in 2013 in the *Asia Pacific Journal of Clinical Nutrition*, researchers from South Korea wanted to learn if Korean red ginseng would improve the insulin sensitivity of healthy overweight or obese men and women who did not have diabetes or hypertension. The researchers enrolled 68 overweight or obese participants; about one-quarter of the subjects were overweight and three-quarters were obese. For 12 weeks, they either consumed 6 g per day of Korean red ginseng or a similar looking placebo. Each participant was told to visit the clinic after 1, 4, and 12 weeks; blood samples were administered at baseline and at 12 weeks. At baseline, both groups had similar insulin sensitivity levels; during the course of the trial, ginseng did not significantly improve insulin sensitivity levels. The researchers concluded that Korean red ginseng "does not improve insulin sensitivity in overweight and obese adults who do not have diabetes or hypertension."[10]

Ginseng May Help Lower Fasting Glucose Levels

In a single-center, randomized, double-blind, placebo-controlled clinical trial published in 2018 in the *Journal of Ginseng Research*, researchers from South Korea examined the ability of ginseng to improve glycemic control in people with fasting glucose levels between 100 mg/dL and 140 mg/dL. The cohort consisted of 72 participants, who had the required levels of fasting glucose and were between the ages of 20 and 75 years. For 12 weeks, they consumed either ginseng berry extract at a dose of 1 g per day or a placebo, which was identical in appearance and flavor. Sixty-three participants completed the trial; there were 29 participants in the ginseng group and 34 in the placebo group. Trial data were collected during individual interviews, and various assessments were conducted. By the end of the trial, the researchers learned that ginseng berry extract significantly reduced serum concentrations of fasting glucose in people with fasting glucose levels of 110 mg/dL or higher. The participants in the placebo group did not exhibit a statistically significant reduction. In addition, the trial demonstrated "that there was no safety concern with the long-term consumption of ginseng berry extract."[11]

Ginseng May or May Not Improve Cognition

In an analysis published in 2010 in the *Cochrane Database for Systematic Reviews*, researchers from China evaluated studies on the efficacy and safety of ginseng when used to improve cognition. The cohort consisted of nine randomized, double-blind, placebo-controlled trials that met the inclusion criteria of the researchers. Eight of the trials enrolled healthy participants, while one included participants with age-related memory impairment. The trials varied in outcome measures, trial duration, and ginseng dosage. All the trials had relatively small sample sizes. The researchers found some evidence that ginseng may improve aspects of cognitive function, behavior, and quality of life; no serious adverse effects were associated with ginseng. Still, they failed to locate convincing evidence demonstrating that ginseng has cognitive enhancing effects in healthy participants and "no high quality evidence" that it is useful for people with dementia. The researchers concluded that "given the potential efficacy of ginseng suggested by laboratory studies," there is a need for better designed trials "on this important issue."[12]

NOTES

1. Arring, N. M., D. Millstine, L. A. Marks, and L. M. Nail. "Ginseng as a Treatment for Fatigue: A Systematic Review." *Journal of Alternative and Complementary Medicine* 24, no. 7 (July 2018): 624–683.

2. Barton, Debra L., Heshan Liu, Shaker R. Dakhil, et al. "Wisconsin Ginseng (*Panax quinquefolius*) to Improve Cancer-Related Fatigue: A Randomized, Double-Blind Trial, N07C2." *Journal of the National Cancer Institute* 105, no. 16 (August 21, 2013): 1230–1238.

3. Yennurajalingam, S., A. Reddy, N. M. Tannir, et al. "High-Dose Asian Ginseng (*Panax Ginseng*) for Cancer-Related Fatigue: A Preliminary Report." *Integrative Cancer Therapies* 14, no. 5 (September 2015): 419–427.

4. Yennurajalingam, S., N. M. Tannir, J. L. Williams, et al. "A Double-Blind, Randomized, Placebo-Controlled Trial of *Panax Ginseng* for Cancer-Related Fatigue in Patients with Advanced Cancer." *Journal of the National Comprehensive Cancer Network* 15, no. 9 (September 2017): 1111–1120.

5. Lee, E. S., Y. J. Yang, J. H. Lee, and Y. S. Yoon. "Effect of High-Dose Ginsenoside Complex (UG0712) Supplementation on Physical Performance of Healthy Adults during a 12-Week Supervised Exercise Program: A Randomized Placebo-Controlled Clinical Trial." *Journal of Ginseng Research* 42, no. 2 (April 2018): 192–198.

6. Shistar, E., J. L. Sievenpiper, V. Djedovic, et al. "The Effect of Ginseng (The Genus *Panax*) on Glycemic Control: A Systematic Review and Meta-Analysis of Randomized Controlled Clinical Trials." *PLoS ONE* 9, no. 9 (2014): e107391.

7. Mucalo, I., E. Jovanovski, D. D. Rahelić, et al. "Effect of American Ginseng (*Panax quinquefolius* L.) on Arterial Stiffness in Subject with Type-2 Diabetes and Concomitant Hypertension." *Journal of Ethnopharmacology* 150, no. 1 (October 28, 2013): 148–153.

8. Park, Byoung-Jin, Yong-Jae Lee, Hye-Ree Lee, et al. "Effects of Korean Red Ginseng on Cardiovascular Risks in Subjects with Metabolic Syndrome: A Double-Blind Randomized Controlled Study." *Korean Journal of Family Medicine* 33, no. 4 (2012): 190–196.

9. Lee, H. W., J. Choi, Y. Lee, et al. "Ginseng for Managing Menopausal Women's Health: A Systematic Review of Double-Blind, Randomized, Placebo-Controlled Trials." *Medicine* 95, no. 38 (September 2016): e4914.

10. Cho, Y. H., S. C. Ahn, S. Y. Lee, et al. "Effect of Korean Red Ginseng on Insulin Sensitivity in Non-Diabetic Healthy Overweight and Obese Adults." *Asia Pacific Journal of Clinical Nutrition* 22, no. 3 (2013): 365–371.

11. Choi, Han Seok, Sunmi Kim, Min Jung Kim, et al. "Efficacy and Safety of *Panax Ginseng* Extract on Glycemic Control: A 12-Week Randomized, Double-Blind, and Placebo-Controlled Clinical Trial." *Journal of Ginseng Research* 42 (2018): 90–97.

12. Geng, J., J. Dong, H. Ni, M. S. Lee, et al. "Ginseng for Cognition." *Cochrane Database for Systematic Reviews* 12 (December 8, 2010): CD007769.

REFERENCES AND FURTHER READING

Arring, N, M., D. Millstine, L. A. Marks, and L. M. Nail. "Ginseng and Treatment for Fatigue: A Systematic Review." *Journal of Alternative and Complementary Medicine* 24, no. 7 (July 2018): 624–633.

Barton, Debra L., Heshan Liu, Shaker R. Dakhil, et al. "Wisconsin Ginseng (*Panax quinquefolius*) to Improve Cancer-Related Fatigue: A Randomized, Double-Blind

Trial, N07C2." *Journal of the National Cancer Institute* 105, no. 16 (August 21, 2013): 1230–1238.

Cho, Y. H., S. C. Ahn, S. Y. Lee, et al. "Effect of Korean Red Ginseng on Insulin Sensitivity in Non-Diabetic Health Overweight and Obese Adults." *Asia Pacific Journal of Clinical Nutrition* 22, no. 3 (2013): 365–371.

Choi, H. S., S. Kim, M. J. Kim, et al. "Efficacy and Safety of *Panax Ginseng* Berry Extract on Glycemic Control: A 12-Week Randomized, Double-Blind, and Placebo-Controlled Clinical Trial." *Journal of Ginseng Research* 42, no. 1 (January 2018): 90–97.

Geng, J., J. Dong, H. Ni, et al. "Ginseng for Cognition." *Cochrane Database for Systematic Reviews* 12 (December 8, 2010): CD007769.

Lee, E. S., Y. J. Yang, J. H. Lee, and Y. S. Yoon. "Effect of High-Dose Ginsenoside Complex (UG0712) Supplementation on Physical Performance of Health Adults During a 12-Week Supervised Exercise Program: A Randomized Placebo-Controlled Clinical Trial." *Journal of Ginseng Research* 42, no. 2 (April 2018): 192–198.

Lee, H. W., J. Choi, Y. Lee, et al. "Ginseng for Managing Menopausal Women's Health: A Systematic Review of Double-Blind, Randomized, Placebo-Controlled Trials." *Medicine* 95, no. 38 (2016): e4914.

Mucalo, I., E., E. Jovanovski, D. Rahelić, et al. "Effect of American Ginseng (*Panax quinquefolius* L.) on Arterial Stiffness in Subjects with Type-2 Diabetes and Concomitant Hypertension." *Journal of Ethnopharmacology* 150, no. 1 (October 28, 2013): 148–153.

Patk, Byooung-Jin, Yong-Jae Lee, Hye-Ree Lee, et al. "Effects of Korean Red Ginseng on Cardiovascular Risks in Subjects with Metabolic Syndrome: A Double-Blind Randomized Controlled Study." *Korean Journal of Family Medicine* 33, no. 4 (2012): 190–196.

Shishtar, E., J. L. Sievenpiper, V. Djedovic, et al. "The Effect of Ginseng (The Genus *Panax*) on Glycemic Control: A Systematic Review and Meta-Analysis of Randomized Controlled Clinical Trials." *PLoS ONE* 9, no. 9 (2014): e107391.

Yennurajalingam, S., A. Reddy, N. M. Tannir, et al. "High-Dose Asian Ginseng (*Panax Ginseng*) for Cancer-Related Fatigue: A Preliminary Report." *Integrative Cancer Therapies* 14, no. 5 (September 2015): 419–427.

Yennurajalingam, S., N. M. Tannir, J. L. Williams, et al. "A Double-Blind, Randomized, Placebo-Controlled Trial of *Panax Ginseng* for Cancer-Related Fatigue in Patients with Advanced Cancer." *Journal of the National Comprehensive Cancer Network* 15, no. 9 (September 2017): 1111–1120.

Glucosamine and Chondroitin

Glucosamine and chondroitin are natural compounds present in the body's carti-lage. (Cartilage is the connective tissue found in many parts of the body such as joints.) Produced by the body, glucosamine and chondroitin appear to stimulate the body to synthesize more cartilage.

Supplemental glucosamine may be harvested from the shells of shellfish, or it can be prepared in the laboratory; supplemental chondroitin can be prepared from the cartilage of animals, such as cows, pigs, or sharks, or it may also be prepared in a laboratory. People who have specific dietary requirements should check out the source(s) of glucosamine and chondroitin before purchasing any product.

Over the past several decades, glucosamine and chondroitin have become very popular supplements for the treatment of osteoarthritis. It has been estimated that about one in every five Americans takes glucosamine, and about one in every ten Americans takes chondroitin. Obviously, millions of Americans hoping to relieve their painful symptoms are taking these supplements everyday. This has happened because the traditional treatments for osteoarthritis—nonsteroidal anti-inflammatory drugs (NSAIDs)—often have undesirable side effects, such as gastrointestinal upset and bleeding, and an increased risk of heart problems and stroke, especially for those who need to take them for longer periods of time. Moreover, NSAIDs may interfere with other medications people with osteoarthri-tis are already taking.

HEALTH BENEFITS AND RISKS

Most research on glucosamine and chondroitin has focused on the effects of these supplements, individually and in combination, on osteoarthritis, a common type of arthritis that destroys cartilage in the joints. When there are reduced carti-lage levels, the bones rub together, which causes pain and swelling and an inabil-ity to move the joint. The parts of the body most likely to be affected by osteoarthritis are the knees, hips, spine, and hands. However, osteoarthritis may even cause jawbone pain and interfere with jawbone mobility, which is exquisitely painful.

There have been hundreds, maybe thousands, of studies on the use of glucos-amine and/or chondroitin for osteoarthritis and other joint problems with mixed results. The topic is quite controversial, and it is not uncommon for experts to disagree. In addition, there are very few studies on these supplements and other medical concerns.

Because glucosamine and chondroitin may raise blood sugar levels, people with diabetes should discuss the supplement with their medical providers. The same is true for people on blood-thinning medication because glucosamine and chondroitin may increase the risk of bleeding. People who are allergic to shellfish need to avoid glucosamine, which may be extracted from a substance in shellfish. There is at least the possibility of an allergic reaction. However, shellfish-free glucosamine may be prepared in the laboratory. People who are allergic to shellfish should search for this alternative. Whether glucosamine and chondroitin are safe for pregnant women, nursing moms, and children has not been determined yet.

Side effects associated with glucosamine and chondroitin include nausea, diarrhea, constipation, heartburn, headaches, and increased intestinal flatulence.

HOW IT IS SOLD AND TAKEN

Although they may be purchased separately, glucosamine and chondroitin are usually sold together as capsules, tablets, and a liquid. The typical initial daily dose of glucosamine is 1500 mg and 1200 mg of chondroitin. If a response is obtained, after a few months the doses may be lowered to 1000 mg of glucosamine and 800 mg of chondroitin. However, medical providers and supplement manufacturers may vary in their recommendations.

RESEARCH FINDINGS

Glucosamine and/or Chondroitin May or May Not Be Useful for Osteoarthritis of the Knee

In a randomized, parallel-group, double-blind, multicenter trial published in 2016 in the journal *Annals of Rheumatic Diseases*, researches from many countries but based in Baltimore, Maryland (USA), wanted to determine if a supplement containing glucosamine and chondroitin would be useful for people with moderate-to-severe pain from knee osteoarthritis. The initial cohort included 606 patients recruited by physicians from France, Germany, Poland, and Spain; all patients were 40 years old or older and had a diagnosis of primary knee osteoarthritis. For 6 months, they were randomized to receive 400 mg chondroitin plus 500 mg glucosamine three times per day or 200 mg celecoxib (Celebrex), an anti-inflammatory prescription medication. Both treatments had good safety profiles and tolerability. Still, around half of the people in each group had at least one adverse effect. Four hundred and sixty-five participants completed the trial. Levels of pain and other related medical concerns were assessed. The researchers determined that both treatments resulted in significant levels of pain reduction. In fact, both groups had a 50% reduction in pain. Moreover, the glucosamine/chondroitin supplement had "comparable efficacy to celecoxib in reducing pain, stiffness, functional limitation and joint swelling/effusion."[1]

In a systematic review and meta-analysis published in 2015 in the journal *Scientific Reports*, researchers from China compared the use of glucosamine alone, chondroitin alone, and the combination of glucosamine and chondroitin to the medication celecoxib. The study cohort consisted of 54 studies that included 16,427 participants. As expected, the various studies used different scales for assessing pain and function. In addition, 38 studies reported patient withdrawal because of adverse effects. Still, the researchers determined that glucosamine alone, chondroitin alone, glucosamine and chondroitin combined, and celecoxib were more effective than placebos in pain relief. Overall, though celecoxib was the best treatment, it had high rates of gastrointestinal side effects. The combination of glucosamine and chondroitin supplementation exhibited clinically significant improvements in function. The researchers concluded that their analysis "provided evidence for the symptomatic efficacy of glucosamine and chondroitin in the treatment of knee OA [osteoarthritis]."[2]

In a meta-analysis published in 2010 in the journal *Rheumatology International*, researchers from South Korea assessed the ability of glucosamine and chondroitin to slow the progression of knee osteoarthritis. The researchers included six randomly controlled trials that had 1502 participants. There were two studies on glucosamine (1500 mg per day) and four studies on chondroitin (800 mg per day). The mean age of participants in the intervention groups ranged from 61.2 to 66 years and 63.1 to 65.5 years in the control groups. All trials included information on joint space narrowing as an outcome variable. In the glucosamine trials, during the first year of treatment, there were no differences in the joint space narrowing between the supplement and the placebo. However, the trials that continued for at least 3 years demonstrated that glucosamine had a small-to-moderate protective effect on minimum joint space narrowing and a protective effect on severe joint space narrowing. In the chondroitin trials, there were no differences between the supplement and the placebo during the first year. Yet, after 2 years, chondroitin had a small but significant protective effect on minimum joint space narrowing. The researchers concluded that "available data shows that glucosamine and chondroitin sulfate may delay radiological progression of OA of the knee after daily administration for over 2 or 3 years."[3]

In a systematic review and meta-analysis published in 2018 in the journal *Clinical Rheumatology*, researchers from Japan investigated the ability of glucosamine to help people dealing with knee osteoarthritis. The cohort consisted of 18 studies published between 2003 and 2016. Nine of these studies used only glucosamine, and nine studies used supplements containing both glucosamine and other supplements such as chondroitin. Nine of the 18 studies were conducted in Japan. While one study exceeded 1 year of observation, the most common observation period was 12 weeks. All studies included some form of pain scale. In most studies, the daily dose of glucosamine was 1500 mg. Overall, 12 studies (67%) concluded that glucosamine was more effective than a placebo. Four of the six randomly controlled trials, with 100 or more participants, concluded that glucosamine was no better than a placebo. The researchers determined that "the collective effect of glucosamine is small." Yet, they concluded that "clinicians should consider glucosamine as a supplement for patients with OA."[4]

In a multicenter, randomized, double-blind, placebo-controlled trial published in 2017 in the journal *Arthritis & Rheumatology*, researchers from Spain recruited

164 patients from nine rheumatology referral centers and one orthopedic surgery center. All patients had knee osteoarthritis and moderate-to-severe knee pain. For 6 months, the patients were randomly assigned to consume a glucosamine and chondroitin supplement containing 1500 mg glucosamine sulfate and 1200 mg chondroitin sulfate or a placebo. After a baseline visit, clinic visits were scheduled at 4, 12, and 24 weeks. Reported adverse reactions included diarrhea, upper abdominal pain, and constipation. One hundred and nineteen patients completed the trial. The researchers found that the mean pain scores decreased by 33% in the placebo group and by 19% in the supplement group. Thus, the patients in the placebo group had better results than those in the supplement group. The researchers concluded that the glucosamine and chondroitin supplement failed to reduce knee joint pain and functionality more than the placebo.[5]

People Dealing with Knee Osteoarthritis May Benefit by Adding Methysulfonylmethane (MSM) to Their Daily Glucosamine and Chondroitin Supplementation

In a double-blind, randomized, controlled clinical trial published in 2017 in the Indonesian internal medicine journal *Acta Medica Indonesiana*, researchers from Indonesia wanted to learn if adding MSM to glucosamine and chondroitin supplementation would benefit those dealing with grade 1 (early) to 2 (mild) knee osteoarthritis. The cohort consisted of 147 people with grades 1–2 knee osteoarthritis; the diagnosis was made by a clinical examination and X-ray imaging. The mean age of the participants was 61 years, and 67.3% were women. The participants were placed in one of the three groups. The members of one group took a supplement containing 1500 mg of glucosamine and 1200 mg of chondroitin sulfate and 500 mg of saccharumlactis (lactose); the members in the second group took 1500 mg of glucosamine and 1200 of chondroitin sulfate and 500 mg of MSM; the members of the third group took a placebo containing lactose. The supplements and placebos were taken once daily for three consecutive months. Over the course of the trial, several assessments were made. The researchers determined that the participants taking the glucosamine, chondroitin, and MSM supplement had the most improvement and pain relief. Interestingly, those taking the glucosamine and chondroitin supplement did not experience reduced joint pain. The researchers concluded that "glucosamine-chondroitin sulfate may bring significant clinical improvement in patients . . . compared to placebo; however, the supplement could not significantly reduce pain."[6]

Glucosamine May or May Not Be Useful for Osteoarthritis in Jaw Joints

In a trial published in 2011 in the journal *Oral Surgery, Oral Medicine, Oral Pathology, Oral Radiology, and Endodontics*, researchers from Sweden wanted to determine if glucosamine supplementation would help people with osteoarthritis in their temporomandibular (TMJ) joints (jaw joints). Problems with jaw joints are termed temporomandibular joint disorders or TMJ. The cohort consisted of 59 patients who had osteoarthritis of their jaw joints. There were 51 women with a mean age of 60 years, and eight men with a mean age of 57 years. For 6 weeks, the patients were randomly assigned to consume 1200 mg per day of glucosamine sulfate or an identical placebo capsule. Pain levels were assessed at baseline and at the end of the trial. Eight people in the glucosamine group and two in the placebo group did not complete the trial. The researchers found no significant differences between the two groups. The participants in both groups experienced improvements. At least in this trial, there was no evidence that glucosamine supplementation would be useful for osteoarthritis in jaw joints. The researchers concluded that "even if some improvements over time were observed, the differences in the magnitude of responses between the active and control arms were not large enough to establish any advantage for the active medication in this trial."[7]

On the other hand, in a trial published in 2013 in the *Journal of Research in Pharmacy Practice*, researchers from Iran compared the use of glucosamine and ibuprofen, an NSAID, for treating painful TMJ disorders. Sixty patients were randomly placed in either the glucosamine group (1500 mg per day) or the ibuprofen group (400 mg twice daily). The glucosamine group had a mean age of 26.60 years, and the ibuprofen group had a mean age of 27.12 years. The participants were assessed at baseline and at 30, 60, and 90 days. The researchers determined that the participants in both groups had significant improvement in their posttreatment pain and mandibular (jawbone) opening. However, the improvement in the glucosamine group was better than the improvement in the ibuprofen group. Gastrointestinal adverse effects were reported by 53% of the participants on ibuprofen and 16% on glucosamine. Therefore, the participants on glucosamine had better results with fewer adverse effects. The researchers concluded that "glucosamine sulfate is a more effective and safer therapeutic agent for treatment of patients with TMJ."[8]

Glucosamine and Chondroitin Appear to Have Anti-Inflammatory Properties

In a randomized, double-blind, placebo-controlled, crossover trial published in 2015 in the online journal *PLoS ONE*, researchers from Seattle, Washington, Boston, Massachusetts, and Nashville, Tennessee (USA), wanted to learn more about the anti-inflammatory properties of glucosamine and chondroitin. The cohort consisted of nine men and nine women between the ages of 20 and 55 years, who were healthy but overweight. For 28 days, the participants were placed on a combination of glucosamine hydrochloride (1500 mg per day) and chondroitin sulfate (1200 mg per day) or a placebo. No adverse events were reported. Biological samples were taken at baseline and after each 28-day intervention. The researchers determined that the supplement lowered mean serum C-reactive protein concentrations, a marker of inflammation, by 23%. Other indicators of inflammation reduction were also significantly decreased. The researchers concluded that "glucosamine and chondroitin supplementation may lower systematic inflammation and alter other pathways in healthy, overweight individuals."[9]

Chondroitin May Be Useful for Hand Osteoarthritis

In a single-center, randomized, double-blind, placebo-controlled clinical trial published in 2011 in the journal *Arthritis & Rheumatism*, researchers from Switzerland evaluated the ability of chondroitin supplementation to help people dealing with hand osteoarthritis. The cohort consisted of 162 symptomatic patients with radiographic evidence of hand osteoarthritis. For 6 months, the participants who were at least 40 years old took either 800 mg of "highly purified" chondroitin sulfate per day (n = 80) or an identical placebo (n = 82). Clinical assessments were conducted 7 days before enrollment, at baseline, and after 1, 3, and 6 months of the trial. By the end of the trial, the researchers learned that 6 months of treatment with chondroitin was "significantly superior to placebo with regard to improvements in global hand pain and hand function." The participants treated with chondroitin also had significant decreases in morning stiffness. The researchers concluded that chondroitin is "an interesting therapeutic alternative for the management of this frequent condition."[10]

There Appears to Be an Association between Mortality and Supplemental Glucosamine and Chondroitin

In a study published in 2012 in the *European Journal of Epidemiology*, researchers from Seattle, Washington (USA), wanted to learn more about the long-term effects of supplemental glucosamine and chondroitin. The researchers used data from a cohort study of male and female Washington State residents, aged 50–76 years, which were collected between 2000 and 2002. After exclusions, the researchers were able to include 77,510 residents in their analysis. Participants were followed for mortality through 2008. By that point, there were 5362 deaths. The researchers determined that, compared to those who never took the combination supplement, the people currently on supplemental glucosamine and chondroitin had an 18% decreased risk of total mortality. Current use of glucosamine was associated with a significant reduced risk of death from cancer and with a large risk reduction for death from respiratory diseases. Further, they concluded that the "use of glucosamine with or without chondroitin was associated with reduced total mortality and with reduction of several broad causes of death." The researchers commented that "there is a need to continue to evaluate other anti-inflammatory drugs, such as glucosamine and chondroitin, that may have a more favorable safety profile and may provide risk reduction for the range of diseases associated with inflammation."[11]

Supplemental Glucosamine and Chondroitin May or May Not Be Associated with Lower Rates of Colorectal Cancer

In a case-control analysis published in 2018 in *Scientific Reports*, researchers from Spain wanted to learn if supplemental glucosamine and chondroitin had anticolorectal cancer properties. They used data from the MCC–Spain study, a case-control study performed in 12 provinces in Spain that included 2140 cases of colorectal cancer and 3950 population controls. The data included information on sociodemographic factors, lifestyle, family and medical history, and drug use. The reported frequency of use of glucosamine and chondroitin was 0.89% in people with colorectal cancer and 2.03% in controls. While supplement users had a reduced rate of colorectal cancer, when the data were adjusted for the use of NSAIDs, the relationship was no longer significant. The researchers noted that it is possible that "the observed effects of our study could be attributed to NSAIDs concurrent use."[12]

Oral Glucosamine Supplements May Be Associated with Glaucoma

In a small retrospective clinical study published in 2013 in *JAMA Ophthalmology*, researchers from Maine and Virginia (USA) examined the association between glucosamine supplementation and glaucoma. Glaucoma occurs when there is an increase in intraocular pressure or pressure inside the eye. Untreated, this pressure may lead to blindness. The cohort consisted of 17 patients, who ranged in age from 62 to 90 years. Eleven patients had glaucoma prior to beginning glucosamine supplement, and the glaucoma improved after discontinuation of the supplement. Six patients had glaucoma evaluations only after they began taking glucosamine and after discontinuing the supplement when the glaucoma improved. The researchers underscored the need for more research on this potential association. They concluded that "this study shows the reversible effect of these changes, which is reassuring. However, the possibility that permanent damage can result from prolonged use of glucosamine supplementation is not eliminated."[13]

NOTES

1. Hochberg, Marc. C., Johanne Martel-Pelletier, Jordi Monfort, et al. "Combined Chondroitin Sulfate and Glucosamine for Painful Knew Osteoarthritis: A Multicentre, Randomised, Double-Blind, Non-Inferiority Trial versus Celecoxib." *Annals of Rheumatic Diseases* 75 (2016): 37–44.

2. Zeng, C., J. Wei, H. Li, et al. "Effectiveness and Safety of Glucosamine, Chondroitin, the Two in Combination, or Celecoxib in the Treatment of Osteoarthritis of the Knee." *Scientific Reports* 5 (November 18, 2015): 16827.

3. Lee, Y. H., J. H. Woo, S. J. Choi, et al. "Effect of Glucosamine or Chondroitin Sulfate on the Osteoporosis Progression: A Meta-Analysis." *Rheumatology International* 30, no. 3 (January 2010): 357–363.

4. Ogata, T., Y. Ideno, M. Akai, et al. "Effects of Glucosamine in Patients with Osteoarthritis of the Knee: A Systematic Review and Mata-Analysis." *Clinical Rheumatology* 39, no. 9 (September 2018): 2479–2487.

5. Roman-Blas, J. A., S. Castañeda, O. Sánchez-Pernaute, et al. "Combined Treatment with Chondroitin Sulfate and Glucosamine Sulfate Shows No Superiority over Placebo for Reduction of Joint Pain and Functional Impairment in Patients with Knee Osteoarthritis: A Six-Month Multicenter, Randomized, Double-Blind, Placebo-Controlled Clinical Trial." *Arthritis & Rheumatology* 69, no. 1(January 2017): 77–85.

6. Lubis, A. M. T., C. Siagian, E. Wonggokusuma, et al. "Comparison of Glucosamine-Chondroitin Sulfate with and without Methylsulfonylmethane in Grade

I–II Knee Osteoarthritis: A Double-Blind, Randomized Controlled Trial." *Acta Medica Indonesiana* 49, no. 2 (April 2017): 105–111.

7. Cahlin, Birgitta Johansson and Lars Dahlström. "No Effect of Glucosamine Sulfate on Osteoarthritis in the Temporomandibular Joints—A Randomized, Controlled, Short-Term Study." *Oral Surgery, Oral Medicine, Oral Pathology, Oral Radiology, and Endodontics* 112 (2011): 760–766.

8. Haghighat, A., A. Behnia, N. Kaviani, and B. Khorami. "Evaluation of Glucosamine Sulfate and Ibuprofen Effects in Patients with Temporomandibular Joint Osteoarthritis Symptom." *Journal of Research in Pharmacy Practice* 2, no. 1 (January 2013): 34–39.

9. Navarro, S. L., E. White, E. D. Kantor, et al. "Randomized Trial of Glucosamine and Chondroitin Supplementation on Inflammation and Oxidative Stress Biomarkers and Plasma Proteomics in Healthy Humans." *PLoS ONE* 10, no. 2 (February 26, 2015): e0117534.

10. Gabay, C., C. Medinger-Sadowski, D. Gascon, et al. "Symptomatic Effects of Chondroitin 4 and Chondroitin 6 Sulfate on Hand Osteoarthritis: A Randomized, Double-Blind, Placebo-Controlled Clinical Trial at a Single Center." *Arthritis & Rheumatism* 63, no. 11 (November 2011): 3383–3391.

11. Bell, Griffith A., Elizabeth D. Kantor, Johanna W. Lampe, et al. "Use of Glucosamine and Chondroitin in Relation to Mortality." *European Journal of Epidemiology* 27, no. 8 (August 2012): 593–603.

12. Ibáñez-Sanz, G., A. Diez-Villaneuva, L. Vilorio-Marqués, et al. "Possible Role of Chondroitin Sulphate and Glucosamine for Primary Prevention of Colorectal Cancer. Results from the MCC-Spain Study." *Scientific Reports* 8, no. 1 (February 1, 2018): 2040.

13. Murphy, Ryan K., Lecea Ketzler, Robert D. E. Rice, et al. "Oral Glucosamine Supplements as a Possible Ocular Hypertensive Agent." *JAMA Ophthalmology* 132, no. 7 (July 2013): 955–957.

REFERENCES AND FURTHER READING

Cahlin, Birgitta Johansson and Lars Dahlström. "No Effect of Glucosamine Sulfate on Osteoarthritis in the Temporomandibular Joints—A Randomized, Controlled, Short-Term Study." *Oral Surgery, Oral Medicine, Oral Pathology, Oral Radiology, and Endodontics* 112 (2011): 760–766.

Ell, Griffith A., Elizabeth D. Kantor, Johanna W. Lampe, et al. "Use of Glucosamine and Chondroitin in Relation to Mortality." *European Journal of Epidemiology* 27, no. 8 (August 2012): 593–603.

Gabay, C., C. Medinger-Sadowski, D. Gascon, et al. "Symptomatic Effects of Chondroitin 4 and Chondroitin 6 Sulfate on Hand Osteoarthritis: A Randomized, Double-Blind, Placebo-Controlled Clinical Trial at a Single Center." *Arthritis & Rheumatism* 63, no. 11 (November 2011): 3383–3391.

Haghighat, A., A. Behnia, N. Kaviani, and B. Khorami. "Evaluation of Glucosamine Sulfate and Ibuprofen Effects in Patients with Temporomandibular Joint Osteoarthritis Symptom." *Journal of Research in Pharmacy Practice* 2, no. 1 (January 2013): 34–39.

Hochberg, Marc C., Johanne Martel-Pelletier, Jordi Monfort, et al. "Combined Chondroitin Sulfate and Glucosamine for Painful Knee Osteoarthritis: A Multicentre, Randomised, Double-Blind, Non-Inferiority Trial versus Celecoxib." *Annals of Rheumatic Diseases* 75 (2016): 37–44.

Ibáñez-Sanz, G., A. Diez-Villanueva, L. Vilorio-Marués, et al. "Possible Role of Chondroitin Sulphate and Glucosamine for Primary Prevention of Colorectal Cancer.

Results from the MCC-Spain Study." *Scientific Reports* 8, no. 1 (February 1, 2018): 2040.

Lee, Y. H., J. H. Woo, S. J. Choi, et al. "Effect of Glucosamine or Chondroitin Sulfate on the Osteoarthritis Progression: A Meta-Analysis." *Rheumatology International* 30, no. 3 (January 2010): 357–363.

Lubis, A. M. T., C. Siagian, E. Wonggokusuma, et al. "Comparison of Glucosamine-Chondroitin Sulfate with and without Methylsulfonylmethane in Grade I–II Knee Osteoarthritis: A Double Blind Randomized Controlled Trial." *Acta Medica Indonesiana* 49, no. 2 (April 2017): 105–111.

Murphy, Ryan K., Lecea Ketzler, Robert D. E. Rice, et al. "Oral Glucosamine Supplements as a Possible Ocular Hypertensive Agent." *JAMA Ophthalmology* 131, no. 7 (July 2013): 955–957.

Navarro, S. L., E. White, E. D. Kantor, et al. "Randomized Trial of Glucosamine and Chondroitin Supplementation on Inflammation and Oxidative Stress Biomarkers and Plasma Proteomics Profiles in Healthy Humans." *PLoS ONE* 10, no. 2 (February 26, 2015): e0117534.

Ogata, T., Y. Ideno, M. Akai, et al. "Effects of Glucosamine with Osteoarthritis of the Knee: A Systematic Review and Meta-Analysis." *Clinical Rheumatology* 39, no. 9 (September 2018): 2479–2487.

Roman-Blas, J. A., S. Castañeda, O. Sánchez-Pernaute, et al. "Combined Treatment with Chondroitin Sulfate and Glucosamine Sulfate Shows No Superiority over Placebo for Reduction of Joint Pain and Functional Impairment in Patients with Knee Osteoarthritis: A Six-Month Multicenter, Randomized, Double-Blind, Placebo-Controlled Clinical Trial." *Arthritis & Rheumatology* 69, no. 1 (January 2017): 77–85.

Zeng, C., J. Wei, H. Li, et al. "Effectiveness and Safety of Glucosamine, Chondroitin, the Two in Combination, or Celecoxib in the Treatment of Osteoarthritis of the Knee." *Scientific Reports* 5 (November 18, 2015): 16827.

Green Tea

It is believed that the green tea plant originated during ancient times in Tibet, western China, and northern India. Green tea is extracted from the leaves of the plant, *Camellia sinensis*, which has a shrub-like appearance. To grow properly, green tea plants need a semi-tropical environment with heavy rainfall; they are placed in rows or on terraces.

In general, green tea leaves are picked by hand, and then steamed, rolled, dried, and packed in chests, which preserves the tea's aroma and prevents the absorption of any unwanted outside substances or scents.

Green tea contains active compounds from a group of polyphenols called catechins. Probably the best known catechin is epigallocatechin gallate. Catechins protect cells and reduce the formation of free radicals in the body, thus supporting health and antiaging. In addition, green tea contains carotenoids, tocopherols, the amino acid L-theanine, ascorbic acid, and minerals, such as chromium, magnesium, selenium, and zinc. Unless caffeine has been removed, green tea has about half the amount of caffeine as coffee; however, the actual amount varies according to the specific type of tea.

HEALTH BENEFITS AND RISKS

Green tea is useful for a wide variety of medical concerns. It is thought to support cardiovascular health, boost immunity, kill cancer cells and bacteria, and help weight loss. In fact, green tea supplements are advertised and sold as a weight loss tool, metabolic rate booster, and a natural fat burner, especially for fat in the abdominal area. It is believed to have anti-inflammatory properties and to improve bone density, cognition, and depression. Some contend that green tea increases physical performance and improves nonalcoholic fatty liver disease and inflammatory bowel disease. Because it may prevent sudden increases in blood sugar levels, people who have diabetes may start drinking green tea and/or purchase supplements to help control their sugar levels.

On the other hand, green tea has been associated with some potential side effects. Because it contains caffeine, those who are sensitive to caffeine should avoid green tea. Moreover, green tea may increase the risk of stomach upset and bleeding problems, especially in people on blood-thinning medications. Other side effects associated with green tea include headache, nervousness, sleep problems, vomiting, diarrhea, irritability, irregular heartbeat, tremor, heartburn, dizziness, ringing in ears, and reduced iron absorption. Green tea is known to interact with a host of different medications including chemotherapy, lithium, monoamine oxidase inhibitors, clozapine, ephedrine, aspirin, beta-blockers, antibiotics, adenosine, oral contraceptives, and phenylpropanolamine. It is best to check with a medical provider before initiating supplementation.

HOW IT IS SOLD AND TAKEN

As expected, green tea may be purchased as a dried leaf tea. The best way to obtain catechins and other benefits is to drink freshly brewed green tea in water that has not yet reached the boiling point. Typically, the recommended consumption is three or four cups per day. However, some people suggest higher amounts.

Green tea may also be purchased in capsules, tablets, powder, and liquid extract. Recommendations vary widely. It is best to follow the directions on the label or discuss supplementation with a medical provider.

RESEARCH FINDINGS

Consumption of Tea Appears to Improve Some Types of Mortality

In a meta-analysis published in 2015 in the *British Journal of Nutrition*, researchers from China investigated the association between tea consumption and overall mortality. The researchers found 18 relevant and eligible studies. Of these, six were from the United States, four from Europe, and eight from Asian countries. Eight of the studies involving 12,221 cases among 163,854 individuals described the association between tea consumption and all-cancer mortality. Ten studies involving 11,306 cases among 240,637 individuals described the association between tea consumption and cardiovascular disease (CVD) mortality. Fifteen studies involving 55,528 cases among 440,297 individuals reported the association between tea consumption and all-cause mortality. The researchers learned that green tea consumption was inversely associated with mortality from CDV and all-cause mortality, but was not associated with all-cancer mortality. The inverse association between green tea consumption and CVD mortality was more apparent in women than in men. The researchers concluded that "the dose-response analysis indicated that one cup per d [day] increment of green tea consumption was associated with five percent lower risk of CVD mortality and with four percent lower risk of all-cause mortality."[1]

In a study published in 2015 in the journal *Annals of Epidemiology*, researchers from Japan examined the association between green tea consumption and all-cause mortality, cancer, heart disease, cerebrovascular disease, respiratory disease, injuries, and other causes. The cohort consisted of 90,914 Japanese men (n = 42,836) and women (n = 48,078) between the ages of 40 and 69 years who were recruited between 1990 and 1994. During 18.7 years of follow-up, there were 12,874 reported deaths. Of these, 5327 deaths were caused by cancer, 1577 deaths were caused by heart disease, 1264 deaths were caused by cerebrovascular disease, 783 deaths were caused by respiratory disease, 992 deaths were caused by injuries, and 2931 deaths were caused by other causes. When the researchers compared those who drank less than a cup of green tea per day to those who drank five cups or more per day, they found that the men in the latter group had a 13% lower risk of dying from all causes and the women in the latter group had a 17% lower risk from dying from all causes. In addition, the researchers learned that green tea consumption was inversely associated with mortality from heart disease, cerebrovascular disease, and respiratory disease. They concluded that "because green tea is regularly consumed throughout life, the health effects of these compounds may accumulate to make a large effect on the longevity of the general population."[2]

Green Tea May Play a Role in the Prevention of CVD

In an analysis published in 2013 in the *Cochrane Database of Systematic Reviews,* researchers from the United Kingdom examined the ability of green and black tea to help prevent CVD. The researchers identified a total of 11 randomized controlled trials that included 821 participants. Seven trials addressed green tea and four investigated black tea. Doses of the teas differed between the trials. The researchers learned that green tea produced statistically significant reductions in total cholesterol and blood pressure. Yet, the researchers cautioned that there are few long-term studies addressing the use of green and black tea to prevent cardiovascular problems, concluding that "the limited evidence suggests that tea has favourable effects on CVD risk factors, but due to the small number of trials contributing to each analysis, the results should be treated with some caution."[3]

In a study published in 2017 in the *American Journal of Medicine*, researchers from many locations in the United States, but based in Bethesda, Maryland (USA), evaluated the association between tea and coffee consumption and coronary artery calcium and major adverse cardiovascular events. The researchers obtained data on 6508 ethnically diverse participants from the Multi-Ethnic Study of Atherosclerosis. The average age was 62.3 years and included 52.9% women. The participants completed a 120-item food frequency questionnaire. Follow-up interviews were conducted every 9 to 12 months. There was a median follow-up of 5.3 years for coronary artery calcium and 11.1 years for cardiovascular events. Compared to people who never drank tea, people who drank at least a cup of tea each day had a slower progression of coronary artery calcium and a lower incidence of cardiovascular events. The researchers commented that their findings "supported regular tea consumption as part of a heart healthy diet as recommended by the American Heart Association."[4]

Green Tea May Be a Good Addition to the Diet of Overweight Women

In a 12-week randomized, double-blind, placebo-controlled trial published in 2017 in the journal *Clinical Nutrition ESPEN*, researchers from Brazil evaluated the use of green tea and metformin, a type 2 diabetes medication, both individually and in combination, in nondiabetic overweight women. Specifically, they wanted to determine the impact, if any, on lipid profile, glycemic control, and body composition. The cohort consisted of 120 overweight women between the ages of 20 and 45 years, who were recruited between June and August 2014. They were assigned to one of four groups: control (1 g of cellulose per day), green tea (1 g per day), metformin (1 g per day), or metformin and green tea (1 g of each per day). All capsules had the same appearance. During the trial, 32 women withdrew, and 88 completed the trial. The researchers found that the green tea treatment alone was better at improving glycemic control and lipid profile in nondiabetic overweight women. However, the women in the metformin group lost weight, though there was no change in their lipid levels. The researchers concluded that "green tea extract is a promising alternative for reducing type 2 diabetes risk in overweight women."[5]

Then Again, It May or May Not Help People at Risk for Type 2 Diabetes

In a systematic review and meta-analysis published in 2014 in the *Journal of Human Nutrition and Dietetics*, researchers from China examined the usefulness of green tea and green tea extract for people at risk for type 2 diabetes. They identified seven randomly controlled trials that included 510 participants. Four trials were conducted in Asia, and the median length of follow-up was 4 weeks to 6 months. The researchers learned that, in populations at risk for type 2 diabetes, neither green tea nor green tea extract produced any significant and clinically meaningful changes in fasting plasma glucose levels, fasting serum insulin levels, plasma glucose in oral glucose tolerance test, as well as other related tests. The researchers emphasized the need for more studies with larger samples sizes and longer durations, and concluded that "comparing different doses of green tea and of high methodological quality, particularly in allocation concealment and blinding, are warranted, and these should help to determine the effects of green tea or green tea extract on insulin sensitivity and plasma glucose homeostasis in populations at risk of type 2 diabetes mellitus."[6]

In a meta-analysis published in 2013 in the *American Journal of Clinical Nutrition*, researchers from China reviewed studies on the effect of green tea or green tea extract on glucose control and insulin sensitivity. The researchers located 17 randomly controlled trials with a total of 1133 participants. The number of participants included in each trial ranged from 34 to 240, and the study duration ranged from 2 weeks to 6 months. Nine of the trials focused on overweight and obese adults, four trials had participants with type 2 diabetes, two trials had participants with borderline diabetes, and two trials had healthy participants. Seven trials were deemed "high quality." The researchers learned that green tea consumption significantly reduced fasting glucose and hemoglobin A1c, another measure of blood sugar. At the same time, when the researchers used data only from the high-quality trials, green tea consumption significantly reduced fasting insulin concentrations. The researchers underscored the need for more high-quality randomly controlled trials "to evaluate the effects of green tea on glucose control and insulin sensitivity . . . to further evaluate and confirm these findings."[7]

Green Tea May or May Not Help People Lose Weight and/or Maintain Their Weight

In an analysis published in 2012 in the *Cochrane Database of Systematic Reviews*, researchers based in Canada examined the ability of green tea to help overweight and obese people lose weight and not add additional pounds. Fourteen randomly controlled trials met their inclusion criteria and were judged to be at low risk for bias. The six trials conducted outside of Japan, with 532 participants, showed a very small, statistically insignificant mean difference in weight loss from green tea. The eight trials conducted in Japan, with 1030 participants, found that those in the green tea group lost an average of 0.2–3.5 kg more than those in the control group. The most common reported adverse effects were hypertension and constipation. The amount of weight loss was so small that it would likely not have any clinical relevance. Further, green tea did not play any role in helping people maintain their weight. They concluded that "green tea preparations appeared to induce a small, statistically non-significant loss in overweight or obese adults."[8]

In a meta-analysis published in 2009 in the *International Journal of Obesity*, researchers from the Netherlands analyzed the association between catechins in green tea, weight loss, and weight maintenance. They identified 11 randomized controlled trials that met their inclusion criteria and compared catechins in green tea or green tea supplements with no catechins or different doses of catechins on weight loss and weight maintenance for at least 12 weeks. The baseline body mass index of the participants varied from 18.5 to 35 kg/m. The trials usually included males and females aged 16–65 years. Most participants were Asian—Japanese, Thai, Taiwanese, and Chinese—but four trials were conducted on Caucasians. The researchers learned that catechins had a significant positive effect on weight loss and weight maintenance. They concluded that "catechins or an epigallocatechin gallate (EGCG)-caffeine mixture have a small but positive effect on WL [weight loss] and WM [weight maintenance]."[9]

Green Tea Appears to Lower Plasma Nadolol Levels, an Important Medication for Hypertension

In a randomized crossover trial published in 2014 in the journal *Clinical Pharmacology & Therapeutics*, researchers from Germany, Japan, and Italy evaluated the effects of green tea on the serum levels of the beta-blocker, high blood pressure medication, nadolol, in healthy people. Eight males and two females between the ages of 20 and 30 years were included in the study. After 14 days of repeated consumption of green tea or water, ten healthy volunteers received a single oral dose of 30 mg nadolol. The researchers found that green tea significantly decreased the effects of nadolol on systolic blood pressure. Additional laboratory testing determined that green tea significantly inhibited OATP1A2-mediated nadolol uptake in the intestine. Plasma concentrations and urinary excretion of nadolol were markedly reduced by 85% and 81.6%, respectively. Therefore, people who take nadolol for their high blood pressure and who also drink green tea or take green tea supplements may have insufficient amounts of this medication in their blood. Although they acknowledged the need for more studies, the researchers advised people on nadolol to avoid green tea.[10]

Green Tea May Have Some Antiprostate Cancer Properties

In a systematic review published in 2017 in the journal *Nature and Cancer*, researchers based in Malaysia examined studies on the potential association between green tea and prostate cancer. They included a total of 15 studies with 11 reporting the consumption of green tea and the prevention of prostate cancer and four reporting the effect of green tea as a treatment for prostate cancer. Three studies were randomly controlled trials, three were single-arm, phase-2, open-label studies, four were case-control studies, and five were cohort studies. While the amount of green tea consumed varied from study to study, most studies were considered "moderate to high quality." The researchers learned that green tea appeared to be an effective chemopreventive agent, especially in men with high-grade prostate intraepithelial neoplasia. However, there is no evidence that green tea is useful as a treatment. The researchers underscored the need for more well-designed randomly controlled trials "to determine if green tea indeed has a role in the prevention and treatment of PCa [prostate cancer]."[11]

Green Tea May Have Antipancreatic Cancer Properties

In a population-based, case-controlled trial published in 2012 in the journal *Cancer Epidemiology*, researchers from China and New Haven, Connecticut (USA), examined the association between green tea consumption and risk of pancreatic cancer in urban Shanghai, China. Their cohort consisted of 908 people with pancreatic cancer and 1067 healthy controls. All participants were between the ages of 35 and 79 years. Among the participants, 68.7% of the men and 26.9% of the women were tea drinkers, of whom 94.7% and 86.8% were green tea drinkers, respectively. The researchers compiled information on tea drinking, including types of tea, amount of tea consumption, temperature of tea, and duration of regular tea drinking. The researchers learned that female green tea drinkers had a reduced risk of pancreatic cancer. Regular drinking of green tea, increased consumption, longer duration of tea drinking, and lower temperatures of tea were associated with a 30%–40% reduction in pancreatic cancer risk. This association was not evident in men. Their risk only dropped when they drank tea at lower temperatures. The researchers commented that their findings have "potential implications for preventing pancreatic cancer through a modifiable factor and merits further research."[12]

Green Tea May Reduce the Risk of Colorectal Cancer

In a study published in 2011 in the journal *Carcinogenesis*, researchers from China and Nashville, Tennessee (USA), evaluated the association between green tea consumption and the risk of colorectal cancer. Data were obtained from the

Shanghai Men's Health Study, a population-based prospective cohort study, which included 60,567 Chinese men aged 40 to 74 years at baseline. During a mean follow-up of 4.6 years, 243 cases of colorectal cancer were identified. Of these, 123 had early-stage tumors and 93 had late-stage tumors. The mean age at diagnosis was 66.4 years, however, the age at diagnosis ranged from 45 to 79 years. The researchers learned that nonsmoking men who drank green tea at least three times per week for more than six consecutive months had a reduced risk of colorectal cancer. In fact, the risk reduction was directly related to the amount of green tea consumption. The more green tea the men drank, the lower their risk. The researchers noted that their "findings are consistent with data from both in vitro and in vivo experiments, indicating that green tea may serve as an effective chemopreventive agent."[13]

Green Tea May Reduce the Risk of Chronic Obstructive Lung Disease

In a study published in 2018 in the *Journal of Nutrition*, researchers from South Korea analyzed the association between green tea and chronic obstructive lung disease. They used data from the Korean National Health and Education Survey (KNHANES) collected between 2008 and 2015. (KNHANES is a nationwide cross-sectional survey of the entire Korean population.) The cohort consisted of 13,570 participants who were at least 40 years old. The researchers determined that most participants either did not drink green tea or drank green tea less than one time per day. Only 1,082 (8%) participants drank green tea one time per day and 506 (3.7%) consumed green tea two or more times per day. The mean age of the participants was 54.4 years, and those who consumed more green tea tended to be younger than those who did not consume green tea. Of those who consumed green tea, men were twice as likely as women to do so. The researchers learned that the consumption of green tea at least two times per day was associated with an increase in pulmonary function and lower risk of developing chronic obstructive lung disease. They concluded that "considering the antioxidant effects of green tea, the results of the present study agree with those of previous studies."[14]

NOTES

    1. Tang, J., J. S. Zheng, L. Fang, et al. "Tea Consumption and Mortality of All Cancers, CVD and All Causes: A Meta-Analysis of Eighteen Prospective Cohort Studies." *British Journal of Nutrition* 114, no. 5 (September 14, 2015): 673–683.

    2. Saito, E., M. Inoue, N. Sawada, et al. "Association of Green Tea Consumption with Mortality Due to All Causes and Major Causes of Death in a Japanese Population: The Japan Public Health Center-Based Prospective Study (JPHC Stud)." *Annals of Epidemiology* 25, no. 7 (July 2015): 512–518.

    3. Hartley, L., N. Flowers, J. Holmes, et al. "Green and Black Tea for the Primary Prevention of Cardiovascular Disease." *Cochrane Database of Systematic Reviews* 6 (June 18, 2013): CD009934.

4. Miller, P. E., D. Zhao, A. C. Frazier-Wood, et al. "Associations between Coffee, Tea, and Caffeine Intake with Coronary Artery Calcification and Cardiovascular Events." *American Journal of Medicine* 130, no. 2 (February 2017): 188–197.

5. Alves Ferreira, M., A. P. Oliveira Gomes, A. P. Guimarães de Moraes, et al. "Green Tea Extract Outperforms Metformin in Lipid Profiles and Glycaemic Control in Overweight Women: A Double-Blind. Placebo-Controlled, Randomized Trail." *Clinical Nutrition ESPEN* 22 (December 2017): 1–6.

6. Wang, X., J. Tian, J. Jiang, et al. "Effects of Green Tea or Green Tea Extract on Insulin Sensitivity and Glycaemic Control in Populations at Risk of Type 2 Diabetes Mellitus: A Systematic Review and Meta-Analysis of Randomised Controlled Trials." *Journal of Human Nutrition and Dietetics* 5 (October 2014): 501–512.

7. Liu, K., R. Zhou, B. Wang, et al. "Effect of Green Tea on Glucose Control and Insulin Sensitivity: A Meta-Analysis of 17 Randomized Controlled Trials." *American Journal of Clinical Nutrition* 98, no. 2 (August 2013): 340–340.

8. Jurgens, T. M., A. M Whelan, L. Killian, et al. "Green Tea for Weight Loss and Weight Maintenance in Overweight or Obese Adults." *Cochrane Data of Systematic Reviews* 12 (December 12, 2012): CD 008650.

9. Hurseel, R., W. Viechtbauer, and M. S. Westerterp-Plantenga. "The Effects of Green Tea and Weight Maintenance: A Meta-Analysis." *International Journal of Obesity* 33, no. 9 (September 2009): 956–961.

10. Misaka, S., J. Yatabe, F. Müller, et al. "Green Tea Ingestion Greatly Reduces Plasma Concentrations of Nadolol in Healthy Subjects." *Pharmacology & Therapeutics* 95, no. 4 (April 2014): 432–438.

11. Jacob, Sabrina Anne, Tahir Mehmood Khan, and Learn-Han Lee. "The Effect of Green Tea Consumption on Prostate Cancer Risk and Progression: A Systematic Review." 69, no. 3 (2017): 353–364.

12. Wang, Jing, Wei Zhang, Lu Sun, et al. "Green Tea Drinking and Risk of Pancreatic Cancer: A Large-Scale, Population-Based Case-Control Study in Urban Shanghai." *Cancer Epidemiology* 36 (2012): e354–e358.

13. Yang, Gong, Wei Zheng, Wong-Bing Xiang, et al. "Green Tea Consumption and Colorectal Cancer Risk: A Report from the Shanghai's Men's Health Study." *Carcinogenesis* 32, no. 11 (2011): 1684–1688.

14. Oh, Chang-Mo, In-Hwan Oh, Bong-Keun Choe, et al. "Consuming Green Tea At Least Twice Each Day is Associated with Reduced Odds of Chronic Obstructive Lung Disease in Middle-Aged and Older Korean Adults." *Journal of Nutrition* 148 (2018): 70–76.

REFERENCES AND FURTHER READING

Alves Ferreira, M., A. P. Oliveira Gomes, A. P. Guimarães de Moraes, et al. "Green Tea Extract Outperforms Metformin in Lipid Profile and Glycaemic Control in Overweight Women: A Double-Blind, Placebo-Controlled, Randomized Trial." *Clinical Nutrition ESPEN* 22 (2017): 1–6.

Hartley, L., N. Flowers, J. Holmes, et al. "Green and Black Tea for the Primary Prevention of Cardiovascular Disease." *Cochrane Database of Systematic Reviews* 6 (June 18, 2013): CD009934.

Hursel, R., W. Viechtbauer, M. S. Westerterp-Plantenga. "The Effects of Green Tea on Weight Loss and Weight Maintenance: A Meta-Analysis." *International Journal of Obesity* 33, no. 9 (September 2009): 956–961.

Jacob, Sabrina Anne, Tahir Mehmood Khan, and Learn-Han Lee. "The Effect of Green Tea Consumption on Prostate Cancer Risk and Progression: A Systematic Review." *Nutrition and Cancer* 69, no. 3 (2017): 353–364.

Jurgens, T. M., A. M. Whelan, L. Killian, et al. "Green Tea for Weight Loss and Weight Maintenance in Overweight or Obese Adults." *Cochrane Database of Systematic Reviews* 12 (December 12, 2012): CD008650.

Liu, K., R. Zhou, B. Wang, et al. "Effect of Green Tea on Glucose Control and Insulin Sensitivity: A Meta-Analysis of 17 Randomized Controlled Trials." *American Journal of Clinical Nutrition* 98, no. 2 (August 2013): 340–348.

Miller, P. E., D. Zhao, A. C. Frazier-Wood, et al. "Associations between Coffee, Tea, and Caffeine Intake with Coronary Artery Calcification and Cardiovascular Events." *American Journal of Medicine* 130, no. 2 (February 2017): 188–197.

Misaka, S., J. Yatabe, F. Müller, et al. "Green Tea Ingestion Greatly Reduces Plasma Concentrations of Nadolol in Healthy Subjects." *Clinical Pharmacology & Therapeutics* 95, no. 4 (April 2014): 432–438.

Oh, Chang-Mo, In-Hwan Oh, Bong-Keun Choe, et al. "Consuming Green Tea At Least Twice Each Day Is Associated with Reduced Odds of Chronic Obstructive Lung Disease in Middle-Aged and Older Korean Adults." *Journal of Nutrition* 148 (2018): 70–76.

Saito, E., M. Inoue, N. Sawada, et al. "Association of Green Tea Consumption with Mortality Due to all Causes and Major Causes of Death in a Japanese Population: The Japan Public Health Center-Based Prospective Study (JPHC Study)." *Annals of Epidemiology* 25 (2015): 512–518.

Tang, J., J. S. Zheng, L. Fang, et al. "Tea Consumption and Mortality of All Cancers, CVD and All Causes: A Meta-Analysis of Eighteen Prospective Cohort Studies." *British Journal of Nutrition* 114, no. 5 (September 14, 2015): 673–683.

Wang, Jing, Wei Zhang, Lu Sun, et al. "Green Tea Drinking and Risk of Pancreatic Cancer: A Large-Scale, Population-Based Case-Control Study in Urban Shanghai." *Cancer Epidemiology* 36 (2012): e354–e358.

Wang, X., J. Tian, J. Jiang, et al. "Effects of Green Tea or Green Tea Extract on Insulin Sensitivity and Glycaemic Control in Populations at Risk of Type 2 Diabetes Mellitus: A Systematic Review and Meta-Analysis of Randomised Controlled Trials." *Journal of Human Nutrition and Dietetics* 27, no. 5 (October 2014): 501–512.

Yang, Gong, Wei Zheng, Yong-Bing Xiang, et al. "Green Tea Consumption and Colorectal Cancer Risk: A Report from the Shanghai Men's Health Study." *Carcinogenesis* 32, no. 11 (2011): 1684–1688.

Hyaluronic Acid

Hyaluronic acid, also known as hyaluronan, is a clear substance naturally produced by the human body. It is primarily found in the joints and connective tissue, tendons, cartilage, skin, and eyes. Hyaluronic acid helps the body retain water, enabling tissues to remain moist and lubricated.

Though people may add oral hyaluronic acid supplements to their diets, creams, serums, and ointments are also widely available. Likewise, medical providers frequently use injectable hyaluronic acid to treat osteoarthritis and eye disorders. In addition, it may be injected into the skin and lips, reducing the signs of aging.

The human body can obtain hyaluronic acid from certain foods including grass-fed meats, especially pork, poultry, and beef. Prepared from bones, cartilage, and ligaments, bone broth is a great source of hyaluronic acid. In addition, some foods help the body synthesize hyaluronic acid including foods containing high amounts of vitamin C, such as citrus fruits, and magnesium-rich foods, such as nuts, avocados, and bananas. However, as the body ages, it loses its ability to synthesize its own hyaluronic acid. Therefore, it is not uncommon for the elderly experiencing joint pain to consume hyaluronic acid supplements as joints that are well lubricated are less likely to be painful.

HEALTH BENEFITS AND RISKS

Although hyaluronic acid is probably best known for helping people with joint problems, such as osteoarthritis, it is widely recognized for its antiaging properties, such as reducing skin wrinkles. In addition, hyaluronic acid is said to have wound healing and antibacterial properties. It may even be useful for acid reflux, dry eye discomfort, and preserving bone strength.

Though hyaluronic acid supplementation is generally considered safe for most people, some may be advised to avoid adding it to the diet. These include people who are allergic or cannot tolerate meats, poultry, and eggs, people on blood-thinning medications, or those suffering from blood-clotting disorders. People who develop an infection near an affected joint should not take hyaluronic acid, at least until the infection is resolved. Pregnant and breastfeeding women should probably avoid this supplement, and it should not be given to children under the age of 18 years. The use of the supplement in these groups has not been properly researched. There is some very limited evidence that hyaluronic acid may facilitate the growth of cancer cells. People dealing with cancer or who have a history of cancer may wish to avoid the supplementation. Whether hyaluronic acid is associated with cancer risk is extremely controversial and quite contentious.

The only known side effect associated with topical hyaluronic acid is dryness. True allergic reactions to hyaluronic acid are believed to be rare.

HOW IT IS SOLD AND TAKEN

Hyaluronic acid is sold as a liquid, ointment, cream, and serum. In addition, it may be purchased in capsules, tablets, and as an extract. Though dosage recommendations vary, a dose of 50 mg twice each day with meals is frequently recommended. Others advise 80 to 200 mg daily. Medical providers often suggest higher doses or oral supplementation with injections. Be aware that most hyaluronic acid supplements are made from chickens. Hence, vegetarians and vegans who want to take this supplement need to search for a nonanimal source. Hyaluronic acid may be prepared from bacteria. For dry eyes, a frequent recommendation is 0.2% hyaluronic acid eye drop three or four times per day for 3 months.

RESEARCH FINDINGS

Hyaluronic Acid Oral Supplementation Appears to Be Useful for People with Osteoarthritis

In a double-blind, randomized, placebo-controlled study published in 2015 in the journal *Rheumatology International*, researchers from Michigan and California (USA) as well as Spain evaluated a supplement containing hyaluronic acid on obese people who had knee osteoarthritis for at least 10 months. The researchers recruited 51 male and female participants between the ages of 40 and 75 years, and placed them on the supplement (80 mg per day) or placebo for 3 months. Forty participants (78%) completed the trial. Compared to those taking the placebo, the participants on hyaluronic acid supplementation had improvements in pain, function, and inflammation. The researchers concluded that their hyaluronic acid supplementation "holds promise for a safe and effective agent for the treatment of patients with knee osteoarthritis and who are overweight."[1]

Oral Hyaluronic Acid Appears to Be Useful for Chronic Joint Pain

In a randomized, double-blind, placebo-controlled trial published in 2015 in the *Journal of Medicinal Food*, researchers from Klamath Falls, Oregon (USA), wanted to determine if the daily oral intake of a liquid product containing high-molecular-weight hyaluronic acid would be useful for chronic joint pain. The initial cohort consisted of 78 people between the ages of 19 and 71 years. For 2 weeks, they took either 45 mL of the product each day or a placebo; then, for the last 2 weeks of the trial, they took either 30 mL per day of the product or a placebo.

Seventy-two people completed the 4-week trial. While the researchers learned that the participants in both groups experienced reductions in pain, the reductions in the supplement group were "more robust." The participants in both groups used less pain medication during the day; however, the reduction in the supplement group was, again, "more robust." The participants in the supplement group had a significant increase in sleep quality and physical energy levels. The researchers commented that "the data presented here suggest that high-molecular-weight HA [hyaluronic acid] offers a noninvasive method for pain management in situations involving moderate chronic joint pain affecting mobility."[2]

In a 12-month, prospective, randomized, double-blind, placebo-controlled trial published in 2012 in *Scientific World Journal*, researchers from Japan assigned 60 participants with knee osteoarthritis to 200 mg per day of hyaluronic acid or a placebo, which contained corn starch. All participants were told to complete a quadriceps strengthening exercise with straight leg raising, which is believed to be useful for knee osteoarthritis. Further, the participants were asked to maintain a daily exercise log. The researchers completed periodic assessments. By the end of 12 months, there were 18 participants in the supplement group and 20 in the placebo group. Although the participants in both groups experienced improvements in their knee osteoarthritis conditions, the improvements in the supplement group were more "obvious." The supplement appeared to be more effective for those between the ages of 50 and 70 than those over the age of 70 years. The researchers concluded that "Oral administration of HA [hyaluronic acid] may improve the symptoms of knee OA [osteoarthritis] in patients 70 years or younger when combined with the quadriceps strengthening exercise."[3]

Topical Hyaluronic Acid Has Wound Healing Properties

In a double-blind, randomized, multicenter trial published in 2012 in the *Journal of Wound Care*, researchers from France and Poland evaluated the wound healing properties of hyaluronic acid. The trial was conducted between June 2007 and November 2009; all the study participants had at least one leg ulcer. The initial cohort consisted of 101 participants. The hyaluronic acid group had 50 participants, whereas the control group had 51 participants. The trial continued for 60 days or until the wound was completely healed. In participants with multiple ulcers, one ulcer was selected to be included in the trial. The applications were applied daily by a nurse at the participant's home or in various care facilities. The cream was applied with sterile gauze directly on the wound. More than 79% of the participants did not miss any daily applications of their allocated treatments. Yet, 27 participants did not complete the trial (11 from the treatment group and 16 from the control group). Additionally, 77 adverse events were reported, of which 39 were considered related to the treatment. There was no statistical difference in adverse events between the two groups. The researchers learned that on day 45 of the treatment, the percentage reduction in ulcer surface was significantly greater in the hyaluronic acid group than the control group. Similar results were obtained at other times when the wounds were evaluated. In addition, the participants in the hyaluronic acid group had significantly lower levels of pain. Yet, considering other factors, such as the rate of complete healing and wound characteristics, there were no significant differences between the two treatments. The researchers concluded that "hyaluronic acid cream was significantly more effective than the neutral vehicle in the local treatment of leg ulcers of venous or mixed aetiology, in terms of wound size reduction and reducing the burden of pain, with a good safety profile."[4]

Oral Hyaluronic Supplement Benefits the Skin

In a study published in 2017 in the *Journal of Evidence-Based Complementary & Alternative Medicine*, researchers from Germany examined the effect of the oral intake of hyaluronic supplement, Regulatpro Hyaluron, on several aspects of the skin. The cohort consisted of 20 female participants with healthy skin between the ages of 45 and 60 years. At baseline, all participants were examined by a dermatologist. The participants drank the hyaluronic acid supplement followed by a glass of water in the morning. The participants were assessed again after 20 and 40 days. The researchers learned that the intake of the supplement solution led to a significant increase in skin elasticity and hydration as well as a significant decrease in skin roughness and wrinkle depths. By the end of the trial, 70% of the participants noted that they would recommend the supplement, and 60% were willing to purchase the product. During the course of the trial, no side effects or unwanted skin changes were noted. Hence, the researchers concluded that "the impact of HA [hyaluronic acid] over a longer period of time seems to have a positive impact on skin health."[5]

In a pilot open-label trial published in 2012 in the journal *Clinical Interventions in Aging*, researchers from Port Chester, New York and Newport Beach, California (USA), investigated the effect on the skin of a dietary supplement containing low-molecular-weight hyaluronic acid, hydrolyzed collagen type II, and chondroitin sulfate. The cohort consisted of 26 healthy females between the ages of 35 and 59 years, who had visible signs of skin aging. They had mild-to-moderate photodamaged skin and mild-to-moderate fine lines and wrinkles. Approximately half of the participants were Caucasian. During the trial, the participants were instructed to take two capsules (1 g) daily, and were told to refrain from using any other product that would affect the skin. The participants were assessed at baseline, at 6 weeks, at 12 weeks, and when the trial ended. No adverse effects were reported. The researchers learned that the supplement triggered a significant decrease in facial lines, wrinkles, dryness, and scaling. They concluded that the dietary supplement "elicited several physiological events which can be harnessed to counteract natural photoaging processes to reduce visible aging signs in the human face."[6]

Hyaluronic Acid Cream Has Antiaging Skin Properties

In a study published in 2011 in *Journal of Drugs in Dermatology*, researchers from Germany and Denmark tested the ability of topical applications of 0.1%

hyaluronic acid of different molecular weights to relax wrinkles. The cohort consisted of 76 participants between the ages of 30 and 60 years. For 60 days, the participants applied one of the creams to one side of the face twice a day; a placebo cream was applied to the other side of the face. During the trial, the participants were instructed not to use other products in the tested areas and to avoid exposure to ultraviolet radiation. The researchers assessed a number of factors such as skin hydration, skin elasticity, and wrinkles. They found that all the creams containing hyaluronic acid resulted in improvements in skin hydration and overall elasticity values compared to the placebo. Application of low-molecular-weight hyaluronic acid was associated with significant reduction of wrinkle depth. These changes were sometimes seen as early as 1 month of application. Further, "objective measurement methods were used to document the effects" in this study.[7]

Hyaluronic Acid Foam Is Useful for Treating Mild-to-Moderate Atopic Dermatitis

In a single-center, double-blind, randomized trial published in 2011 in the *Journal of Cosmetic Dermatology*, a researcher from North Carolina (USA) examined the use of a hyaluronic acid foam and a ceramide-containing emulsion cream for the treatment of mild-to-moderate atopic dermatitis (red and itchy skin). The researcher enrolled 20 participants aged 18 years or older. The participants were told to place the hyaluronic acid foam on one limb and the ceramide cream on the opposite limb twice daily. The researcher only evaluated treatments on the arms or legs. The participants reported appearance of redness, peeling, drying, stinging/burning, and overall skin irritation. After 4 weeks of treatment with both products, 18 participants completed the trial. The researcher learned that by the end of the trial both treatments achieved statistically significant improvement in all clinical signs and symptoms of atopic dermatitis. However, after 2 weeks, the hyaluronic acid foam achieved statistically significant improvement in overall eczema severity, whereas the ceramide cream did not. Furthermore, in all studied areas, such as ease of use, odor, and better efficacy, the hyaluronic acid foam was statistically preferred over the ceramide cream. The participants indicated that they would purchase the hyaluronic acid foam over the ceramide cream. If people prefer a product, they are more likely to continue to use it. The researcher concluded that "an emollient with excellent esthetics may improve compliance and enhance efficacy when applied with topical corticosteroids, standard initial therapy for managing the inflammation associated with an atopic dermatitis flare."[8]

Hyaluronic Acid Is Useful for Dry Eye Syndrome, and When Combined with the Common Sugar Trehalose, It Works Even Better

In a phase III, randomized, active-controlled, investigator-masked, multicenter trial published in 2017 in the *European Journal of Ophthalmology*, researchers from France and Tunisia compared the efficacy and safety of an eye drop containing hyaluronic acid to an eye drop containing hyaluronic acid and the common sugar trehalose. The cohort consisted of 105 adults who were 18 years old or older from France and Tunisia. All participants had moderate-to-severe dry eye disease. (Dry eye disease is characterized by ocular discomfort, visual disturbance, and tear film instability.) For 84 days, 53 participants were treated with hyaluronic acid eye drops, and 52 were treated with hyaluronic acid and trehalose eye drops. Periodic assessments were conducted. The researchers found that the hyaluronic acid–trehalose eye drop was well-tolerated and had fewer adverse effects than the hyaluronic acid eye drop. By day 35 of the trial, the researchers saw a clear benefit of the combination eye drop and a very evident improvement in the quality of life of the participants. The researchers concluded that "hyaluronic acid-trehalose is effective and safe, with better patient satisfaction than existing HA-only eyedrops particularly from the first month of treatment, and offers a therapeutic advancement in the treatment of moderate to severe DED [dry eye disease]."[9]

Hyaluronic Acid May Be Useful for Nonerosive Reflux Disease

In a multicenter, randomized, double-blind trial published in 2017 in the journal *Alimentary Pharmacology and Therapeutics*, researchers from Italy wanted to determine if a medication that combined hyaluronic acid and chondroitin sulfate (Esoxx) would help people with nonerosive reflux disease (NERD). The cohort, which was drawn from 16 Italian hospitals, consisted of 154 participants suffering from NERD; all participants, who ranged in age from 18 to 75 years, received the supplement (n = 76) or a placebo (n = 78). During the 14-day treatment period, all participants also took a standard dose of an acid suppressant with standard-dose proton pump inhibitors. At baseline and at the end of the trial, the researchers assessed the degree of heartburn, acid regurgitation, retrosternal pain, acid taste in the mouth, and health-related quality of life. Additionally, the participants maintained daily symptom diaries. Eighteen participants did not complete the trial. The researchers determined that a significantly higher proportion of the participants taking the combined supplement rather than the placebo obtained symptom relief. They concluded that "the results of this study show that, when mucosal protection is added to acid suppression, a significantly higher number of NERD patients obtained symptoms relief with combination therapy."[10]

Hyaluronic Acid Oral Supplementation May or May Not Foster the Growth of Cancer Cells

In an article published in 2015 in the journal *Clinical Drug Investigation*, researchers from Italy acknowledged the possible benefits of oral hyaluronic acid for people suffering from osteoarthritis. Yet, they noted that there are now many oral hyaluronic products on the market, some of which may expose people with a history of cancer to an increased risk of recurrence. According to the researchers, oral hyaluronic acid may "interact with specific receptors and promote cell proliferation." In people with a history of cancer, this interaction may be harmful. People who take oral hyaluronic acid supplementation for osteoarthritis tend to do so for longer periods of time. In addition, to obtain the relief they want, people may take higher doses; there is no proof that such a higher intake is safe. The researchers advised people who have been diagnosed with cancer within the previous 5 years to avoid taking oral hyaluronic acid supplementation. They commented that "this interaction may be potentially hazardous in cancer patients for which these oral formulations should be contraindicated."[11]

On the other hand, in an article published in 2014 in the *Journal of Food Science*, researchers from Japan came to a very different conclusion. In their various in vitro tests on cells and in vivo tests on mice, they found that oral hyaluronic acid "has little effect on the proliferation of several cancer cell lines." In their in vitro studies, they used two types of hyaluronic acid, neither of which altered several cancer cell lines. In their in vivo study, supplementation with oral hyaluronic did not change "tumor proliferation, metastasis, or angiogenesis." The researchers concluded "that exogenously administered HA, including HA administered orally, has little effect on cancer."[12]

NOTES

1. Nelson, F. R., R. A. Zvirbulis, B. Zonca, et al. "The Effects of an Oral Preparation Containing Hyaluronic Acid (Oralvisc®) on Obese Knee Osteoarthritis Patients Determined by Pain, Function, Bradykinin, Leptin, Inflammatory Cytokines, and Heavy Water Analysis." *Rheumatology International* 35, no. 1 (January 2015): 43–52.

2. Jensen, Gitte S., Victoria L. Attridge, Miki R. Lenninger, and Kathleen F. Bensen. "Oral Intake of a Liquid High-Molecular-Weight Hyaluronan Associated with Relief of Chronic Pain and Reduced Use of Pain Medication: Results of a Randomized, Place-Controlled Double-Blind Pilot Study." *Journal of Medicinal Food* 18, no. 1 (2015): 95–101.

3. Tashiro, T., S. Seino, T. Sato, et al. "Oral Administration of Polymer Hyaluronic Acid Alleviates Symptoms of Knee Osteoarthritis: A Double-Blind, Placebo-Controlled Study over a 12-Month Period." *Scientific World Journal* 2012 (2012): Article ID: 167928.

4. Dereure, O., M. Czubek, and P. Combemale. "Efficacy and Safety of Hyaluronic Acid in Treatment of Leg Ulcers: A Double-Blind RCT." *Journal of Wound Care* 21, no. 3 (March 2012): 131–132, 134–136, and 138–139.

5. Göllner, I., W. Voss, U. von Hehn, and S. Kammerer. "Ingestion of an Oral Hyaluronan Solution Improves Skin Hydration, Wrinkle Reduction, Elasticity, and Skin Roughness: Results of a Clinical Study." *Journal of Evidence-Based Complementary & Alternative Medicine* 22, no. 4 (October 2017): 816–823.

6. Schwartz, S. R. and J. Park. "Ingestion of BioCell Collagen®, a Novel Hydrolyzed Chicken Sternal Cartilage Extract; Enhanced Blood Microcirculation and Reduced Facial Aging Signs." *Clinical Interventions in Aging* 7 (2012): 267–273.

7. Pavicic, T., G. G. Gauglitz, P. Lersch, et al. "Efficacy of Cream-Based Novel Formations of Hyaluronic Acid of Different Molecular Weight in Anti-Wrinkle Treatment." *Journal of Drugs in Dermatology* 10, no. 9 (September 2011): 990–1000.

8. Draelos, Z. D. "A Clinical Evaluation of the Comparable Efficacy of Hyaluronic Acid-Based Foam and Ceramide-Containing Emulsion Cream in the Treatment of Mild-to-Moderate Dermatitis." *Journal of Cosmetic Dermatology* 10, no. 3 (September 2011): 185–188.

9. Chiambaretta, F., S. Doan, M. Labetoulle, et al. "A Randomized, Controlled Study of the Efficacy and Safety of a New Eyedrop Formulation for Moderate to Severe Dry Eye." *European Journal of Ophthalmology* 27, no. 1 (January 19, 2017): 1–9.

10. Savarino, V., F. Pace, and C. Scarpignato. "Randomised Clinical Trial: Muvosal Protection Combined with Acid Suppression in the Treatment of Non-Erosive Reflux Disease–Efficacy of Esoxx, a Hyaluronic Acid-Chondroitin Sulphate Based Bioadhesive Formulation." *Alimentary Pharmacology and Therapeutics* 45 (2017): 631–642.

11. Simone, P., and M. Alberto. "Caution Should Be Used in Long-Term Treatment with Oral Compounds of Hyaluronic Acid in Patients with a History of Cancer." *Clinical Drug Investigation* 35, no. 11 (November 2015): 689–692.

12. Seino, S., F. Takeshita, A. Asari, et al. "No Influence of Exogenous Hyaluronan on the Behavior of Human Cancer Cells or Endothelial Cell Capillary Formation." *Journal of Food Science* 79, no. 7 (July 2014): T1469–T1475.

REFERENCES AND FURTHER READING

Chiambaretta, F., S. Doan, M. Labetoulle, et al. "A Randomized, Controlled Study of the Efficacy and Safety of a New Eyedrop Formulation for Moderate to Severe Dry Eye Syndrome." *European Journal of Ophthalmology* 27, no. 1 (January 19, 2017): 1–9.

Dereure, O., M. Czubek, and P. Combemale. "Efficacy and Safety of Hyaluronic Acid in Treatment of Leg Ulcers: A Double-Blind RCT." *Journal of Wound Care* 21, no. 3 (March 2012): 131–132, 134–136, and 138–139.

Draelos, Z. D. "A Clinical Evaluation of the Comparable Efficacy of Hyaluronic Acid-Based Foam and Ceramide-Containing Emulsion Cream in the Treatment of Mild-to-Moderate Atopic Dermatitis." *Journal of Cosmetic Dermatology* 10, no. 3 (September 2011): 185–188.

Göllner, I., W. Voss, U. von Hehn, and S. Kammerer. "Ingestion of an Oral Hyaluronan Solution Improved Skin Hydration, Wrinkle Reduction, Elasticity, and Skin Roughness: Results of a Clinical Study." *Journal of Evidence-Based Complementary and Alternative Medicine* 22, no. 4 (October 2017): 816–823.

Jensen, Gitte S., Victoria L. Attridge, Miki R. Lenninger, and Kathleen F. Benson. "Oral Intake of a Liquid High-Molecular-Weight Hyaluronan Associated with Relief of Chronic Pain and Reduced Use of Pain Medication: Results of a Randomized, Placebo-Controlled Double-Blind Pilot Study." *Journal of Medicinal Food* 18, no. 1 (2015): 95–101.

Nelson, F. R., R. A. Zvirbulis, B. Zonca, et al. "The Effects of an Oral Preparation Containing Hyaluronic Acid (Oralvisc®) on Obese Knee Osteoarthritis Patients Determined by Pain, Function, Bradykinin, Leptin, Inflammatory Cytokines, and Heavy Water Analyses." *Rheumatology International* 35 (2015): 43–52.

Pavicic, T., G. G. Gauglitz, P. Lersch, et al. "Efficacy of Cream-Based Novel Formulations of Hyaluronic Acid of Different Molecular Weights in Anti-Wrinkle Cream." *Journal of Drugs in Dermatology* 10, no. 9 (September 2011): 990–1000.

Savarino, V., F. Pace, and C. Scarpignato. "Randomised Clinical Trial: Mucosal Protection Combined with Acid Suppression in the Treatment of Non-Erosive Reflux Disease–Efficacy of Esoxx, a Hyaluronic Acid–Chondroitin Sulphate Based Bioadhesive Formulation." *Alimentary Pharmacology and Therapeutics* 45 (2017): 631–642.

Schwartz, S. R. and J. Park. "Ingestion of BioCell Collagen®, a Novel Hydrolyzed Chicken Sternal Cartilage Extract: Enhanced Blood Microcirculation and Reduced Facial Aging Signs." *Clinical Interventions in Aging* 7 (2012): 267–273.

Seino, S., F. Takeshita. A. Asari, et al. "No Influence of Exogenous Hyaluronan on the Behavior of Human Cancer Cells or Endothelial Cell Capillary Formation." *Journal of Food Science* 79, no. 7 (July 2014): T1469–T1475.

Simone, P. and M. Alberto. "Caution Should Be Used in Long-Term Treatment with Oral Compounds of Hyaluronic Acid in Patients with a History of Cancer." *Clinical Drug Investigation* 35, no. 11 (November 2015): 689–692.

Tashiro, T., S. Seino, T. Sato, et al. "Oral Administration of Polymer Hyaluronic Acid Alleviates Symptoms of Knee Osteoarthritis: A Double-Blind, Placebo-Controlled Study over a 12-Month Period." *Scientific World Journal* 2012 (2012): Article ID: 167928.

Krill Oil

Krill oil is a supplement prepared from krill, a small, shrimp-like crustacean. Situated at the bottom of the food chain, krill feed primarily on phytoplankton, also known as microscopic marine algae.

Krill oil is often compared to fish oil, both of which have beneficial omega-3 fatty acids including eicosapentaenoic acid (EPA) and docosahexaenoic acid (DHA). Thus, they both support cardiovascular health, skin health, and have anti-inflammatory properties. However, the phospholipid-derived fatty acids in krill oil allow it to be better absorbed than fish oil. Moreover, krill oil contains astaxanthin, a carotenoid with strong antioxidant properties, enabling it to fight free radicals in the body. In addition, because krill eat algae, they are thought to be purer than other types of fish, which may have heavy metals and/or mercury. Because krill are an incredibly abundant animal species, they are said to be a more sustainable source of omega-3 fatty acids.

HEALTH BENEFITS AND RISKS

Krill oil is thought to reduce the risk of chronic illnesses such as cardiovascular disease and cancer. Other benefits include antiaging properties, brain health, strengthening bones and joints, aiding in weight loss, and maintaining glowing skin.

Potential side effects of krill oil supplementation include bad breath, belching, fishy aftertaste, heartburn, nausea, indigestion, and stomach upset. People on blood-thinning medication should not consume krill oil as it may trigger excessive bleeding. People who have an allergy to seafood or shellfish should also not consume krill oil.

HOW IT IS SOLD AND TAKEN

Most krill oil is sold in softgels and capsules. Recommendations vary from 250 to 500 mg per day to 1000 to 3000 mg per day. In most instances, it is best to begin with a lower dose, gradually increasing it over time. It is important to discuss krill oil supplementation with a medical provider.

RESEARCH FINDINGS

Krill Oil Supplementation Appears to Be Useful for Mild Knee Joint Pain

In a randomized, double-blind trial published in 2016 in the online journal *PLoS ONE*, researchers from Japan investigated the ability of krill oil supplementation to benefit those with mild knee joint pain. The cohort consisted of 50 adults between the ages of 38 and 85 years, with mild knee pain. The participants were seen at the Fukushima Orthopedic Clinic in Tochigi, Japan between September 2014 and March 2015. All of the subjects complained of knee pain but did not require pain medication. For 30 days, the participants took either 2 g per day of a krill oil supplement or an identical appearing placebo. The researchers assessed the levels of knee pain. Forty-seven participants completed the intervention and examinations. The researchers learned that, though the participants in both groups experienced significant improvement in knee pain, the improvement in the krill oil group was better than that in the placebo group. When the researchers controlled for age, sex, weight, smoking, and drinking habits, they found that krill oil significantly lowered knee pain during sleeping, standing, and range of motion for both right and left knees compared to the placebo. The researchers concluded that their findings "demonstrated that krill oil could mitigate the subjective symptoms of mild knee pain."[1]

Krill Oil Supplementation May or May Not Lower Serum Triglyceride Levels

In a double-blind, randomized, multicenter, placebo-controlled trial published in 2014 in the journal *Nutrition Research*, researchers from Norway and Canada tested the ability of krill oil to lower the levels of fasting serum triglycerides in participants with a low fish intake and borderline high or high levels of fasting serum triglyceride (150–499 mg/dL). The cohort of 300 male and female participants was divided into five groups—placebo (olive oil), 0.5 g per day, 1 g per day, 2 g per day, or 4 g per day of krill oil. Serum lipid levels were measured at baseline, at 6 weeks, at 12 weeks, when the trial ended. Data on 267 participants were included in the analysis. Compared to the placebo group, the participants in the krill oil groups, who were pooled for the analysis, had a statistically significant reduction in serum triglyceride levels. Moreover, krill oil lowered triglyceride levels in people with borderline or high levels of triglycerides without increasing the levels of low-density lipoprotein cholesterol (LDL) or "bad" cholesterol. The findings suggest that "krill oil is effective in reducing a cardiovascular risk factor."[2]

In a trial published in 2018 in the *Journal of Nutritional Science*, researchers from Norway compared the cardiovascular benefits of taking krill oil supplements to the benefits of consuming lean and fatty fish. The cohort consisted of 36 healthy participants between the ages of 18 and 70 years who had slightly elevated triglyceride levels. For 8 weeks, they were randomized to consume lean or fatty fish or take a krill oil supplement or a placebo. The 12 people in the fish group ate three weekly fish meals. The 12 people in the krill oil group and the 12 people in the placebo (high-oleic sunflower oil) group took a total of 4 g per day of oil. Blood samples were drawn at baseline and at the end of the trial. The researchers found that the intake of krill oil or lean and fatty fish do not significantly reduce serum triglyceride levels, though all but two people in the krill group had reduced fasting triglyceride levels. Krill oil supplements significantly reduced blood glucose levels, and fish intake increased vitamin D levels, a "clinically relevant" finding.[3]

Krill Oil Seems to Have Several Properties That Support Cardiovascular Health, But It May or May Not Trigger Small Elevations in Cholesterol

In a systematic review and meta-analysis published in 2017 in the journal *Nutrition Reviews*, researchers from many different countries examined the lipid modifying effects of krill oil in humans. They focused on randomly controlled trials that investigated the impact of at least 2 weeks of krill oil supplementation on a minimum of one lipid parameter. The researchers located seven relevant trials with 427 participants in the krill oil supplement groups and 235 participants in control groups. The number of participants in these trials ranged from 20 to 267. Krill oil doses ranged from 500 mg per day to 4 g per day, and the duration of supplementation ranged from 4 weeks to 3 months. The researchers determined that krill oil supplementation caused a significant reduction in LDL and triglyceride levels. Additionally, it significantly increased high-density lipoprotein cholesterol (HDL) or "good" cholesterol. A reduction in total cholesterol levels was notable, but did not reach statistical significance. The researchers concluded that "the favorable effects of krill oil on the lipid profile found in the current meta-analysis suggest the use of this marine product as an interesting add-on therapy in dyslipidemic patients."[4]

On the other hand, in a pilot trial published in 2015 in the journal *Lipids in Health and Disease*, researchers from Norway assembled a cohort of 18 healthy volunteers with a mean age of 23 years. All participants took nine 500 mg krill oil capsules per day for 28 days, and a number of different assessments were conducted. Seventeen participants (15 females and two males) were included in the analysis. The researchers found that krill oil supplementation reduced several parameters linked to cardiovascular risk, such as plasma levels, lipoprotein particle concentrations, fatty acid compositions, and redox status. However, there were small elevations in cholesterol levels. The researchers concluded that "krill oil had beneficial biological effects in persons with a normal lipid profile and may prevent the development of several risk factors related to CVD [cardiovascular disease]."[5]

Krill Oil Supplementation Does Not Appear to Influence Exercise Performance

In a trial published in 2015 in *PLoS ONE*, researchers from Scotland wanted to learn more about the association between krill oil supplementation and exercise performance. The cohort consisted of 19 males and 18 females with a mean age of 25.8 years. The participants were randomly assigned to consume 2 g of krill oil each day (n = 18) or a placebo (n = 19) for six weeks. At baseline and at the end of the trial, the participants completed a maximal incremental exercise test (a test that increases in intensity) and a cycling time trial (tests riders against the clock). Blood samples were collected before and after supplementation and at three points after exercising. The researchers determined that krill oil supplementation did not increase or alter exercise performance in the young and healthy volunteers.

Likewise, krill oil did not affect time trial performance, nor were heart rates or oxygen consumption altered. But, the researchers added that krill oil, and other fish oils, may be useful for other populations, such as older people, or in other exercise forms, such as strength training. They also commented that it may be true that krill and other fish oil "simply do not alter endurance exercise performance."[6]

But Krill Oil May Support Resistance Exercise

In a double-blind, placebo-controlled trial published in 2018 in the *Journal of Nutrition and Metabolism*, researchers from Wisconsin and North Carolina (USA) wanted to determine if krill oil has any effect on muscle growth and recovery after resistance exercise. The cohort consisted of 21 male participants between the ages of 18 and 30 years. They were divided into a krill oil supplementation group (3 g krill oil per day) or a placebo group (olive oil). The krill oil dosage delivered 240 mg of DHA and 393 mg of EPA, as well as a small amount of astaxanthin. All participants took part in an 8-week resistance training program. At baseline and again at the end of the trial, body composition, maximal strength, peak power, and the rate of perceived recovery were assessed. Other assessments included complete blood counts, urinalyses, and measurements of safety parameter and cognitive performance. Eighteen participants completed the trial; there were nine participants in each group. The researchers learned that exercise-induced lean body mass significantly increased among participants in the krill oil group. The researchers concluded that "krill oil supplementation in athletes is safe and while no significant effect on cognition and strength were observed, its effects on body composition with resistance exercise deserves further research."[7]

Krill Oil and Fish Oil May or May Not Have Different Levels of Bioavailability

In an analysis published in 2015 in the journal *Vascular Health and Risk Management*, researchers from Norway examined 14 original studies on the bioavailability levels of krill oil and fish oil supplements. Seven studies were clinical trials (five double-blind and two open-label) and seven were animal studies. Three clinical studies included healthy participants between the ages of 20 and 50; two studies included healthy overweight or obese participants between the ages of 35 and 64 years; and two studies included healthy participants with normal or slightly elevated lipid levels and patients with hyperlipidemia, with mean ages between 40 and 50 years. All but one study included both males and females. According to the researchers, the clinical studies suggested that there was a difference in bioavailability between krill oil and fish oil supplements. Two of the human studies found that the bioavailability of EPA and DHA were better from krill oil than fish oil. However, the researchers stressed the need for "better-designed clinical studies" that clarify "the beneficial health effects" of krill oil compared to fish oil. The animal studies found very little differences between the health effects of krill oil and fish oil supplements.[8]

It Is Not Clear If Krill Oil Is Useful for Depression in Adults

In an analysis published in 2015 in the *Cochrane Database of Systematic Reviews*, researchers from the United Kingdom examined randomized controlled trials on the use of omega-3 fatty acids, such as krill oil, for depression in adults. The researchers identified 26 relevant studies. Twenty-five studies with a total of 1438 participants compared omega-3 fatty acids to a placebo, and one study compared the use of omega-3 fatty acids to antidepressant treatment. For the placebo comparison, the researchers found a small-to-modest benefit for depressive symptomology, which was unlikely to be "clinically meaningful." Unfortunately, most studies were small and had a high risk of bias on several measures. The researchers noted that their analysis was likely influenced by three large trials. One study that compared omega-3 fatty acids to antidepressant medication had only 40 participants and found no difference in the treatments in depressive symptomology, rates of response to treatment, or failure to complete. The researchers concluded that they "do not have sufficient high quality evidence to determine the effects" of omega-3 fatty acids for major depressive disorder. Finally, concluding that "more evidence and more complete evidence are required."[9]

People with Type 2 Diabetes May Benefit from Krill Oil Supplementation

In a randomized, double-blind, controlled, crossover trial published in 2015 in the journal *BMJ Open Diabetes Research & Care*, researchers from Danbury, Connecticut (USA), evaluated the effects of krill oil supplementation on cardiovascular risks in people with type 2 diabetes. The 47 participants, with a mean age of 64.8 years, had confirmed type 2 diabetes; 66% of the participants were males. Seventy-two percent had high blood pressure; 74% had elevated cholesterol levels; and 81% were taking a statin to lower cholesterol levels. The participants were placed on krill oil (100 mg per day) or olive oil supplementation for 4 weeks. After a 2-week washout period, they were placed on the other supplement. All participants were offered an optional 17 weeks of krill oil supplementation. Testing took place at baseline, after completing the first supplement, after completing the second supplement, and after the additional 17 weeks of krill oil. A total of 34 participants completed the additional 17-week supplementation. The researchers determined that krill oil supplementation improved endothelial functioning and increased HDL. Why is this important? The researchers noted that cardiovascular disease is the most common cause of death in people with type 2 diabetes. The researchers concluded that "krill oil may lead to moderate improvement of cardiovascular risks, specifically endothelial dysfunction and HDL in patients with type 2 diabetes."[10]

Krill Oil Appears to Support Human Brain Function in the Elderly

In a randomized, double-blind, parallel-group trial published in 2013 in the journal *Clinical Interventions in Aging*, researchers from Japan wanted to determine if krill oil supplement would benefit brain function in the elderly. The cohort consisted of 45 healthy men between the ages of 61 and 72 years. A psychiatrist confirmed that none of the participants had cognitive impairment. For 12 weeks, they were placed on krill oil, sardine oil, or a placebo oil; each group included 15 participants. Various tests were conducted at periodic intervals. A food frequency questionnaire evaluated the participants' diet. By the end of the trial, there were 13 participants in the krill oil group, 14 in the sardine oil group, and 15 in the placebo group. The cognitive benefits were best among men in the krill oil group, and the intake of krill oil was associated with enhanced performance of calculations. The participants in the krill and sardine oil groups performed better on the working memory tasks than those in the placebo group. Still, the researchers added that "krill oil demonstrated effects that were equivalent to or better than those of sardine oil." They also underscored the need for future trials with larger sample sizes and the inclusion of women.[11]

When Combined with Salmon Oil, Krill Oil Supplementation Appears to Lower Insulin Sensitivity in Overweight Men

In a randomized, double-blind, controlled, crossover trial published in 2015 in the *American Journal of Clinical Nutrition*, researchers from New Zealand and Australia wanted to learn how a supplement containing krill and salmon oil would affect overweight men. The cohort consisted of 47 men with a mean age of 46.5 years, who were all overweight but otherwise healthy. For 8 weeks, the participants took krill oil supplementation (five 1 g capsules per day) or a placebo. After an 8-week washout period, they switched to the other treatment for an additional 8 weeks. The supplementation was 88% krill oil and 12% salmon oil; the placebo group was given canola oil. The researchers conducted periodic assessments. They learned that insulin sensitivity was 14% lower among men on supplementation than those in the placebo group. Further, when they controlled for the likely positive effects of blood EPA and DHA, the reduction in insulin sensitivity was 27% lower than the control oil. As a result, the krill and salmon oil supplementation "may increase [the] risk of developing type 2 diabetes and cardiovascular disease." Moreover, they "cautioned against the use of krill oil in individuals at increased risk of type 2 diabetes or cardiovascular disease."[12]

NOTES

1. Suzuki, Y., M. Fukushima, K. Sakuraba, et al. "Krill Oil Improves Mild Knee Joint Pain: A Randomized Control Trial." *PLoS ONE* 11, no. 10 (October 4, 2016): e0162769.

2. Berge, K., K. Musa-Velsos, M. Harwood, et al. "Krill Oil Supplementation Lowers Serum Triglycerides without Increasing Low-Density Lipoprotein Cholesterol in Adults with Borderline High or High Triglyceride Levels." *Nutrition Research* 34, no. 2 (February 2014): 126–133.

3. Rundblad, A., K. B. Holven, I. Bruheim, et al. "Effects of Krill Oil and Lean and Fatty Fish on Cardiovascular Risk Markers: A Randomised Controlled Trial." *Journal of Nutritional Science* 7 (2018): e3:11.

4. Ursoniu, S., A. Sahebkar, M. C. Serban, et al. "Lipid-Modifying Effects of Krill Oil in Humans: Systematic Review and Meta-Analysis of Randomized Controlled Trials." *Nutrition Reviews* 75, no. 5 (May 1, 2017): 361–373.

5. Berge, R. K., M. S. Ramsvik, P. Bohov, et al. "Krill Oil Reduces Plasma Triacylglycerol Level and Improves Related Lipoprotein Particle Concentration, Fatty Acid Composition and Redox Status in Healthy Young Adults–A Pilot Study." *Lipids in Health and Disease* 14 (2015): 163.

6. Da Boit, Mariasole, Ina Mastalurova, Goda Brazaite, et al. "The Effect of Krill Oil Supplementation on Exercise Performance and Markers of Immune Function." *PLoS ONE* 10, no. 9 (September 25, 2015): e0139174.

7. Georges, John, Matthew H. Sharp, Ryan P. Lowery, et al. "The Effects of Krill Oil on mTOR Signaling and Resistance Exercise: A Pilot Study." *Journal of Nutrition and Metabolism* 2018 (2018): Article ID: 7625981.

8. Ulven, S. M. and K. B. Holven. "Comparison of Bioavailability of Krill Oil versus Fish Oil and Health Effect." *Vascular Health and Risk Management* 11 (August 28, 2015): 511–524.

9. Appleton, K. M., H. M. Sallis, R. Perry, et al. "Omega-3 Fatty Acids for Depression in Adults." *Cochrane Database of Systematic Reviews* 11 (November 5, 2015): CD004692.

10. Lobraico, J. M., L. C. DiLello, A. D Butler, et al. "Effects of Krill Oil on Endothelial Function and Other Cardiovascular Risk Factors in Participants with Type 2 Diabetes, A Randomized Controlled Trial." *BMJ Open Diabetes Research & Care* 3 (2015): e000107.

11. Konagai, C., K. Yanagimoto, K. Hayamizu, et al. "Effects of Krill Oil Containing n-3 Polyunsaturated Fatty Acids in Phospholipid Form on Human Brain Function: A Randomized Controlled Trial in Healthy Elderly Volunteers." *Clinical Interventions in Aging* 8 (2013): 1247–1257.

12. Albert, B. B., J. G. Derraik, C. M. Brennan, et al. "Supplementation with a Blend of Krill and Salmon Oil Is Associated with Increased Metabolic Risk in Overweight Men." *American Journal of Clinical Nutrition* 102, no. 1 (July 2015): 49–57.

REFERENCES AND FURTHER READING

Albert, B. B., J. G. Derraik, C. M. Brennan, et al. "Supplementation with a Blend of Krill and Salmon Oil Is Associated with Increased Metabolic Risk in Overweight Men." *American Journal of Clinical Nutrition* 102, no. 1 (July 2015): 49–57.

Appleton, K. M., H. M. Sallis, R. Perry, et al. "Omega-3 Fatty Acids for Depression in Adults." *Cochrane Database of Systematic Reviews* 11 (November 5, 2015): CD004692.

Berge, K., K. Musa-Veloso, M. Harwood, et al. "Krill Oil Supplementation Lowers Serum Triglycerides without Increasing Low-Density Lipoprotein Cholesterol in Adults with Borderline High or High Triglyceride Levels." *Nutrition Research* 34, no. 2 (February 2014): 126–133.

Berge, R. K., M. S. Ramsvik, P. Bohov, et al. "Krill Oil Reduces Plasma Triacylglycerol Level and Improves Related Lipoprotein Particle Concentration, Fatty Acid Composition and Redox Status in Healthy Young Adults–A Pilot Study." *Lipids in Health and Disease* 14 (2015): 163.

Da Boit, Mariasole, Ina Mastaluriva, Goda Brazaite, et al. "The Effect of Krill Oil Supplementation on Exercise Performance and Markers of Immune Function." *PLoS ONE* 10, no. 9 (September 25, 2015): e0139174.

Georges, John, Matthew H. Sharp, Ryan P. Lowery, et al. "The Effects of Krill Oil on mTOR Signaling and Resistance Exercise: A Pilot Study." *Journal of Nutrition and Metabolism* 2018 (2018): Article ID: 7625981.

Konagai, C., K. Yanagimoto, K. Hayamizu, et al. "Effects of Krill Oil Containing n-3 Polyunsaturated Fatty Acids in Phospholipid Form on Human Brain Function: A Randomized Controlled Trial in Healthy Elderly Volunteers." *Clinical Interventions in Aging* 8 (2013): 1247–1257.

Lobraico, J. M., L. C. DiLello, A. D. Butler, et al. "Effects of Krill Oil on Endothelial Function and Other Cardiovascular Risk Factors in Participants with Type 2 Diabetes, a Randomized Controlled Trial." *BMJ Open Diabetes Research & Care* 3 (2015): e000107.

Rundblad, A., K. B. Holven, I. Bruheim, et al. "Effects of Krill Oil and Lean and Fatty Fish on Cardiovascular Risk Markers: A Randomised Controlled Trial." *Journal of Nutritional Science* 7 (January 17, 2018): e3: 11 pages.

Suzuki, Y., M. Fukushima, K. Sakuraba, et al. "Krill Oil Improves Mild Knee Joint Pain: A Randomized Control Trial." *PLoS ONE* 11, no. 10 (October 4, 2016): e0162769.

Ulven, S. M., and K. B. Holven. "Comparison of Bioavailability of Krill Oil versus Fish Oil and Health Effect." *Vascular Health and Risk Management* 11 (August 28, 2015): 511–524.

Ursoniu, S., A. Sahebkar, M. C. Serban, et al. "Lipid-Modifying Effects of Krill Oil in Humans: Systematic Review and Meta-Analysis of Randomized Controlled Trials." *Nutrition Reviews* 75, no. 5 (May 1, 2017): 361–373.

L-Theanine

L-theanine is an amino acid found in tea leaves, especially green and black tea leaves, and some mushrooms. First identified by Japanese scientists in 1949, L-theanine is similar in structure to glutamate, a naturally occurring amino acid that helps transmit nerve impulses.

L-theanine is a psychoactive substance that can cross the blood–brain barrier. In fact, within 30 min of oral ingestion, it crosses the barrier, and is able to do so at relatively low doses. Researchers have determined that L-theanine supplementation elevates levels of gamma-aminobutyric acid (GABA), serotonin, and dopamine—neurotransmitters that regulate several cognitive functions, such as mood and alertness. Moreover, GABA lowers stress signals in the brain, and serotonin and dopamine support improvements in mood and a sense of well-being.

There are two forms of theanine: L-theanine and D-theanine. However, almost all of theanine—about 98%—is L-theanine. This entry only addresses L-theanine.

HEALTH BENEFITS AND RISKS

L-theanine is thought to be useful to promote relaxation, reduce stress, and improve sleep. At the same time, it is believed to increase concentration and alertness and relieve fatigue. People also use L-theanine for anxiety, depression, schizophrenia, attention deficit hyperactivity disorder (ADHD), elevated blood pressure, as well as to prevent flu and Alzheimer's disease. It may even have anticancer properties, and it appears to support immunity and cardiovascular health. There is some evidence that L-theanine reduces menstrual discomfort.

There are no known confirmed or direct side effects of L-theanine. However, people who obtain L-theanine from drinking large amounts of tea may experience nausea, upset stomach, and irritability. People on blood pressure lowering medications should use L-theanine with caution as it may reduce blood pressure levels considerably. L-theanine should not be combined with other stimulant medications, such as pseudoephedrine (Sudafed) as the nervous system may become overstimulated.

HOW IT IS SOLD AND TAKEN

An extremely popular supplement, L-theanine is sold as capsules, powder, tablets, gummies, and liquids. It is also found in tea; an average cup has about 25 mg of L-theanine. Though there are no L-theanine dosage guidelines, most supplements range from 100 to 400 mg per dose. Still, people may take higher doses. It is probably best not to exceed 400 mg per day for a limited period without discussing with a medical provider.

RESEARCH FINDINGS

L-Theanine Supplementation Seems to Improve Cognitive Functioning

In a placebo-controlled, five-way crossover trial published in 2017 in the journal *Nutritional Neuroscience*, researchers from Sri Lanka and Lubbock, Texas (USA), wanted to determine if L-theanine alone and L-theanine combined with caffeine had positive effects on cognition and neurophysiological measures of attention. The cohort consisted of 20 healthy male volunteers who were undergraduates at a university in Sri Lanka, with age ranging from 21 to 23 years and a mean age of 21.9 years. The participants were given either 200 mg of L-theanine or 160 mg of caffeine or 200 mg of L-theanine and 160 mg of caffeine or 150 ml cup of Ceylon black tea or a placebo. None of the participants had any adverse effects from the treatments. After the treatments, the researchers waited between 30 and 60 min before administering various tests. The researchers found that a dose of L-theanine equivalent to eight cups of black tea improved cognitive and neurophysiological measures of selective attention to a degree that was comparable to that of caffeine. Therefore, it took a higher dose of L-theanine to experience "acute effects of improving attention." Even better results were obtained when L-theanine was combined with caffeine. However, when only one cup of tea was consumed, there was no significant effect on measures of attention. The researchers concluded that "this suggests that if tea is to be used as 'functional food' to enhance selective attention, enrichment of tea with theanine and/or caffeine is necessary."[1]

L-Theanine Supplementation Appears to Have Antistress Properties

In a double-blind, placebo-controlled, balanced, crossover trial published in 2016 in the journal *Nutrients*, researchers from Australia and Santa Monica, California (USA), investigated the ability of L-theanine supplement to help people deal with stress. The initial cohort consisted of 36 healthy adults between the ages of 18 and 40 years. After baseline assessments were conducted during the first visit to the testing site, there were two testing days, separated by at least a 48-h washout period. Before the stressful testing began, the participants consumed a drink containing 200 mg of L-theanine or one without the supplement. During their second day of testing, they consumed the opposite drink. The researchers determined that 1 h after the administration of the drink containing L-theanine there were significant reductions in the "subjective stress response to a cognitive stressor." In addition, an analysis of salivary cortisol, a measure of stress response, revealed significantly decreased salivary cortisol. The researchers concluded that their findings "further support the anti-stress effects of L-theanine."[2]

L-Theanine Supplementation Helps Control Blood Pressure and Anxiety in People Dealing with High-Stress Mental Tasks

In a randomized, placebo-controlled, crossover trial published in 2012 in the *Journal of Physiological Anthropology*, researchers based in Japan examined the use of L-theanine or caffeine to control blood pressure in people undergoing stressful mental and physical tasks. The initial cohort consisted of 16 healthy volunteers, including eight men and eight women with an average age of 22.8 years. In total, three separate trials were performed in which the participants consumed either 200 mg L-theanine plus placebo, 100 mg caffeine plus placebo, or a placebo. Fourteen participants completed the entire trial. The researchers found that L-theanine significantly changed both diastolic and systolic blood pressures in participants whose blood pressure increased more than average. They noted that their findings "demonstrated the possibility that L-theanine can attenuate blood pressure elevation induced by mental tasks," while it also reduced anxiety. Further, L-theanine did not have any effect on decreasing elevations in blood pressure caused by strong physical stress.[3]

L-Theanine Supplementation Helped People Maintain Vigilance during a Sustained Attention Task

In a double-blind, randomized, crossover trial published in 2012 in the journal *Neuropharmacology*, researchers from New York (USA), the United Kingdom, and the Netherlands investigated the ability of L-theanine and caffeine to help people remain focused on monotonous tasks over protracted time periods. The initial cohort consisted of 27 healthy participants between the ages of 18 and 40 years, with a mean age of 26 years. Eight of the participants were female. The 5-day trial began on the first day with the administration of questionnaires and a sample 1-h training session. This was followed by 4 days of treatments and the recording of electrical activity via high-density electrophysiology. The treatments given were 100 mg L-theanine, 50 mg caffeine, 100 mg L-theanine and 50 mg caffeine, and a placebo. The final analyses used data from 21 participants. The researchers learned that, when the participants consumed only L-theanine, there were significant reductions in both commission and omission errors. Similar results were obtained when L-theanine was combined with caffeine, which is an unexpected finding. Apparently, 100 mg of L-theanine or the 50 mg of caffeine "already provide a maximal effect on sustained attention."[4]

L-Theanine Supplementation May Help People Dealing with Major Depressive Disorder

In an open-label, clinical trial published in 2016 in the journal *Acta Neuropsychiatrica*, researchers from Japan wanted to learn if L-theanine supplementation would benefit people dealing with debilitating major depressive disorder. The cohort consisted of four men, with a mean age of 41 years, and 16 women, with a mean age of 42.9 years; all participants suffered from major depressive disorder. While they continued to take their regular medication, the participants were placed on 250 mg per day of oral L-theanine supplementation, which was taken at bedtime. Assessments were conducted at baseline, at 4 weeks, at 8 weeks, and when the trial ended. All participants completed the entire trial, "suggesting a high tolerability of L-theanine." The researchers found that L-theanine supplementation resulted in reductions in clinical symptoms, such as overall depression, anxiety, and sleep problems. In addition, there were improvements in cognitive functions. The researchers concluded that "L-theanine could be a useful natural compound in the treatment of MDD [major depressive disorder]."[5]

L-Theanine Supplementation May Improve the Quality of Sleep in Boys with Attention Deficit Hyperactivity Disorder (ADHD)

In a 6-week, randomized, double-blind, placebo-controlled trial published in 2011 in the journal *Alternative Medicine Review*, researchers from Canada and Japan wanted to learn if L-theanine supplementation would improve the sleep quality of boys with ADHD. Apparently, between 25% and 50% of children and teens with ADHD have sleep disturbances. The cohort consisted of 98 boys between the ages of 8 and 12 years who were diagnosed with ADHD. They were placed on 400 mg per day of a L-theanine chewable tablet or an identical appearing placebo chewable tablet. Using wrist actigraphy, the participants were evaluated for five consecutive nights at baseline and at the end of the trial. Parents completed a questionnaire at baseline and the end of the trial. The findings from the actigraph watches indicated that the participants who consumed L-theanine had significantly higher sleep percentage and sleep efficiency scores, and a non-significant trend for less activity during sleep. Other factors, such as sleep latency, remained unchanged. Interestingly, the parents' questionnaire did not correlate significantly with the data collected, "suggesting that parents were not particularly aware of their children's sleep quality." Still, the "findings indicate that L-theanine does indeed appear to be an effective agent in positively influencing the quality of sleep among male children who have been diagnosed with ADHD."[6]

L-Theanine Supplementation May Help Deal with Symptoms of Schizophrenia and Schizoaffective Disorder

In an 8-week, randomized, double-blind, placebo-controlled, two-center trial published in 2011 in the *Journal of Clinical Psychiatry*, researchers from Israel wanted to learn if L-theanine supplementation would be useful for people with schizophrenia and schizoaffective disorder. The initial cohort consisted of 60 participants who had been diagnosed with schizophrenia or schizoaffective disorder. There were 48 men and 12 women, with a mean age of 36.4 years. Thirty participants were placed on 400 mg per day of L-theanine supplementation, and 30 were placed on a placebo. All participants were taking at least one antipsychotic medication. Assessments were made during five visits. Neurocognitive tests were performed at baseline and after 4 and 8 weeks. Forty-eight men and nine women completed the trial. The researchers learned that L-theanine supplementation was associated with a reduction in anxiety as well as positive and general psychopathology scores; however, it did not relieve other associated problems, such as negative and depressive symptoms and quality of life impairments. Still, L-theanine was "safe and well-tolerated." The researchers concluded that "L-theanine augmentation of antipsychotic therapy can ameliorate positive, activation, and anxiety symptoms in schizophrenia and schizoaffective disorder patients."[7]

L-Theanine Supplementation May Have Properties against the Common Cold

In a randomized, double-blind, pilot trial published in 2010 in the *Journal of Amino Acids*, researchers from Japan wanted to learn if a supplement containing L-theanine and cystine, an oxidized dimeric form of the amino acid cysteine, would be useful against the common cold. The cohort consisted of 176 healthy males. During a 5-week duration (January–February), the participants took four tablets per day of 70 mg of L-theanine and 175 mg of L-cystine or placebos. The participants recorded any cold-related symptoms, such as runny and/or stuffy nose, sneezing, sore throat, and cough, as well as the number of days that they experienced these symptoms. The final analyses used data from 88 participants in the supplement group and 85 in the placebo group. The researchers learned that for all but one of the cold-related symptoms the incidences were lower in the supplement group, although not all of the differences were statistically significant. At the same time, the supplement did not have any effect on the duration of colds. The researchers predicted that, in the future, the supplement will be used for cold prevention and symptom relief.[8]

L-Theanine May Have Positive Effects for People Prone to Anxiety

In a double-blind, repeated-measurement design trial published in 2011 in the *Journal of Functional Foods*, researchers based in Japan examined the use of L-theanine supplementation for attention, reaction time, and anxiety. The cohort consisted of 18 normal healthy university students. The students were divided into two groups—a "high anxiety propensity" group (n = 8) and a "minimal anxiety propensity" group (n = 10). During different testing periods, the groups were given one dose of 200 mg L-theanine or a placebo. Sixty minutes after supplementation, the researchers measured reaction time responses, heart rate, and alpha brain waves. They also conducted a test measuring anxiety levels. The researchers found that the students in the high-anxiety group had significant differences in responses to L-theanine and placebo. When the high-anxiety students took L-theanine, they experienced slowing of heart rate, improved attentional performance, and better reaction times. When the same students took the placebo, these responses did not occur. There were no significant differences in responses between L-theanine and placebo supplementation in the low-anxiety group. The researchers concluded that "results evidently demonstrated that L-theanine clearly has a pronounced effect on attention performance and reaction time in normal healthy subjects prone to high anxiety."[9]

L-Theanine Supplementation Seems to Affect Cerebral Blood Flow, Attention, and Mood

In a double-blind, placebo-controlled, counterbalanced, crossover trial published in 2015 in the journal *Psychopharmacology*, researchers based in the United Kingdom investigated the effects of L-theanine and caffeine, both separately and together, on cerebral blood flow, cognition, and mood. The cohort consisted of 12 habitual users of caffeine and 12 nonhabitual users of caffeine. The participants age ranged from 18 to 35 years, with a mean age of 21.8 years. The habitual users consumed more than 150 mg of caffeine per day in their tea drinks. During four separate testing visits, the participants received 75 mg caffeine or 50 mg L-theanine, 50 mg L-theanine and 75 mg caffeine, or a placebo. Various assessments were conducted at baseline and 30 min after the dose was administered. As expected, the researchers determined that caffeine made the body's blood vessels smaller, thereby temporarily increasing blood pressure. When L-theanine was combined with caffeine, these blood pressure effects were reduced. There was also improvement in performance on attention tasks and increase in overall mood ratings. According to the researchers, "this supports previous findings of an interaction between these substances."[10]

L-Theanine Does Not Appear to Be Useful for Generalized Anxiety Disorder

In a randomized, double-blind, placebo-controlled, multicenter pilot trial published in 2019 in the *Journal of Psychiatric Research*, researchers from Australia examined the ability of L-theanine supplementation to assist people dealing with generalized anxiety disorder. All the initial 46 participants were on medications that were not effectively treating their psychiatric disorder. For 8 weeks, they were placed on L-theanine (initially 450 mg per day which was sometimes increased to 900 mg per day) or a placebo, which was matched for appearance, taste, and scent. Nineteen participants in the supplement group and 18 in the placebo group completed the trial. When the researchers conducted assessments of anxiety, sleep quality, and cognition, they were unable to find differences between the supplement and placebo. The L-theanine supplement failed to outperform the placebo in measures of anxiety, mood, worry, or cognition. There was some indication that L-theanine supplementation may improve self-reported sleep satisfaction and mild insomnia symptoms. The researchers concluded that "while this preliminary study did not support the efficacy of L-theanine in the treatment of anxiety symptoms in GAD [generalized anxiety disorder], further studies to explore the application of L-theanine in sleep disturbance are warranted."[11]

NOTES

1. Kahathuduwa, Chanaka N., Tharaka L. Dassanayake, A. M. Tissa Amarakoon, and Vajira S. Weerasinghe. "Acute Effects of Theanine, Caffeine and Theanine–Caffeine Combination on Attention." *Nutritional Neuroscience* 20, no. 6 (July 2017): 369–377.

2. White, David J., Suzanne de Klerk, William Woods, et al. "Anti-Stress, Behavioural and Magnetoencephalography Effects of an L-Theanine-Based Nutrient Drink: A Randomised, Double-Blind, Placebo-Controlled, Crossover Trial." *Nutrients* 8, no. 1 (January 2016): 53.

3. Yoto, Ai, Mao Motoki, Sato Murao, and Hidehiko Yokogoshi. "Effects of L-Theanine or Caffeine Intake on Changes in Blood Pressure under Physical and Psychological Stresses." *Journal of Physiological Anthropology* 31 (2012): 28.

4. Foxe, J. J., K. P. Morie, P. J. Laud, et al. "Assessing the Effects of Caffeine and Theanine on the Maintenance of Vigilance during a Sustained Attention Task." *Neuropharmacology* 62, no. 7 (June 2012): 2320–2327.

5. Hidese, S., M. Ota, C. Wakabayashi, et al. "Effects of Chronic L-Theanine Administration in Patients with Major Depressive Disorder: An Open-Label Study." *Acta Neuropsychiatrica* 29, no. 2 (April 2017): 72–79.

6. Lyon, M. R., M. P. Kapoor, and L. R. Juneja. "The Effects of L-Theanine (Suntheanine®) on Objective Sleep Quality in Boys with Attention Deficit Hyperactivity Disorder (ADHD): A Randomized, Double-Blind, Placebo-Controlled Trial." *Alternative Medicine Review* 16, no. 4 (December 2011): 348–354.

7. Ritsner, M. S., C. Miodownik, Y. Ratner, et al. "L-Theanine Relieves Positive, Activation and Anxiety Symptoms in Patients with Schizophrenia and Schizoaffective Disorder: An 8-Week, Randomized, Double-Blind, Placebo-Controlled, 2-Center Study." *Journal of Clinical Psychiatry* 72, no. 1 (January 2011): 34–42.

8. Kurihara, Shigekazu, Takenori Hiraoka, Masahisa Akutsu, et al. "Effects of L-Cystine and L-theanine Supplementation on the Common Cold: A Randomized, Double-Blind, and Placebo-Controlled Trial." *Journal of Amino Acids* 2010 (2010): Article ID: 307475.

9. Higashiyama, Akiko, Hla Hla Htay, Makoto Ozebi, et al. "Effect of L-Theanine on Attention and Reaction Time Response." *Journal of Functional Foods* 3, no. 3 (July 2011): 171–178.

10. Dodd, F. L., D. O. Kennedy, L. M. Riby, and C. F. Haskell-Ramsay. "A Double-Blind, Placebo-Controlled Study Evaluating the Effects of Caffeine and L-Theanine Both Alone and in Combination on Cerebral Blood Flow, Cognition and Mood." *Psychopharmacology* 232 (2015): 2563–2576.

11. Sarris, Jerome, Gerard J. Byrne, Lachlan Cribb, et al. "L-Theanine in the Adjunctive Treatment of Generalized Anxiety Disorder: A Double-Blind, Randomised, Placebo-Controlled Trial." *Journal of Psychiatric Research* 110 (2019): 31–37.

REFERENCES AND FURTHER READING

Dodd, F. L., D. O. Kennedy, L. M. Riby, and C. F Haskell-Ransay. "A Double-Blind, Placebo-Controlled Study Evaluating the Effects of Caffeine and L-Theanine Both Alone and in Combination on Cerebral Blood Flow, Cognition and Mood." *Psychopharmacology* 232 (2015): 2563–2576.

Foxe, J. J., K. P. Morie, P. J. Laud, et al. "Assessing the Effects of Caffeine and Theanine on the Maintenance of Vigilance during a Sustained Attention Task." *Neuropharmacology* 62, no. 7 (June 2012): 2320–2327.

Hidese, S., M. Ota, C. Wakabayashi, et al. "Effects of Chronic L-Theanine Administration in Patients with Major Depressive Disorder: An Open-Label Study." *Acta Neuropsychiatrica* 29, no. 2 (April 2017): 72–79.

Higashiyama, Akiko, Hla Hla Htay, Makoto Ozeki, et al. "Effects of L-Theanine on Attention and Reaction Time Response." *Journal of Functional Foods* 3, no. 3 (July 2011): 171–178.

Kahathuduwa, Chanaka N., Tharaka L. Dassanayake, A. M. Tissa Amarakoon, and Vajira S. Weerasinghe. "Acute Effects of Theanine, Caffeine and Theanine–Caffeine Combination on Attention." *Nutritional Neuroscience* 20, no. 6 (July 2017): 369–377.

Kurihara, Shigekazu, Takenori Hiraoka, Masahisa Akutsu, et al. "Effects of L-Cystine and L-Theanine Supplementation on the Common Cold: A Randomized, Double-Blind, and Placebo-Controlled Trial." *Journal of Amino Acids* 2010 (2010): Article ID: 307475.

Lyon, M. R., M. P. Kapoor, and L. R. Juneja. "The Effects of L-Theanine (Suntheanine®) on Objective Sleep Quality in Boys with Attention Deficit Hyperactivity Disorder (ADHD): A Randomized, Double-Blind, Placebo-Controlled Clinical Trial." *Alternative Medicine Review* 16, no. 4 (December 2011): 348–354.

Ritsner, M. S., C. Miodownik, Y. Ratner, et al. "L-Theanine Relieves Positive, Activation, and Anxiety Symptoms in Patients with Schizophrenia and Schizoaffective Disorder: An 8-Week, Randomized, Double-Blind, Placebo-Controlled, 2-Center Study." *Journal of Clinical Psychiatry* 72, no. 1 (January 2011): 34–42.

Sarris, J., G. J. Byrne, L. Cribb, et al. "L-Theanine in the Adjunctive Treatment of Generalized Anxiety Disorder: A Double-Blind, Randomised, Placebo-Controlled Trial." *Journal of Psychiatric Research* 110 (March 2019): 31–37.

White, David J., Suzanne de Klerk, William Woods, et al. "Anti-Stress, Behavioural and Magnetoencephalography Effects of an L-Theanine-Based Nutrient Drink: A Randomised, Double-Blind, Placebo-Controlled, Crossover Trial." *Nutrients* 8, no. 1 (January 2016): 53.

Yoto, Ai, Mao Motoki, Sato Murao, and Hidehiko Yokogoshi. "Effects of L-Theanine or Caffeine Intake on Changes in Blood Pressure under Physical and Psychological Stress." *Journal of Physiological Anthropology* 31 (2012): 28.

Lutein and Zeaxanthin

Lutein and zeaxanthin are two carotenoids located in the eyes. Because they filter high-energy blue wavelengths, they help protect the eyes, especially the lens, macula, and retina, as well as maintain healthy eye cells. Lutein and zeaxanthin are the only two carotenoids found in large quantities in the eyes; higher levels in the eyes appear to be associated with better vision.

The human body is unable to synthesize all the required lutein (pronounced loo-teen) and zeaxanthin (pronounced zee-uh-zan-thin). Therefore, lutein and zeaxanthin, which are antioxidants, must be obtained from food and/or supplements. Foods that contain lutein and zeaxanthin include green leafy vegetables, such as kale, spinach, collards and turnip greens, egg yolks, green beans, and oranges.

The amount of lutein and zeaxanthin in the macular region of the retina is measured as the macular pigment optical density (MPOD). Medical professionals use MPOD as a biomarker for predicting disease and visual function.

HEALTH BENEFITS AND RISKS

As antioxidants, lutein and zeaxanthin neutralize free radicals associated with oxidative stress and retinal damage. Therefore, people believe that lutein and zeaxanthin help prevent eye problems, such as cataracts and age-related macular degeneration (AMD). There are no known risks associated with lutein and zeaxanthin, although consuming large amounts of carotenoids may give the skin a yellowish tone. There are no known reactions between lutein and zeaxanthin and prescription medications. Using the fat substitute Olestra may lower blood lutein concentrations in healthy people. Pregnant and breastfeeding women should check with a medical provider before taking lutein and zeaxanthin supplementation.

HOW IT IS SOLD AND TAKEN

Lutein and zeaxanthin are frequently sold together in a tablet, capsule, or softgel. They may be combined with other nutrients such as vitamin C or vitamin E. Multivitamins may or may not contain lutein and zeaxanthin. If they do, they tend to have lower amounts, which are insufficient to make a notable difference.

There are no specific recommendations for the daily intake of lutein and zea-xanthin. However, some suggests that health benefits may be obtained from 10 mg per day of lutein and 2 mg per day of zeaxanthin.

RESEARCH FINDINGS

High Intake of Lutein and Zeaxanthin Is Associated with a Reduced Long-Term Risk of Advanced AMD

In a prospective cohort study published in 2015 in *JAMA Ophthalmology*, researchers from Boston, Massachusetts, Providence, Rhode Island, Bethesda, Maryland, and Salt Lake City, Utah (USA), examined the association between the intake of lutein and zeaxanthin and the long-term risk of advanced AMD. With AMD, people lose central vision. Data were obtained from the Nurses' Health Study and the Health Professionals Follow-Up Study in the United States. The cohort consisted of 63,443 women and 38,603 men. All the participants were at least 50 years old, and, at baseline, were free of AMD, diabetes mellitus, cardio-vascular disease, and cancer. Carotenoid intake scores were computed from food frequency questionnaires, both at the beginning and during follow-up. Follow-up was 26 years for the Nurses' survey and 24 years for the Health Professional sur-vey. The researchers found 1361 intermediate and 1118 advanced cases of AMD; at onset of AMD, the median age was 73 years for women and 76 years for men. The researchers learned that a higher intake of lutein and zeaxanthin was associ-ated with a 40% lower risk of advanced AMD. Higher intakes of other carotenoids were also associated with a reduced risk of the advanced illness. In contrast, there did not appear to be an association between carotenoids and intermediate AMD. According to the researchers, this suggested an effect on the "progression" of the illness rather than the "initiation." The researchers concluded that their findings "lend further support to the causal role of lutein/zeaxanthin in protecting against the development of advanced AMD."[1]

Supplementation with Lutein and Zeaxanthin Appears to Benefit Those with Early AMD

In a randomized, double-blind, placebo-controlled trial published in 2015 in the *British Journal of Ophthalmology*, researchers from China wanted to learn if sup-plementation with lutein and zeaxanthin would benefit people with early AMD. For 2 years, 112 people from Beijing, China with early AMD were placed on one of four daily treatments—10 mg lutein, 20 mg lutein, 10 mg lutein and 10 mg zea-xanthin, or a placebo. Testing was conducted at baseline, at 48 weeks, and when the trial ended. Four participants were excluded from the final analysis. The researchers learned that supplementation with lutein or lutein and zeaxanthin sig-nificantly increased levels of MPOD, and supplementation with either of the lutein supplements enhanced retinal sensitivity in people with early AMD. No signifi-cant changes were observed in the placebo group. The researchers concluded "that the change in MPOD is responsible for the change in retinal sensitivity," which is "consistent with other studies."[2]

Maybe Lutein and Zeaxanthin Do Not Provide Any Notable Protection against Early AMD

In a prospective study published in 2008 in the *American Journal of Clinical Nutrition*, researchers from different locations but based in Boston, Massachusetts (USA), evaluated the association between the intake of lutein and zeaxanthin and AMD. The initial cohort consisted of 71,494 women and 41,564 men who were 50 years or older and had no diagnosis of AMD or cancer. During 18 years of follow-up, the researchers documented 673 incident cases of early AMD and 442 incident cases of neovascular AMD with a visual loss of 20/30 or worse, primarily from the illness. The researchers found no association between intake of lutein and zeaxanthin and early AMD, and found a statistically nonsignificant and non-linear inverse association between lutein and zeaxanthin intake and neovascular AMD. The researchers commented that there is a need for more research into their second finding, and that "the suggestion of inverse association related to the risk of neovascular AMD needs to be examined further."[3]

There Appears to Be an Association between Plasma Levels of Lutein and Zeaxanthin and the Risk of Age-Related Nuclear Cataracts

In a cross-sectional study published in 2012 in the *British Journal of Nutrition*, researchers from Finland evaluated the association between plasma levels of lutein and zeaxanthin and the risk of age-related nuclear cataracts. Data were obtained from the Kuopio Ischaemic Heart Disease Risk Factor (KIHD) Study. The cohort consisted of 1689 elderly participants (1130 men and 559 women) between the ages of 61 and 80 years. Carotenoids were analyzed from plasma samples. A total of 113 cases of incident age-related cataracts was confirmed, of which 108 were nuclear cataracts. The researchers learned that the participants with cataracts had significantly lower levels of plasma lutein and zeaxanthin levels than those without cataracts. They concluded that "high plasma concentrations of lutein and zeaxanthin were associated with a decreased risk of age-related nuclear cataract in the elderly population."[4] This finding was consistent with previous epidemiological studies.

Lutein Supplements Appear to Be Useful for People Who Spend a Good Deal of Time in Front of Computer Screens

In a trial published in 2009 in the *British Journal of Nutrition*, researchers from China investigated the use of lutein supplementation for people who spend a lot of time in front of computer screens. The cohort consisted of 37 healthy participants whose age ranged from 22 to 30 years. All participants had long-term exposure to the light of computer monitors. For 12 weeks, they took either 6 mg per day of lutein or 12 mg per day of lutein or a placebo. As might be expected, at the end of the trial, the participants in both lutein groups had increased levels of serum lutein. In addition, both lutein groups had improvements in measures of contrast sensitivity, with the improvement reaching significance in the high-dose group. Moreover, the participants in the high-dose group had improvements in visual acuity. Still, in contrast to other studies, no changes were observed in the sensitivity to glare. According to the researchers, "this was probably because the subjects in previous studies were hospital patients with ocular diseases."[5]

Lutein and Zeaxanthin Supplementation May Improve Cognition in Older Adults

In a double-masked, randomized, placebo-controlled trial published in 2017 in the journal *Frontiers of Aging Neuroscience*, researchers from Athens, Georgia (USA), investigated the ability of supplemental lutein and zeaxanthin to improve cognition in older adults living in the community. The initial cohort consisted of 62 older adults. Forty-two participants were placed in the supplement group, who took a daily supplement with 10 mg lutein and 2 mg zeaxanthin. Twenty participants took placebos, which were visually identical to the active supplement. At the end of 1 year, during which there was periodic testing, data from 51 participants, with a mean age of 73.7 years, were available for analysis. The researchers learned that the participants taking the supplements had statistically significant increases in "complex attention and cognitive flexibility." When male and female participants were analyzed separately, the male participants who took the supplement had significant improvement in the composite memory domain. The researchers concluded that the supplement had "a positive effect on higher level functions of the brain" and it "improved cognitive function in community-dwelling, older men and women."[6]

In a trial published in 2018 in the journal *Ophthalmology & Visual Science*, researchers from France and Germany examined the association between plasma lutein and zeaxanthin, MPOD, and cognitive functioning in 184 adults, with an average age of 82.3 years. All participants, who were from the French cities of Bordeaux, Dijon, or Montpellier, underwent complete eye examinations at the University Hospital of Bordeaux that included measurements of best-corrected visual acuity and MPOD in both eyes. Plasma levels of lutein and zeaxanthin were assessed, and cognitive performances were measured. Almost 70% of the participants were women, and 84.2% had high blood pressure. More than half of the participants had already undergone cataract surgery, and 21.7% had a nuclear cataract. The researchers learned that higher MPOD levels were significantly associated with higher cognitive function, specifically higher verbal fluency abilities and visual memory. A positive association was found between crude concentrations of lutein and zeaxanthin and verbal fluency ability. Meanwhile, a higher lutein plus zeaxanthin over total triglycerides plus total cholesterol ratio (L + Z/ TG + TC) was significantly associated with global cognitive z-score, episodic memory, and verbal fluency. The researchers concluded that their findings "suggested that both higher MPOD and L + Z concentrations were significantly associated with higher cognitive performances."[7]

Higher Levels of Dietary Lutein and Zeaxanthin May Improve Cognition in Preadolescents

In a study published in 2018 in the journal *Nutrients*, researchers from Athens, Georgia, Champaign, Illinois, and Boston, Massachusetts (USA), evaluated the dietary intake of lutein and zeaxanthin in 51 children between the ages of 7 and 13 years. Forty-nine percent were female. The majority of the children were white and from well-educated families. MPOD measurements were taken, and cognitive functioning was assessed. Testing was conducted by two experimenters who had "extensive experience" working with children. The researchers found an association between higher carotenoid status and improvements in several types of cognitive functioning. The researchers commented that their findings are consistent with studies of lutein and zeaxanthin in adults, and they "highlight the importance of diet in supporting cognitive health in preadolescent children."[8]

High Levels of Lutein Appear to Be Inversely Associated with the Risk for Dementia and Alzheimer's Disease

In a study published in 2016 in *Journal of Gerontology, Series A: Biological Sciences and Medical Sciences*, researchers from France and Switzerland evaluated the association between plasma carotenoids and the risk of dementia and Alzheimer's disease in French elders. The cohort consisted of 1,092 nondemented older participants, with an average age of 74.4 years, who were followed for up to 10 years. To determine plasma concentrations of carotenoids, baseline tests were administered. A committee of neurologists diagnosed dementia and Alzheimer's disease; there were 199 dementia cases, including 132 cases of Alzheimer's disease. The researchers learned that only the higher concentrations of lutein were significantly inversely associated with dementia and Alzheimer's disease. They concluded that "this large cohort of older participants suggests that maintaining higher concentrations of lutein in respect to plasma lipids may moderately decrease the risk of dementia and AD."[9]

High Serum Carotenoids Appear to Be Associated with Improvement in Nonalcoholic Fatty Liver Disease

In a prospective study published in 2019 in the *European Journal of Nutrition*, researchers from China examined the association between levels of serum carotenoids and nonalcoholic fatty liver disease. Data were obtained from the Guangzhou Nutrition and Health Study. The initial cohort consisted of 3336 Chinese adults between the ages of 40 and 75 years. Blood tests were used to assess the levels of serum carotenoids and other factors, and abdominal ultrasonography was employed to determine the presence and degree of nonalcoholic fatty liver disease at 3 and 6 years. Trained researchers conducted face-to-face interviews with structured questionnaires, and a validated food frequency questionnaire was used to estimate daily food intake. The final analysis included 2687 participants (1833 women and 854 men). The researchers found that improvement in nonalcoholic fatty liver disease was associated with higher serum concentrations of carotenoids, including lutein and zeaxanthin. The researchers concluded that their finding "added solid evidence to support the hypothesis that carotenoids might have a beneficial role in the control of NAFLD [non-alcoholic fatty liver disease]."[10]

Higher Dietary Carotenoid Intake Appears to Be Associated with Reduced Hip Fractures

In a study published in 2014 in the *Journal of Bone and Mineral Research*, researchers from Singapore and Pittsburgh, Pennsylvania (USA), examined the association between dietary carotenoids and hip fractures in men. The researchers used data from the Singapore Chinese Health Study, a prospective cohort of 63,257 men and women aged 45 to 74 years between 1993 and 1998. At baseline, participants were interviewed on lifestyle factors and medical history. Usual dietary foods were measured using a food frequency questionnaire. The final analysis, which came after a mean follow-up of 9.9 years, included a total of 61,524 participants who did not have hip fractures and 1630 who had hip fractures. The mean age at fracture was 74.4 years; women accounted for 72.4 of all hip fractures. The men had a 5% higher intake of carotenoids than the women. The researchers noted that they found a statistically significant inverse relationship between intake of carotenoids and hip fracture. The higher the intake of carotenoids, the lower the risk, which was most evident in thin, elderly men. The researchers concluded that their findings indicated "that adequate intake of vegetables may reduce risk of osteoporotic fractures among elderly men and that the antioxidant effects of carotenoids may counteract the mechanism of osteoporosis related to leanness."[11]

In a case-control study published in 2018 in the journal *Bone*, researchers from China reviewed the association between intake of dietary carotenoids and risk of hip fractures in people who were middle-aged or elderly. The cohort consisted of 1070 patients between the ages of 52 and 83 years, with hip fractures and 1070 age and gender-matched controls. Information on dietary carotenoid intake was assessed with a 79-item food frequency questionnaire administered during face-to-face interviews. The study was conducted between June 2009 and August 2015 in Guangdong Province, China. The researchers learned that higher intake of total carotenoids and specific carotenoids, such as lutein and zeaxanthin, was associated with significantly lower risk of hip fractures in both men and women. According to the researchers, these findings "support the hypothesis that these carotenoids may be protective against fracture."[12]

In a meta-analysis published in 2017 in the journal *Oncotarget*, researchers from China also evaluated the association between intake of carotenoids and risk of hip fractures. Their cohort consisted of five prospective and two case-control studies with 140,265 participants and 4324 fracture cases. All participants were 50 years or older. The five prospective studies assessed the association between dietary carotenoid levels and hip fracture risk. The two case-control studies focused on the association between circulating carotenoid levels and any fracture risk. The researchers learned that the hip fracture risk among the participants with a high dietary intake of carotenoids was 28% lower than the risk of participants with a low dietary intake of carotenoids. Almost 80% of the participants were women, and all women were postmenopausal. The follow-up of the prospective studies ranged from 3.7 to 18 years. Dietary carotenoids were assessed by validated food frequency questionnaires, and circulating carotenoid concentrations were determined by a laboratory technique known as high-performance liquid chromatography. The researchers commented that their findings indicated that a higher intake of dietary carotenoids may reduce the risk of hip fractures. They concluded that "future well-designed prospective cohort studies and randomized controlled trials are warranted to specify the associations between carotenoids and fracture."[13]

Lutein and Zeaxanthin Do Not Appear to Offer Any Protection from Prostate Cancer

In a retrospective, case-control study published in 2018 in *Nutrients*, researchers from Vietnam and Australia attempted to learn more about an association between the intake of carotenoids and prostate cancer. The cohort consisted of 652 participants, of whom 244 were incident prostate cancer patients aged 64 to 75 years and 408 were matched controls. The participants were recruited in Ho Chi Minh City during 2013–2015. Diets were reviewed with an 89-item food frequency questionnaire during face-to-face interviews. The researchers estimated intake of several carotenoids including lutein and zeaxanthin. While the researchers found that higher intakes of lycopene, tomato, and carrots were significantly associated with a reduced risk of prostate cancer, no statistically significant associations existed between prostate cancer and lutein and zeaxanthin. The researchers acknowledged that one of the limitations of the study was that the men came from the same general area in Ho Chi Minh City, and that the findings "may not be generalizable to the entire Vietnamese population."[14]

NOTES

1. Wu, j., E. Cho, W. C. Willett, et al. "Intakes of Lutein, Zeaxanthin, and Other Carotenoids and Age-Related Macular Degeneration during 2 Decades of Prospective Follow-Up." *JAMA Ophthalmology* 133, no. 12 (December 2015): 1415–1424.

2. Huang, Y. M., H. L. Dou, F. F. Huang, et al. "Changes Following Supplementation with Lutein and Zeaxanthin in Retinal Function in Eyes with Early Age-Related Macular Degeneration: A Randomised, Double-Blind, Placebo-Controlled Trial." *British Journal of Ophthalmology* 99, no. 3 (March 2015): 371–375.

3. Cho, Eunyoung, Susan E. Hankinson, Bernard Rosner, et al. "Prospective Study of Lutein/Zeaxanthin Intake and Risk of Age-Related Macular Degeneration." *American Journal of Clinical Nutrition* 87 (2008): 1837–1843.

4. Karppi, Jouni, Jari A. Laukkanen, and Sudhir Kurl. "Plasma Lutein and Zeaxanthin and the Risk of Age-Related Nuclear Cataract among the Elderly Finnish Population." *British Journal of Nutrition* 108 (2012): 148–154.

5. Ma, L., X. M. Lin, Z. Y. Zou, et al. "A 12-Week Lutein Supplementation Improves Visual Function in Chinese People with Long-Term Computer Display Light Exposure." *British Journal of Nutrition* 102, no. 2 (July 2009): 186–190.

6. Hammond, B. R., Jr., L. S. Miller, M. O. Bello, et al. "Effects of Lutein/Zeaxanthin Supplementation on the Cognitive Function of Community Dwelling Older Adults: A Randomized, Double-Masked, Placebo-Controlled Trial." *Frontiers in Aging Neuroscience* 9 (August 3, 2017): Article 254.

7. Ajana, S., D. Weber, C. Helmer, et al. "Plasma Concentrations of Lutein and Zeaxanthin, Macular Pigment Optical Density, and Their Associations with Cognitive Performances among Older Adults." *Investigative Ophthalmology & Visual Science* 59 (April 2018): 1828–1835.

8. Saint, S. E., L. M. Renzi-Hammond, N. A. Khan, et al. "The Macular Carotenoids Are Associated with Cognitive Function in Preadolescent Children." *Nutrients* 10, no.2 (February 10, 2018): 193.

9. Feart, C., L. Leterreur, C. Helmar, et al. "Plasma Carotenoids Are Inversely Associated with Dementia Risk in an Elderly French Cohort." *Journal of Gerontology, Series A: Biological Sciences and Medical Sciences* 71, no. 5 (May 2016): 683–688.

10. Xiao, M. L., G. D. Chen, F. F. Zeng, et al. "Higher Serum Carotenoids Associated with Improvement of Non-Alcoholic Fatty Liver Disease on Adults: A Prospective Study." *European Journal of Nutrition* 58, no. 2 (March 2019): 721–730.

11. Dai, Z., R. Wang, L.W. Ang, et al. "Protective Effects of Dietary Carotenoids on Risk of Hip Fracture in Men: The Singapore Chinese Health Study." *Journal of Bone and Mineral Research* 29, no. 2 (February 2014): 408–417.

12. Cao, W. T., F. F. Zeng, B. L. Li, et al. "Higher Dietary Carotenoid Intake Associated with Lower Risk of Hip Fracture in Middle-Aged and Elderly Chinese: A Matched Case-Control Study." *Bone* 111 (June 2018): 116–122.

13. Xu, Jiuhong, Chunli Song, Xiaochao Song, et al. "Carotenoids and Risk of Fracture: A Meta-Analysis of Observational Studies." *Oncotarget* 8, no. 2 (2017): 2391–2399.

14. Van Hoang, D., N. M. Pham, A. H. Lee, et al. "Dietary Carotenoid Intakes and Prostate Cancer Risk: A Case-Control Study from Vietnam." *Nutrients* 10 (2018): 70.

REFERENCES AND FURTHER READING

Ajana, S., D. Weber, C. Helmer, et al. "Plasma Concentrations of Lutein and Zeaxanthin, Macular Pigment Optical Density, and Their Associations with Cognitive Performances among Older Adults." *Investigative Ophthalmology & Visual Science* 59 (April 2018): 1828–1835.

Cao, W. T., F. F. Zeng, B. L. Li, et al. "Higher Dietary Carotenoid Intake Associated with Lower Risk of Hip Fracture in Middle-Aged and Elderly Chinese: A Matched Case-Control Study." *Bone* 111 (June 2018): 116–122.

Cho, Eunyoung, Susan E. Hankinson, Bernard Rosner, et al. "Prospective Study of Lutein/Zeaxanthin Intake and Risk of Age-Related Macular Degeneration." *American Journal of Clinical Nutrition* 87 (2008): 1837–1843.

Dai, Z., R. Wang, L. W. Ang, et al. "Protective Effects of Dietary Carotenoids on Risk of Hip Fracture in Men: The Singapore Chinese Health Study." *Journal of Bone and Mineral Research* 29, no. 2 (February 2014): 408–417.

Feart, C., L. Letenneur, C. Helmer et al. "Plasma Carotenoids are Inversely Associated with Dementia Risk in an Elderly French Cohort." *Journal of Gerontology, Series A: Biological Sciences and Medical Sciences* 71, no. 5 (May 2016): 683–688.

Hammond, B. R., Jr., L. S. Miller, M. O. Bello, et al. "Effects of Lutein/Zeaxanthin Supplementation on the Cognitive Function of Community Dwelling Older Adults: A Randomized, Double-Masked, Placebo-Controlled Trial." *Frontiers in Aging Neuroscience* 9 (August 3, 2017): Article 2654.

Huang, Y. M., H. L. Dou, F. F. Huang, et al. "Changes Following Supplementation with Lutein and Zeaxanthin in Retinal Function in Eyes with Early Age-Related Macular Degeneration: A Randomised, Double-Blind, Placebo-Controlled Trial." *British Journal of Ophthalmology* 99, no. 3 (March 2015): 371–375.

Karppi, Jouni, Jari A. Laukkanen, and Sudhir Kurl. "Plasma Lutein and Zeaxanthin and the Risk of Age-Related Nuclear Cataract among the Elderly Finnish Population." *British Journal of Nutrition* 108 (2012): 148–154.

Ma, L., X. M. Lin, Z. Y. Zou, et al. "A 12-Week Lutein Supplementation Improves Visual Function in Chinese People with Long-Term Computer Display Light Exposure." *British Journal of Nutrition* 102, no. 2 (July 2009): 186–190.

Saint, S. E., L. M. Renzi-Hammond, N. A. Khan, et al. "The Macular Carotenoids Are Associated with Cognitive Function in Preadolescent Children." *Nutrients* 10, no. 2 (February 10, 2018): 193.

Van Hoang, D., N. M. Pham, A. H. Lee et al. "Dietary Carotenoid Intake and Prostate Cancer Risk: A Case-Control Study from Vietnam." *Nutrients* 10, no. 1 (2018): 70.

Wu, J., E. Cho, W. C Willett, et al. "Intakes of Lutein, Zeaxanthin, and Other Carotenoids and Age-Related Macular Degeneration during 2 Decades of Prospective Follow-Up." *JAMA Ophthalmology* 133, no. 12 (December 2015): 1415–1424.

Xiao, M. L., G. D. Chen, F. F. Zeng, et al. "Higher Serum Carotenoids Associated with Improvement of Non-Alcoholic Fatty Liver Disease in Adults: A Prospective Study." *European Journal of Nutrition* 58, no. 2 (March 2019): 721–730.

Xu, Jiuhong, Chunli Song, Xiaochao Song, et al. "Carotenoids and Risk of Fracture: A Meta-Analysis of Observational Studies." *Oncotarget* 8, no. 2 (2017): 2391–2399.

Melatonin

Melatonin (N-acetyl-5-methoxytryptamine) is a hormone responsible for maintaining the sleeping and waking cycle of the body—the body's circadian rhythm or internal 24-h clock. Melatonin is secreted by the pineal gland in the brain, which is the size of a pea. The synthesis and release of melatonin are stimulated by darkness and suppressed by light. During night, the body produces more melatonin; however, during the day, the amount of melatonin produced is sharply reduced. The pineal gland starts producing melatonin around 9 pm, and their levels remain higher during the night. By 9 am, there is very little melatonin in the body. Normally, the levels remain low throughout the day.

The body's circadian rhythm may be easily undone when one is not exposed to light during the day, as may be the case with people who have poor vision or who are blind. Likewise, the circadian rhythm may be compromised when one sees light during the night, as is the case with people who work in the night shift.

Melatonin is a strong antioxidant and plays a powerful role in fighting free radicals and preventing and delaying debilitating illnesses and the aging process.

While the body naturally produces melatonin, the actual amount in the body is easily disrupted by the consumption of caffeine-containing products, alcohol, and tobacco.

Because it controls the timing and release of female reproductive hormones, melatonin plays a key role in female reproductive health. It helps determine when a female starts to menstruate, the frequency and length of menstrual cycles, and when menopause occurs.

Young children have the highest amounts of nighttime melatonin. It is generally considered that melatonin levels diminish with age, which explains, in part, why older people tend not to sleep as well as younger people.

HEALTH BENEFITS AND RISKS

Melatonin is thought to be useful for a wide variety of health problems. Melatonin is best known for its role in the sleep/wake cycle. Hence, melatonin is often recommended for sleep problems, such as insomnia and jet lag. It is not uncommon for adults and children who have problems falling asleep or staying asleep to take melatonin supplements. Melatonin may be recommended to those with a condition known as delayed sleep phase, in which the sleep pattern is delayed by 2 h or more from a conventional sleep pattern. Children on the autism spectrum often have low levels of serum melatonin and sleep disturbances and may benefit from supplementation.

In addition to sleep problems, melatonin may be useful for headaches, especially cluster headaches, certain cancers, such as breast and prostate cancer, symptoms of menopause, Alzheimer's disease, fibromyalgia, a weakened immune system, overactive bladder, high blood pressure, amyotrophic lateral sclerosis, tinnitus or ringing in the ear, and gallbladder stones.

Side effects associated with melatonin include headaches, nausea, dizziness, drowsiness, irritability, restless legs, skin pigmentation, and blood clots. Because melatonin regulates female reproduction, it is recommended that pregnant or breastfeeding women avoid it.

People on blood pressure or anticlotting medications should avoid melatonin, as well as those with diabetes or suffering from a seizure disorder. Melatonin should not be used by anyone taking an ACE inhibitor medication, and it may interfere with other medications, such as benzodiazepines. People with a bleeding disorder or who have received a transplant should refrain from using this supplement. In certain people, melatonin may worsen the symptoms of depression. A selective serotonin reuptake inhibitor, known as fluvoxamine (Luvox), may increase melatonin levels in the body causing excessive drowsiness.

HOW IT IS SOLD AND TAKEN

Melatonin is a hugely popular supplement that is sold in many forms such as tablets, capsules, gummies, sublingual lozenges, liquids, patches, lotions, and creams.

Currently, there are no recommended doses for melatonin supplements. The optimum daily dose for different medical problems is a highly debatable and controversial topic. It is usually best to start with a low dose of 0.3 mg or 0.5 mg before bedtime. However, people have been known to take higher doses of 10 and 40 mg, or even higher. Unless under the supervision of a medical provider, it is best to not exceed 5 mg per day. It is recommended to consult an appropriate medical provider before giving melatonin to a child.

RESEARCH FINDINGS

Melatonin Appears to Be Useful for Sleep Disorders

In a meta-analysis published in 2013 in the online journal *PLoS ONE*, researchers based in New Haven, Connecticut (USA), searched the literature for randomized, placebo-controlled trials regarding the effects of melatonin for the treatment of primary sleep disorders in adults and children. They located 19 studies involving 1683 participants. The researchers learned that melatonin significantly reduced sleep latency or the length of time it takes to transition from full wakefulness to sleep. Participants randomly assigned to melatonin fell asleep minutes earlier than those taking placebos, and they had longer and better sleep quality. These results were statistically significant. According to the researchers, while the benefits of melatonin are smaller than those of the available prescription sleep medications, "melatonin should be considered in clinical practice due to its benign side-effect profile, cost, and limited evidence of habituation and tolerance."[1]

In a meta-analysis published a few years later, in 2017, in the journal *Sleep Medicine Reviews*, researchers from the United Kingdom identified 12 peer-reviewed, randomized, controlled trials with a total of 510 participants. All participants were at least 18 years old, with an established primary sleep disorder. The doses of melatonin ranged from 0.1 to 10 mg, with treatment durations ranging from 2 to 5 weeks. The researchers determined that melatonin supplementation was useful in reducing sleep-onset latency in primary insomnia. Melatonin also helped people with delayed sleep phase syndrome, a disorder in which sleep is delayed by more than 2 h, and it regulated the sleep–wake patterns among people who were blind. The researchers commented that their findings "highlight the potential importance of melatonin in treating certain first degree sleep disorders."[2]

Melatonin Appears to Be Useful for Insomnia in Children with Autism Spectrum Disorders, and When Combined with Cognitive Behavioral Therapy, It Is Even Better

In a randomized, placebo-controlled trial published in 2012 in the *Journal of Sleep Research*, researchers from Italy wanted to determine if controlled-release melatonin would benefit children with autism spectrum disorders who had persistent insomnia. The cohort consisted of 160 children between the ages of 4 and 10 years, all of whom had some degree of autism and ongoing insomnia. They were placed on one of four treatments—a combination of controlled-release melatonin (3 mg per day) and cognitive behavior therapy, controlled-release melatonin (3 mg per day), four sessions of cognitive behavior therapy, or a placebo that looked the same as melatonin. The children were studied at baseline and after 12 weeks of treatment. Each child was monitored for 1 week with an actigraph, a noninvasive method used to study sleep–wake patterns. In addition, parents kept sleep diaries and answered a sleep questionnaire. The final analyses included 134 children, with almost equal numbers of children in each of the groups. More than 72% of the children had symptoms of insomnia for more than 2 years. Yet, the children in the three treatment groups experienced improvements. Melatonin was primarily effective in reducing the symptoms of insomnia; cognitive behavior therapy had "a light positive impact" on sleep latency. The combination treatment outperformed the other treatments. The dose of 3 mg of melatonin proved to be "safe and effective and no adverse effects were reported." The researchers concluded that their "findings indicated that all three treatment options may be recommended, taking into consideration the family's treatment preferences, treatment availability, cost and time burden."[3]

Melatonin Helps the Sleep Problems of Children with Autism Spectrum and May Be Used for Longer Periods of Time

In a randomized, double-blind placebo-controlled, multicenter trial published in 2017 in the *Journal of the American Academy of Child & Adolescent Psychiatry*, researchers from the United Kingdom, Israel, and Baltimore, Maryland (USA), wanted to determine if prolonged-release melatonin supplementation would help the sleep problems associated with autism spectrum disorder in children. Moreover, they also wanted to learn if prolonged-release melatonin could be used for longer periods of time. The cohort consisted of 125 children and adolescents between the ages of 2 and 17.5 years. In all cases, behavioral therapy had failed to improve sleep disturbances. For 13 weeks, the children took melatonin (2 mg escalated to 5 mg) or a placebo. A total of 95 participants finished the double-blind phase. The completion rate was higher in the treatment group (85%) than the placebo group (67.7%), and the results were dramatic. By the end of the trial, the participants on melatonin slept an average of 57.5 min longer at night, while those on the placebo slept 9.14 min longer. Sleep latency decreased by 39.6 min, on average, with melatonin and 12.5 min with the placebo. Adverse effects were "few and mild." Some of the participants experienced headaches, fatigue, and daytime sleepiness. The researchers concluded that melatonin was "efficacious and safe for treatment of insomnia in children and adolescents."[4]

There Is No Universal Agreement That Melatonin Is Safe for Children

In an article published on 2015 in the *Journal of Paediatrics and Child Health*, a researcher from Australia outlined some potential problems with treating children with melatonin. The researcher noted that melatonin is being increasingly recommended for children and adolescents who have difficulty initiating and maintaining sleep. Yet, early research on melatonin found that it had effects on the reproductive systems of both males and females. Initially, the use of melatonin was recommended only for children with "severe neurodevelopmental disorders." Many of the early studies were small and uncontrolled and relied on assessments from the parents. As time progressed, melatonin doses were increased. Additional studies have found that melatonin acts on other systems including cardiovascular, immune, and metabolic. Yet, there are insufficient long-term studies in children. They concluded that "if melatonin is to be used for treatment of sleep disorders in children, it is important that appropriate rigorous follow-up studies are conducted into early adulthood."[5]

One Type of Melatonin May Help People with Elevated Nocturnal Blood Pressure

In a meta-analysis published in 2011 in the journal *Vascular Health and Risk Management*, researchers from Israel investigated the ability of melatonin to lower elevated levels of nocturnal (nighttime) blood pressure. The researchers noted that people with nocturnal high blood pressure are at an increased risk for cardiovascular complications. They found seven relevant trials with 221 participants. Six studies involved 200 adults, and one study had 21 adolescents. Three of the trials used controlled-release melatonin and four trials used fast-release melatonin. In their initial analysis, the researchers did not find any significant differences in nocturnal blood pressure between the people who took melatonin and those who took placebos. However, during subgroup analyses, they found that controlled-release melatonin significantly reduced nocturnal blood pressure, whereas fast-release melatonin appeared to have no effect. The researchers concluded that "it is necessary that larger trials of longer duration be conducted in order to determine the long-term beneficial effects of controlled-release melatonin in patients with nocturnal hypertension [high blood pressure]."[6]

Melatonin May Be Useful for Chronic Tinnitus

In a prospective, randomized, double-blind, crossover clinical trial published in 2011 in the journal *Annals of Otology, Rhinology & Laryngology*, researchers from Columbus, Ohio (USA), wanted to learn if melatonin would help symptoms of tinnitus, the perception of ringing, buzzing, or other sounds in the ears in the absence of actual noise. Participants who have been dealing with chronic tinnitus for at least 6 months received a daily 3 mg melatonin supplement for 30 days or a placebo. After a 30-day washout period, they were placed on the alternative treatment. Sixty-one participants completed the trial and the periodic testing and assessments. The participants on melatonin had improved scores on several standardized measures. The response was better among men, among participants with a history of noise exposure, without depression or anxiety, with more severe and bilateral tinnitus, and those who had not undergone prior tinnitus therapy. The researchers concluded that "melatonin is associated with a statistically significant decrease in tinnitus intensity and improved sleep quality in patients with chronic tinnitus."[7]

Melatonin May Help with the Symptoms of Fibromyalgia

In a double-blind, placebo-controlled trial published in 2011 in the *Journal of Pineal Research*, researchers from Baghdad, Iraq wanted to learn if melatonin could play a useful role in the treatment of fibromyalgia, a chronic musculoskeletal disorder characterized by generalized muscular pain accompanied by fatigue and tenderness at specific sites called tender points. The trial examined the use of different doses of melatonin alone or in combination with fluoxetine (Prozac) for the treatment of fibromyalgia. The cohort consisted of 95 women and six men who fulfilled the criteria of the American College of Rheumatology for fibromyalgia. They were placed in one of four groups: group A (n = 24) was treated with 20 mg per day of fluoxetine, group B (n = 27) was treated with 5 mg per day of melatonin, group C (n = 27) was treated with 20 mg per day of fluoxetine plus 3 mg melatonin, and group D (n = 23) was treated with 20 mg per day of fluoxetine and 5 mg per day of melatonin. Each participant was clinically evaluated at baseline and after 8 weeks. The researcher found that either dose of melatonin combined with fluoxetine resulted in significant reductions in the symptoms associated with fibromyalgia. The researchers commented that "although melatonin is approved as a sleep aid, it has a variety of other beneficial effects that may account for its potential role in the treatment of fibromyalgia."[8]

While Not as Effective as the Amitriptyline, Melatonin May Be Used for Migraines in Children

In a parallel, single-blind, randomized, open-label clinical trial published in 2018 in the *Iranian Journal of Child Neurology*, researchers from Iran tested the use of amitriptyline, an antidepressant, and melatonin to prevent migraines in children. The cohort consisted of 41 girls and 39 boys between the ages of 5 and 15 years, with a mean age of 10.44 years. All children had migraines, with and without aura. Therefore, they were referred to a neurology clinic between June 2013 and January 2014. For 90 days, they were placed on either amitriptyline (1 mg/kg/day) or melatonin (0.3 mg/kg/day). The supplements and placebos were administered at bedtime. Every 2 weeks, the parents were asked for updates on the headaches. The researchers found good responses in 82.5% in the amitriptyline group and 62.5% in the melatonin group. Although both amitriptyline and melatonin reduced the frequency, severity, duration, and disability of the headaches, amitriptyline was more effective. However, 7.5% of the melatonin group had daily sleepiness as a side effect and 22.5% of the amitriptyline group had side effects, such as daily sleepiness, constipation, and fatigue. Melatonin was deemed safer than amitriptyline. The researchers concluded that "prophylactic migraine therapy should be considered in children with frequent and functional disabling headaches."[9]

Melatonin May Benefit Postmenopausal Women

In a trial published in 2018 in the *Journal of Physiology and Pharmacology*, researchers from Poland noted that the decrease in estrogen production in postmenopausal women is associated with various psychosomatic disorders, such as sleep disorder, heart palpitations, sweating, and headaches. They wanted to determine whether melatonin supplementation would improve some of these symptoms. The cohort included 60 postmenopausal women between the ages of 51 and 64 years. For 12 months, half of the participants were placed on 3 mg melatonin in the morning and 5 mg melatonin at bedtime, and the other half took placebos. During the trial, there were periodic assessments. The researchers learned that the majority of the women on melatonin supplementation found that their symptoms disappeared or were significantly reduced. In addition, the women had significant reductions in their body mass index. The melatonin was well-tolerated; only three women reported increased fatigue in the morning during the first week. The researchers commented that melatonin improved most psychosomatic symptoms experienced by the women "regardless of the deficiency of female gonadal steroid hormones." They concluded that "melatonin supplementation therapy exerts a positive effect on psychosomatic symptoms in postmenopausal women and can be recommended as the useful adjuvant therapeutic option in treatment of these disorders."[10]

Melatonin May or May Not Be Useful in the Prevention of Delirium in the Elderly

In a systematic review and meta-analysis published in 2016 in the journal *Molecular Neurobiology*, researchers from China and Loma Linda, California

(USA) wanted to learn if melatonin could help prevent the development of delirium, a life-threatening neuropsychiatric syndrome, in the elderly. At present, there are no effective treatments available for this condition. The researchers located four relevant randomly controlled trials with 669 elderly patients. Compared to patients not treated with melatonin, patients treated with melatonin had a "tendency to decrease incidence of delirium." However, there were no statistically significant differences between the groups. On subgroup analyses, the results were different. For example, in the medical ward, melatonin supplementation reduced the incidence of delirium by 75%. In the surgical ward, there was no significant difference in the incidence of delirium. Furthermore, melatonin had no effect on the improvement of sleep–wake rhythm. The researchers noted that "the exact mechanism via which melatonin exerts its effects in delirium is not well known and needs to be further investigated."[11]

Melatonin Content of Supplements Varies Widely

In a study published in 2017 in the *Journal of Clinical Sleep Medicine*, researchers from Canada wanted to learn more about the contents of commercially sold melatonin supplements. Hence, they analyzed 31 supplements using ultraperformance liquid chromatography with electrochemical detection. All the products were purchased from grocery stores or pharmacies in Guelph, Ontario, Canada. There were 16 different brands that included "a representative sample of formulations." The researchers found that the melatonin content ranged from less than 83% to more than 478% of the labeled content. Moreover, there was significant variability within a particular product; it differed by as much as 465%. The least variable products had the "simplest" mix of ingredients. The researchers expressed concern that the higher doses of melatonin in some of the supplements "could lead to unpleasant or unexpected side effects." They underscored the need for improvements in the production methods for melatonin supplementation. Interestingly, they were surprised to find that eight of the supplements contained serotonin, "a biosynthetic precursor of melatonin and a potent neurotransmitter." The researchers emphasized "that natural over-the-counter supplements do not always equal zero-risk alternatives to traditional medications."[12]

Melatonin May Increase Reactive Aggression in Humans

In a double-blind, randomized, placebo-controlled trial published in 2017 in the journal *Psychopharmacology*, researchers from China evaluated the ability of melatonin supplementation to support reactive aggression or aggression in response to a provocation. The cohort consisted of 63 healthy male Chinese university students, with a mean age of 21 years. They completed questionnaires before being equally divided into a group that took a 5 mg dose of melatonin and a group that took a placebo. Then, they completed more questionnaires. During four sessions, aggression levels were assessed using a modified version of the Taylor aggression paradigm. In this game, winners exerted high or low-noise punishments against the losers. The researchers found that the participants in the melatonin group selected more "high" punishments than those in the placebo group. This study confirms the results of previous research in animals and humans. The researchers concluded that "the adverse effect of melatonin on human social functions is worth noting given the side use of melatonin in clinical practice."[13]

NOTES

1. Ferracioli-Oda, Eduardo, Ahmad Qawasmi, and Michael H. Bloch. "Meta-Analysis for the Treatment of Primary Sleep Disorders." *PLoS ONE* 8, no. 5 (2013): e63773.

2. Auld, F., E. L. Maschauer, I. Morrison, et al. "Evidence for the Efficacy of Melatonin in the Treatment of Primary Adult Sleep Disorders." *Sleep Medicine Reviews* 34 (August 2017): 10–22.

3. Cortesi, F., F. Giannotti, T. Sebastiani, et al. "Controlled-Release Melatonin, Singly and Combined with Cognitive Behavioural Therapy, for Persistent Insomnia in Children with Autism Spectrum Disorders: A Randomized Placebo-Controlled Trial." *Journal of Sleep Research* 21, no. 6 (December 2012): 700–709.

4. Gringras, Paul, Tali Nir, John Breddy, et al. "Efficacy and Safety of Pediatric Prolong-Release Melatonin for Insomnia in Children with Autism Spectrum Disorder." *Journal of the American Academy of Child & Adolescent Psychiatry* 56, no. 11 (November 2017): 948–957.

5. Kennaway, D. J. "Potential Safety Issues in the Use of Hormone Melatonin in Paediatrics." *Journal of Paediatric and Child Health* 51, no. 6 (June 2015): 584–589.

6. Grossman, Ehud, Moshe Laudon, and Nava Zisapel. "Effect of Melatonin on Nocturnal Blood Pressure: Meta-Analysis of Randomized Controlled Trials." *Vascular Health and Risk Management* 7 (2011): 577–584.

7. Hurtuk, A., C. Dome, C. H. Holloman, et al. "Melatonin: Can It Stop the Ringing?" *Annals of Otology, Rhinology & Laryngology* 120, no. 7 (July 2011): 433–440.

8. Hussain, S. A., I. I. Al-Khalifa, N. A. Jasim, and F. I. Gorial. "Adjuvant Use of Melatonin for Treatment of Fibromyalgia." *Journal of Pineal Research* 50, no. 3 (April 2011): 267–271.

9. Fallah, R., F. Fazelishoroki, and L. Sekhavat. "A Randomized Clinical Trial Comparing the Efficacy of Melatonin and Amitriptyline in Migraine Prophylaxis of Children." *Iranian Journal of Child Neurology* 12, no. 1 (Winter 2018): 47–54.

10. Chojnacki, C., A. Kaczka, and A. Gasiorowska, et al. "The Effect of Long-Term Melatonin Supplementation on Psychosomatic Disorders in Postmenopausal Women." *Journal of Physiology and Pharmacology* 69, no. 2 (April 2018): NA.

11. Chen, Sheng, LiGen Shi, Feng Liang, et al. "Exogenous Melatonin for Delirium Prevention: A Meta-Analysis of Randomized Controlled Trials." *Molecular Neurobiology* 53 (2016): 4046–4053.

12. Erland, Lauren A. E. and Praveen K. Saxena. "Melatonin Natural Health Products and Supplements: Presence of Serotonin and Significant Variability of Melatonin Content." *Journal of Clinical Sleep Medicine* 13, no. 2 (2017): 275–281.

13. Liu, Jinting, Ru Zong, Wei Xiong, et al. "Melatonin Increases Reactive Aggression in Humans." *Psychopharmacology* 234 (2017): 2971–2978.

REFERENCES AND FURTHER READING

Auld, F., E. L. Maschauer, I. Morrison, et al. "Evidence for the Efficacy of Melatonin in the Treatment of Primary Adult Sleep Disorders." *Sleep Medicine Reviews* 34 (August 2017): 10–22.

Chen, Sheng, LiGen Shi, Geng Liang, et al. "Exogenous Melatonin for Delirium Prevention: A Meta-Analysis of Randomized Controlled Trials." *Molecular Neurobiology* 53 (2016): 4046–4053.

Chojnacki, C., A. Kaczka, A. Gasiorowska, et al. "The Effect of Long-Term Melatonin Supplementation on Psychosomatic Disorders in Postmenopausal Women." *Journal of Physiology and Pharmacology* 69, no. 2 (April 2018): NA.

Cortesi, F., F. Giannotti, T. Sebastiani, et al. "Controlled-Release Melatonin, Singly and Combined with Cognitive Behavioural Therapy, for Persistent Insomnia in Children with Autism Spectrum Disorders: A Randomized Placebo-Controlled Trial." *Journal of Sleep Research* 21, no. 6 (December 2012): 700–709.

Erland, Lauren A. E., and Praveen K. Saxena. "Melatonin Natural Health Products and Supplements: Presence of Serotonin and Significant Variability of Melatonin Content." *Journal of Clinical Sleep Medicine* 13, no. 2 (2017): 275–281.

Fallah, R., F. Fazelishoroki, and L. Sekhavat. "A Randomized Clinical Trial Comparing the Efficacy of Melatonin and Amitriptyline in Migraine Prophylaxis of Children." *Iranian Journal of Child Neurology* 12, no. 1 (Winter 2018): 47–54.

Ferracioli-Oda, Eduardo, Ahmad Qawasmi, and Michael H. Bloch. "Meta-Analysis: Melatonin for the Treatment of Primary Sleep Disorders." *PLoS ONE* 8, no. 5 (2013): e63773.

Gringras, P., T. Nir, J. Breddy, et al. "Efficacy and Safety of Pediatric Prolonged-Release Melatonin for Insomnia in Children with Autism Spectrum Disorder." *Journal of the American Academy of Child & Adolescent Psychiatry* 56, no. 11 (November 2017): 948–957.

Grossman, Ehud, Moshe Laudon, and Nava Zisapel. "Effect of Melatonin on Nocturnal Blood Pressure: Meta-Analysis of Randomized Controlled Trials." *Vascular Health and Risk Management* 7 (2011): 577–584.

Hurtuk, A., C. Dome, C. H. Holloman, et al. "Melatonin: Can It Stop the Ringing?" *Annals of Otology, Rhinology, & Laryngology* 20, no. 7 (July 2011): 433–440.

Hussain, S. A., I. I. Al-Khalifa, N. A. Jasim, and F. I. Gorial. "Adjuvant Use of Melatonin for Treatment of Fibromyalgia." *Journal of Pineal Research* 50 (2011): 267–271.

Kennaway, D. J. "Potential Safety Issues in the Use of the Hormone Melatonin in Paediatrics." *Journal of Paediatrics and Child Health* 51, no. 6 (June 2015): 584–589.

Liu, Jinting, Ru Zhong, Wei Xiong, et al. "Melatonin Increases Reactive Aggression in Humans." *Psychopharmacology* 234 (2017): 2971–2978.

Milk Thistle

Milk thistle (*silybum marianum*), also known as Mary thistle and holy thistle, is native to southern Europe, southern Russian, Asia Minor, and northern Africa. Today, it is also grown in North and South America and south Australia. Milk thistle comes from the same family of plants as the daisy. Although the terms milk thistle and silymarin tend to be used interchangeably, as they are in this entry, silymarin is actually the main component of milk thistle seeds.

Milk thistle is known to grow in almost any soil type, and hence, people easily grow it outside. However, as milk thistle may be toxic to livestock, people who have animals that roam their land should avoid cultivating milk thistle at home.

HEALTH BENEFITS AND RISKS

Historically, people have used milk thistle for liver disorders, such as hepatitis, cirrhosis, and jaundice, as well as gallbladder problems. It may also help lower blood sugar levels in people with type 2 diabetes and may improve the symptoms of indigestion. In addition, milk thistle may lower low-density lipoprotein (LDL) or "bad" cholesterol. Milk thistle acts as an antioxidant and reduces the production of free radicals; moreover, it has anti-inflammatory properties.

Side effects associated with milk thistle include gastrointestinal problems, such as diarrhea, itchiness, and headache. Because it may lower blood sugar levels, people with type 2 diabetes should use milk thistle with caution. As it may have estrogenic effects, some people contend that women with estrogen-related cancers, such as breast cancer, uterine cancer, and ovarian cancer, should consider avoiding milk thistle. Further, women dealing with endometriosis or uterine fibroids may want to exclude this supplement. Some strongly disagree with these suggestions, and maintain that milk thistle has been safely used for at least 2000 years.

Milk thistle should not be taken with certain medications. For example, it may reduce the effectiveness of the antibiotic metronidazole (Flagyl) and the hepatitis C medication simeprevir (Olysio). Taking milk thistle with the immunosuppressant sirolimus (Rapamune) may alter the way the body processes the medication.

Milk thistle should not be used by anyone with an allergy to plants in the *Asteraceae* family.

HOW IT IS SOLD AND TAKEN

Milk thistle is sold as capsules, softgels, tablets, powder, and tea. It is also sold as a cream. There is no standard dose of milk thistle. Some suggest that up to 420 mg per day in divided doses is safe for up to 41 months, while others suggest higher doses. Studies use widely varying amounts of milk thistle.

RESEARCH FINDINGS

Silymarin May Be Useful for the Treatment of Nonalcoholic Fatty Liver Disease (NAFLD)

In a meta-analysis published in 2017 in the journal *Medicine,* researchers from China wanted to learn if silymarin would be an effective treatment for NAFLD, a common illness in overweight people and those with type 2 diabetes. According to these researchers, there is a need "to develop [a] promising and potent drug in treatment of NAFLD." The researchers included eight high-quality randomized controlled trials with 587 participants, with a median age of about 40 years; six of the trials were in English and two were in Chinese. The researchers learned that the participants in the silymarin supplementation groups experienced significant reductions in blood serum indicators of NAFLD. The researchers concluded that silymarin "could be a preferential option for NAFLD patients."[1]

In a trial published in 2012 in the journal *Hepatitis Monthly,* researchers from Iran tested silymarin and two drugs used to treat types 2 diabetes (metformin and pioglitazone) on 66 people with NAFLD. Twenty-two people were treated with 140 mg per day of silymarin; 22 people were treated with metformin; and 22 people were treated with pioglitazone. With a mean age of 32.62 years, there were 42 males and 24 females. The participants took one pill every day for 2 months, and all completed the trial. Biochemical markers of NAFLD were assessed. The researchers found that the participants in all three groups improved, concluding that silymarin was "well tolerated and seemed to have no side effects when used for two months."[2]

In another trial, published in 2017 in the *Journal of Herbmed Pharmacology,* researchers from Iran tested the ability of silymarin to treat NAFLD in children. The cohort consisted of 40 children between the ages of 5 and 16 years with NAFLD. For 12 weeks, half the children were randomly divided into a silymarin supplement group and half were randomly placed in a control group. All the children were told to exercise and make lifestyle changes. It was suggested that they walk 150 to 250 min per week and follow a low-fat and low-carbohydrate diet. At baseline, there were no statistically significant differences between the two groups. While no significant changes were observed in the control group, the participants with a higher grade of fatty liver disease who took the supplement improved to a lower grade of fatty liver disease. Further, the participants taking the supplement had improvements in liver function tests and triglyceride levels. The researchers concluded that "silymarin could improve biochemical and sonographic indices of NAFLD in children and adolescents."[3]

Milk Thistle May Support Cardiovascular Health in People with Abnormal Lipid Levels

In a double-blind, randomized, placebo-controlled clinical trial published in 2013 in the journal *Expert Opinion on Biological Therapy*, researchers from Italy wanted to learn if a combination of milk thistle and tree turmeric (Indian berberry), another medicinal herb, would be useful for people with abnormal amounts of lipids in the blood, a condition known as dyslipidemia. The researchers initially enrolled 102 dyslipidemic participants. After a 6-month period of dietary changes and physical activity, the remaining 98 participants were placed on the supplement twice a day for 3 months (n = 51) or a placebo (n = 47). After a 2-month washout period, the trial was restarted for a second 3-month period. Ninety-one participants completed the entire trial. At baseline and during the trial, periodic assessments were conducted. Compared to the placebo group, the participants in the supplement group had a 23.2% reduction in total cholesterol and a 32.2% reduction in LDL or "bad" cholesterol. Increases in high-density lipoprotein or "good" cholesterol were seen after 3 months. When the supplement was discontinued, the lipid profiles worsened, and then improved when the supplement was restarted. The researchers concluded that the combined supplementation proved to be "effective and safe."[4]

Milk Thistle May Also Be Useful for Those at Lower Cardiovascular Risk

Four of the Italian researchers in the previous trial examined the use of a supplement with milk thistle, tree turmeric, and red yeast rice (Berberol® K) in people with low cardiovascular risk. Their findings were published in 2017 in the *International Journal of Molecular Sciences*. The randomized, double-blind, placebo-controlled trial initially included 143 participants. All the participants were already following an adequate diet and were exercising. For 3 months, they took the supplement (n = 73) or a placebo (n = 70) during dinner. Four participants failed to complete the entire study; as a result, the final analyses were conducted on 139 participants. Assessments were made at baseline and at the end of the trial. The researchers determined that those taking the supplement had significant reductions in total cholesterol, triglycerides, LDL cholesterol, fasting plasma glucose, and high sensitivity C-reactive protein, a measure of inflammation. The researchers concluded that "combining different hypocholesterolemic nutraceutical agents such as *Berberis aristata*, *Silybum marianum* and monacolin K and KA could be effective and safe to obtain a reduction of lipid profile and an improvement of inflammatory parameters."[5]

Milk Thistle Appears Useful for Liver Toxicity in Children with Acute Lymphoblastic Leukemia (ALL)

In a randomized, double-blind, placebo-controlled trial published in 2010 in the journal *Cancer*, researchers from North Carolina and New York City (USA) investigated the usefulness of milk thistle for liver toxicity in children with ALL. The chemotherapy given for ALL is associated with increases in liver toxicity. The cohort consisted of 50 children with ALL between the ages of 1 and 21 years. For 28 days, 24 children were placed on various doses of milk thistle supplementation, and 26 took a placebo. One child in the supplement group refused to take the supplement and was eliminated from the analysis. Liver toxicity tests were conducted. The researchers determined that milk thistle supplementation was "associated with a trend toward significant reductions in liver toxicity." Further, they concluded that milk thistle "may be a safe, effective supportive care agent."[6]

Oral Silymarin Supplementation May Be Useful for People Undergoing Radiation Therapy for Head and Neck Cancer

In a randomized, double-blind, placebo-controlled pilot clinical trial published in 2016 in the journal *Phytotherapy Research*, researchers from Iran wanted to learn if silymarin supplements would prevent mucositis (painful inflammation and ulceration of mucous membranes lining the digestive tract) in people undergoing radiation treatment (RT) for head and neck cancer. Mucositis is a "frequent severe complication" of the treatment for head and neck cancer. The cohort consisted of 27 patients with an average age of 58.82 years; on the first day of radiotherapy, they were assigned to take 420 mg per day of silymarin, in three divided doses, or a visually identical placebo for 6 weeks. Mucositis grading scores were recorded at baseline and weekly for the next 6 weeks. The researchers designated stages 1 and 2 mucositis as tolerable and stages 3 and 4 as intolerable. They found that intolerable mucositis was significantly more prevalent in the placebo group. In fact, none of the patients in the silymarin group experienced a grade 4 mucositis. The researchers concluded that the "prophylactic administration of conventional form of silymarin tablets could significantly reduce the severity of radiotherapy induced mucositis and delay its occurrence in patients with head and neck cancer."[7]

A Topical Silymarin-Based Preparation May Be Useful for People Having Radiation Therapy for Breast Cancer

In an observational trial published in 2011 in the journal *Strahlentherapie und Onkologie*, researchers from Germany evaluated the ability of a silymarin-based cream to prevent radiodermatitis, or the dermatitis associated with radiation therapy (RT) for breast cancer, a very common condition. In fact, more than 80% of patients with breast cancer undergoing postsurgical RT develop radiodermatitis. The cohort consisted of 101 patients, of which 51 were treated with the silymarin-based cream (Leviaderm®). The other 50 patients used a panthenol-containing cream if local lesions occurred. The mean age of the women in the treatment group was 58 years, whereas the mean age of the women in the other group was 61 years. The patients using the silymarin-based cream did dramatically better than the patients in the other group. For example, during week 5 of radiation therapy, 9.8% of the patients using the silymarin-based cream had grade 2 toxicity, whereas 52% in the other group had grade 2 toxicity. The researchers commented that "silymarin-based cream Leviaderm (®) may be promising and effective treatment for the prevention of acute skin lesions caused by RT of breast cancer patients."[8]

When Combined with Selenium Supplementation, Silymarin Supplementation May Help Men after Radical Prostatectomy

In a 6-month, double-blind, placebo-controlled trial published in 2010 in the journal *Biomedical Papers of the Medical Faculty of the University Palacky, Olomouc, Czech Republic*, researchers from the Czech Republic wanted to learn if supplementation of silymarin and selenium would be useful for men who have undergone a radical prostatectomy. (A radical prostatectomy is the surgical removal of the prostate gland and the surrounding tissues, such as seminal vessels and the nearby lymph nodes.) The cohort consisted of 37 men between the ages of 51 to 72 years, all of whom began the trial 2 to 3 months after their radical prostatectomy. Nineteen men were in the supplementation group, and 18 men were in the placebo group. The daily dose of silymarin was 570 mg. Assessments were conducted at baseline, at 3 months, and at 6 months. The researchers determined that the combination supplement significantly reduced total cholesterol and LDL, two markers of lipid metabolism known to be associated with the progression of prostate cancer. The researchers concluded that their findings "suggest that a dietary intervention with a SM-SE combination could benefit patients after radical prostatectomy and who are at the risk of PCa progression."[9]

Silymarin May Help People with Rheumatoid Arthritis

In a nonrandomized, single-arm clinical trial published in 2017 in the *Iranian Journal of Allergy, Asthma and Immunology*, researchers from Iran examined the ability of silymarin supplementation to reduce some of the markers of rheumatoid arthritis, a chronic autoimmune disease that may lead to joint destruction and disability. The initial cohort consisted of 57 patients with stable rheumatoid arthritis who were under a standard treatment. For 3 months, all patients took 420 mg of silymarin supplementation each day. Forty-four patients completed the trial; 86.4% were female and 13.6% were male. Participant's age ranged from 20 to 70 years, with a mean age of 47.59 years. Measurements of rheumatoid arthritis symptoms, such as swelling, joint tenderness, and pain, were taken at baseline and at the end of the trial. The researchers suggested that the improvements may be explained by the anti-inflammatory and antioxidative properties associated with silymarin. Further, they concluded that silymarin improved both clinical and laboratory symptoms, and had a significant effect in reducing disease activity.[10]

Silymarin Cream May Be Useful for Melasma

In a double-blind, placebo-controlled trial published in 2012 in the journal *BMC Dermatology*, a researcher from Iraq evaluated the safety and efficacy of silymarin cream for melasma, or increased skin pigmentation on the face primarily in areas exposed to the sun. After testing the silymarin cream on rabbits, the researcher enrolled 96 adults diagnosed with melasma. Eighty of the participants were women and 16 were men aged between 28 and 55 years, with a median age of 41 years. The most frequent precipitating factors were sun exposure and pregnancy. The participants were divided into three groups. Participants in two groups used different doses of silymarin cream, and those in the remaining group used a placebo cream. The creams were applied twice daily for 4 weeks. During the trial, the participants were assessed weekly. According to the researchers, all participants treated with silymarin cream had significant improvement in their melasma. They concluded that "silymarin has the efficacy to treat melasma in a dose dependent manner. It is safe. No side effects were observed. All patients were fully and completely satisfied from the first week of treatment."[11]

Silymarin May Help People with Type 2 Diabetes

In a systematic review and meta-analysis published in 2016 in the *Journal of Diabetes Research*, researchers based in Romania examined the use of silymarin by people with type 2 diabetes. They included five randomized controlled trials with 270 participants. Four of the trials evaluated people with type 2 diabetes, and one trial included people with type 2 diabetes and alcoholic cirrhosis. Follow-up ranged from 45 days to 6 months. Silymarin daily doses ranged from 200 to 600 mg. The researchers found that in four of the five trials silymarin significantly improved glycemic control in people with type 2 diabetes. However, the researchers acknowledged that their sample size was small and the trials varied, emphasizing the need for more studies on the topic, commenting that "this warrants further investigation."[12]

In a double-blind, randomized, placebo-controlled clinical trial published in 2017 in the *Journal of Evidence-Based Complementary & Alternative Medicine*, researchers from Iran wanted to learn if a supplement containing 200 mg silymarin, 200 mg olibanum, and 200 mg nettle would be useful for people with poorly controlled type 2 diabetes. Sixty participants with elevated glucose levels were placed in the supplement group (n = 30) or a placebo group (n = 30). The participants were told to take one capsule three times each day before meals. They were assessed at baseline and after 3 months. The researchers learned that, though the participants taking the supplements had significant improvements in glucose and triglyceride levels, the supplement did not significantly lower cholesterol or blood pressure. The researchers commented that "further studies with larger sample size and without adjuvant use of other hypoglycemic agents should be done to confirm the observed effects."[13]

Silymarin Does Not Appear to Be Useful for Chronic Hepatitis C

In a multicenter, double-blind, placebo-controlled trial published in 2012 in the journal *JAMA*, researchers from many locations in the United States, but based in North Carolina (USA), noted that patients often use silymarin to treat chronic liver disease, "despite scant and conflicting evidence of its efficacy." The researchers decided to test the effect of silymarin on 154 participants who had hepatitis C that did not respond to interferon therapy, the standard treatment at the time for this chronic illness. The participants were placed on 420 mg silymarin, 700 mg silymarin, or a matching placebo administered three times per day for 24 weeks. The silymarin doses were higher than usual. Seventy-one percent of the participants were male, and the median age was 54 years. The participants were seen at baseline and at six follow-up visits. The researchers determined that the participants on supplementation did not experience more improvement or have a better quality of life than those taking the placebo. There were no significant differences in response between the three groups. The researchers concluded that "silymarin did not provide greater benefit than placebo for patients with treatment resistant chronic HCV infection."[14]

NOTES

1. Zhong, Sheng, Yuxiang Fan, Qi Yan, et al. "The Therapeutic Effect of Silymarin in the Treatment of Nonalcoholic Fatty Disease: A Meta-Analysis (PRISMA) of Randomized Control Trials." *Medicine* 96, no. 49 (December 2017): e9061.

2. Hajiaghamohammadi, Al Akbar, Amir Ziaee, Sonia Oveisi, Homa Masroor. "Effects of Metformin, Pioglitazone, and Silymarin Treatment on Non-Alcoholic Fatty Liver Disease: A Randomized Controlled Pilot Study." *Hepatitis Monthly* 12, no. 8 (2012): e6099.

3. Famouri, Fatemeh, Mohammad-Mehdi Salehi, Noushin Rostampour, et al. "The Effect of Silymarin on Non-Alcoholic Fatty Liver Disease of Children." *Journal of Herbmed Pharmacology* 6, no. 1 (2017): 16–20.

4. Derosa, Giuseppe, Aldo Bonaventura, Lucio Bianchi, et al. "*Berberis aristata/Silybum marianum* Fixed Combination on Lipid Profile and Insulin Secretion in Dyslipidemic Patients." *Expert Opinion on Biological Therapy* 13, no. 11 (2013): 1495–1506.

5. Derosa, Giuseppe, Angela D'Angelo, Davide Romano, and Pamela Maffioli. "Effects of a Combination of *Berberis aristata, Silybum marianum* and Monacolin on Lipid Profile in Subjects at Low Cardiovascular Risk: A Double-Blind, Randomized, Placebo-Controlled Trial." *International Journal of Molecular Sciences* 18 (2017): 343.

6. Ladas, E. J., D. J. Kroll, N. H. Oberlies, et al. "A Randomized Controlled, Double-Blind Pilot Study of Milk Thistle for the Treatment of Hepatotoxicity in in Childhood Acute Lymphoblastic Leukemia (ALL)." *Cancer* 116, no. 2 (January 15, 2010): 506–513.

7. Elyasi, S., S. Hosseini, M. R. Niazi Moghadam, et al. "Effect of Oral Silymarin Administration on Prevention of Radiotherapy Induced Mucositis: A Randomized, Double-Blinded, Placebo-Controlled Clinical Trial." *Phytotherapy Research* 30, no. 11 (November 2016): 1879–1885.

8. Becker-Schiebe, M., U. Mengs, M. Schaefer, et al. "Topical Use of a Silymarin-Based Preparation to Prevent Radiodermatitis: Results of a Prospective Study in Breast Cancer Patients." *Strahlentherapie und Onkologie* 187, no. 8 (August 2011): 485–491.

9. Vidlar, A., J. Vostalova, J. Ulrichova, et al. "The Safety and Efficacy of a Silymarin and Selenium Combination in Men after Radical Prostatectomy—A Six Month Placebo-Controlled Double-Blind Clinical Trial." *Biomedical Papers of the Medical Faculty of the University Palacky, Olomouc, Czech Republic* 154, no. 3 (September 2010): 239–244.

10. Shavandi, Mehrdad, Ali Moini, Yadollah Shakiba, et al. "Silymarin (Livergol®) Decreases Disease Activity Score In Patients with Rheumatoid Arthritis:

A Non-Randomized Single-Arm Clinical Trial." *Iranian Journal of Allergy, Asthma and Immunology* 16, no. 2 (April 2017): 99–106.

11. Altaei, Tagreed. "The Treatment of Melasma by Silymarin Cream." *BMC Dermatology* 12, no. 1 (October 2012): 18.

12. Voroneanu, Luminita, Ionut Nistor, Raluca Dumea, et al. "Silymarin in Type 2 Diabetes Mellitus: A Systematic Review and Meta-Analysis of Randomized Controlled Trials." *Journal of Diabetes Research* 2016 (2016): Article ID: 5147468.

13. Khalili, Nahid, Reza Fereydoonzadeh, Reza Mohtashami, et al. "Silymarin, Olibanum, and Nettle, a Mixed Herbal Formulation in the Treatment of Type II Diabetes: A Randomized, Double-Blind, Placebo-Controlled, Clinical Trial." *Journal of Evidence-Based Complementary & Alternative Medicine* 22, no. 4 (2017): 603–608.

14. Fried, Michael W., Victor J. Navarro, Nezam Afdhal, et al. "Effect of Silymarin (Milk Thistle) on Liver Disease in Patients with Chronic Hepatitis C Unsuccessfully Treated with Interferon Therapy." *JAMA* 308, no. 3 (July 18, 2012): 274–282.

REFERENCES AND FURTHER READING

Altaei, Tagreed. "The Treatment of Melasma by Silymarin Cream." *BMC Dermatology* 12, no. 1 (October 2012): 18.

Becker-Schiebe, M., U. Mengs, M. Schaefer, et al. "Topical Use of a Silymarin-Based Preparation to Prevent Radiodermatitis: Results of a Prospective Study in Breast Cancer Patients." *Strahlentherapie und Onkologie* 187, no. 8 (August 2011): 485–491.

Derosa, Giuseppe, Aldo Bonaventura, Lucio Bianchi, et al. "*Berberis aristata/Silybum marianum* Fixed Combination on Lipid Profile and Insulin Secretion in Dyslipidemic Patients." *Expert Opinion on Biological Therapy* 13, no. 11 (2013): 1495–1506.

Derosa, Giuseppe, Angela D'Angelo Angela, Davide Romano, and Pamela Maffioli. "Effects of a Combination of *Berberis aristata, Silybum marianum* and Monacolin on Lipid Profile in Subjects in Low Cardiovascular Risk: A Double-Blind, Randomized, Placebo-Controlled Trial." *International Journal of Molecular Sciences* 18 (2017): 343.

Elyasi, S., S. Hosseini, M. R. Niazi Moghadam, et al. "Effect of Oral Silymarin Administration on Prevention of Radiotherapy Induced Mucositis: A Randomized, Double-Blinded, Placebo-Controlled Clinical Trial." *Phytotherapy Research* 30, no. 11 (November 2016): 1879–1885.

Famouri, Fatemeh, Mohammad-Mehdi Salehi, Noushin Rostampour, et al. "The Effect of Silymarin on Non-Alcoholic Fatty Liver Disease of Children." *Journal of Herbmed Pharmacology* 6, no. 1 (2017): 16–20.

Fried, Michael W., Victor J. Navarro, Nezam Afdhal, et al. "Effect of Silymarin (Milk Thistle) on Liver Disease in Patients with Chronic Hepatitis C Unsuccessfully Treated with Interferon Therapy." *JAMA* 308, no. 3 (July 18, 2012): 274–282.

Hajiaghamohammadi, Ali Akbar, Amir Ziaee, Sonia Oveisi, and Homa Masroor. "Effects of Metformin, Pioglitazone, and Silymarin Treatment on Non-Alcoholic Fatty Liver Disease: A Randomized Controlled Pilot Study." *Hepatitis Monthly* 12, no. 8 (2012): e6099.

Khalili, Nahid, Reza Fereydoonzadeh, Reza Mohtashami, et al. "Silymarin, Olibanum, and Nettle, a Mixed Herbal Formulation in the Treatment of Type II Diabetes: A Randomized, Double-Blind, Placebo-Controlled, Clinical Trial." *Journal of Evidence-Based Complementary & Alternative Medicine* 22, no. 4 (2017): 603–608.

Ladas, E. J., D. J. Kroll, N. H. Oberlies, et al. "A Randomized Controlled, Double-Blind Pilot Study of Milk Thistle for the Treatment of Hepatotoxicity in Childhood Acute Lymphoblastic Leukemia (ALL)." *Cancer* 116, no. 2 (January 15, 2010): 506–513.

Shavandi, Mehrdad, Ali Moini, Yadollah Shakiba, et al. "Silymarin (Livergol®) Decreases Disease Activity Score in Patients with Rheumatoid Arthritis: A Non-Randomized Single-Arm Clinical Trial." *Iranian Journal of Allergy, Asthma and Immunology* 16, no. 2 (April 2017): 96–106.

Vidlar, A., J. Vostalova, J. Ulrichova, et al. "The Safety and Efficacy of a Silymarin and Selenium Combination in Men After Radical Prostatectomy–A Six Month Placebo-Controlled Double-Blind Clinical Trial." *Biomedical Papers of the Medical Faculty of the University Palacky, Olomouc, Czech Republic* 154, no. 3 (September 2010): 239–244.

Voroneanu, Luminita, Ionut Nistor, Raluca Dumea, et al. "Silymarin in Type 2 Diabetes Mellitus: A Systematic Review and Meta-Analysis of Randomized Controlled Trials." *Journal of Diabetes Research* 2016 (2016): Article ID: 5147468.

Zhong, Sheng, Yuxiang Fan, Qi Yan, et al. "The Therapeutic Effect of Silymarin in the Treatment of Nonalcoholic Fatty Disease: A Meta-Analysis (PRISMA) of Randomized Control Trials." *Medicine* 96, no. 49 (December 2017): e9061.

Probiotics

Probiotics are live microorganisms—bacteria and yeasts—that may confer health benefits on the host. Though it is well-known that there are many types of probiotic supplements, probiotics may also be present in foods prepared by bacterial fermentation. Probiotic containing foods include yogurt, kefir, sauerkraut, tempeh, and kimchi.

While there are dozens of different probiotic bacteria that appear to have health benefits, the two most common groups are *Lactobacillus* and *Bifidobacterium*. Each of these groups has many species and each species has many strains. Probiotic supplements contain live organisms. A single dose may have a particular strain of microbe or a blend of microbes. These combined supplements are known as broad-spectrum probiotics or multiprobiotics. Different probiotics may help different health conditions. For example, *Lactobacillus* appears to be useful for diarrhea and help people digest lactose, the sugar present in milk. Probiotic supplements with an abundance of *Bifidobacterium* appear to ease the symptoms associated with irritable bowel syndrome, such as diarrhea, constipation, gas, and bloating.

Probiotics are measured as colony forming units or CFUs. This designation is used because probiotics colonize the digestive tract. Probiotic bacteria are alive and well if they can form colonies. The term CFUs represents the number of live bacteria present in the products.

HEALTH BENEFITS AND RISKS

Most studies involving probiotics address digestive health. Probiotics are said to be useful for diarrhea that often occurs with the use of antibiotics. Antibiotics destroy many of the natural bacteria in the gut, which shifts the balance and allows harmful bacteria to thrive. Some suggest that people with *Helicobacter pylori* or inflammatory bowel diseases, such as Crohn's disease and ulcerative colitis, should try probiotic supplementation. In addition, probiotics may be useful for weight loss, inflammation, depression, anxiety, vaginal infections, infectious diarrhea, urinary tract infections, elevated cholesterol levels, blood pressure, immune function, and skin health.

Generally, probiotic supplements are well-tolerated and safe. However, during the first few days of supplementation, there may be digestive discomfort and pain. Once the body acclimates to probiotics, digestion improves. Probiotics may or may not be safe for people with compromised immune systems. It is best to check with a medical provider before initiating supplementation.

HOW IT IS SOLD AND TAKEN

Probiotics are sold in tablets, capsules, vaginal suppositories, and powder. Look for products indicating that they are able to survive passage through the gastrointestinal tract. There is no standard dose for probiotics, and recommendations for adults vary widely from one billion CFUs per day to 10 or 20 or more billion CFUs per day.

Some probiotics are shelf-stable and can be stored in any reasonable location, while others must be refrigerated. If probiotics are refrigerated in the store, they should be refrigerated at home. It is best to check the label for storing instructions.

RESEARCH FINDINGS

Probiotics May Be Useful for Some People with Irritable Bowel Syndrome

In a systematic review and meta-analysis published in 2016 in the journal *BMC Gastroenterology*, researchers from China assessed the ability of probiotics to reduce some of the symptoms of irritable bowel syndrome, a common gastrointestinal functional disorder. They located 21 relevant randomized controlled trials that compared the use of probiotics to placebos in patients suffering from irritable bowel syndrome. In total, there were 700 participants in the probiotics groups and 575 in the control groups. The overall symptoms response rate was 53.3% in the probiotics groups and 27.7% in the control groups. As a result, the use of probiotics significantly improved the symptoms of irritable bowel syndrome. In addition, single probiotics appeared to be more effective in overall symptoms response than combination probiotics. While both low and high doses of probiotics were associated with improvements, short duration treatments of less than 8 weeks seemed to be more effective than longer treatments of more than 8 weeks. The researchers added that "an appreciable placebo effect was detected in some studies, which may have minimized the effects of probiotics."[1]

In a systematic review published in 2010 in the journal *Gut*, researchers from several locations but based in Canada identified 18 randomized controlled trials with 1650 participants who had irritable bowel syndrome. The researchers only included trials in which there was at least 1 week of treatment. In all trials, the diagnosis of irritable bowel syndrome was based on either a doctor's opinion or symptom-based diagnostic criteria. While the low-quality trials tended to find that probiotics had a strong effect on irritable bowel syndrome, the high-quality trials reported more modest effects. The researchers found that probiotics had a "therapeutic benefit" in improving the symptoms of irritable bowel syndrome. However, their findings were limited by the variety of species, strains, and doses of probiotics used in the various studies. Some of the data suggested that *Lactobacilli* had no impact on symptoms, while *Bifidobacteria* and combination supplements improved symptoms. They commented that "it is therefore possible that *Bifidobacteria* constitute the active treatment in probiotic combinations." The researchers underscored the need to learn which species, strains, and doses of probiotics are most "efficacious" in treating irritable bowel syndrome. They concluded that "while we need more information, this systematic review suggests that probiotic treatment is a promising strategy to treat patients with IBS."[2]

In a systematic review and meta-analysis published in 2018 in the journal *Neurogastroenterology & Motility*, researchers from Indiana (USA) reviewed clinical trials on the use of VSL#3, a specific patented probiotic, for the symptoms of irritable bowel syndrome. The researchers included five randomized controlled trials with 243 participants in their analyses (124 randomized to VSL#3 and 119 randomized to placebo). They focused on abdominal pain relief, stool consistency, abdominal bloating, and quality of life. The mean age of the participants was 38.3 years, and 69% were women. Treatment duration ranged from 4 to 8 weeks. In their evaluations, the researchers found no significant differences between the participants taking the probiotic and those taking the placebos. At the same time, individual trials showed evidence of some of the benefits of VSL#3, and few adverse events were reported. Moreover, the researchers observed a "trend toward improvement in overall response." Finally, they concluded that "additional studies of VSL#3 are warranted before recommendations regarding its potential efficacy in IBS can be made."[3]

Probiotics Appear to Be Useful for Antibiotic-Associated Diarrhea (AAD)

In a systematic review and meta-analysis published in 2012 in *JAMA*, researchers based in Santa Monica, California (USA), assessed the ability of probiotics to serve as a prevention and treatment for AAD. A total of 82 randomized controlled trials were included in the analysis. The majority used *Lactobacillus*-based interventions alone or in a combination supplement. Probiotics were generally used to prevent AAD. After conducting their analyses, the researchers determined that the risk of developing AAD was significantly lower for participants using probiotics. Moreover, subgroup analyses did not significantly alter the overall results. The researchers commented that they had "sufficient evidence" to conclude that the probiotics therapy reduced the risk of AAD. However, "this generalized conclusion likely obscures heterogeneity in effectiveness among the patients, the antibiotics, and the probiotic strains or blends."[4]

There Is Some Evidence That Probiotics Are Useful for Lower Gastrointestinal Symptoms

In a systematic review published in 2013 in the journal *Alimentary Pharmacology and Therapeutics*, researchers from several European countries but based in the United Kingdom examined the ability of probiotics to be useful for lower gastrointestinal symptoms addressed by primary care providers. Thirty-seven randomized clinical trials involving adults were included, all of which had a placebo-controlled group or a placebo-controlled period. Thirty-two different probiotics at varying doses were administered once, twice, or three times each day. The researchers noted that they found evidence that there is a role for probiotics in the treatment of lower gastrointestinal problems. They found "strong evidence" that probiotics are useful for AAD or diarrhea associated with *H. pylori* treatment. On the other hand, the researchers did not find support for the use of probiotics for diarrhea in adults with irritable bowel syndrome or to treat constipation. Yet, specific probiotics appeared to reduce overall symptoms and abdominal pain in adults with irritable bowel syndrome. Moreover, oral probiotics had a favorable safety record as none of the studies identified any significant adverse effects caused by these supplements. The researchers concluded that the trials that they evaluated "support, with a moderate evidence level, a role for specific probiotics in managing overall symptoms in patients with IBS-D [diarrhea predominant]; improving bowel movements and bloating/distension in patients with IBS; and improving some aspects of health-related quality of life."[5]

Probiotics May Offer Some Assistance to People Dealing with Inflammatory Bowel Diseases

In a meta-analysis published in 2014 in the journal *Inflammatory Bowel Diseases*, researchers from China and Chicago, Illinois (USA), wanted to learn if probiotics were useful for people with inflammatory bowel diseases, such as ulcerative colitis and Crohn's disease. Twenty-three randomized controlled trials with 1763 participants met the inclusion criteria. The length of follow-up in these trials ranged from 1 to 24 months. The researchers learned that probiotics demonstrated a "therapeutic benefit" in inducing remission in participants with ulcerative colitis. Probiotics may also help maintain remission in inflammatory bowel disease. There is even some evidence that probiotics may play a role in the prevention or treatment of inflammatory bowel diseases. Nevertheless, the researchers acknowledged that "there is still considerable work to do before probiotics can be considered as part of the standard treatment of IBD."[6]

Probiotics May or May Not Be Useful for Some People with Cancer

In a systematic review published in 2014 in the journal *Annals of Oncology*, researchers from the United Kingdom wanted to determine if probiotics would be useful for people dealing with cancer treatments, which may cause diarrhea and a compromised immune system. Their analyses included 11 randomized controlled trials, with 1557 participants, that assessed the efficacy of probiotics in people who are dealing with cancer and 17 studies, with 1530 participants, that evaluated the safety of probiotics. The researchers learned that the patients taking probiotics had less severe diarrhea than those not on probiotics. In addition, the people taking probiotics tended to experience a shift from liquid stools to soft and semi-solid stools. In terms of safety, a number of different adverse events were reported; however, the researchers were unable to determine those that might be related to probiotics. Still, they noted that probiotics in immune-compromised people may be associated with sepsis. The researchers concluded that their "systematic review demonstrates that there is currently insufficient evidence to claim that probiotics are effective and safe in people with cancer."[7]

Probiotics May Be Useful for Acute Respiratory Infections

In a systematic review and meta-analysis published in 2014 in the *British Journal of Nutrition*, researchers from the United Kingdom and Colorado (USA) evaluated the usefulness of probiotics for acute respiratory infections. The researchers found 20 relevant randomized controlled trials, of which 12 were considered to have a low risk of bias. The studies included both children and adults, and the probiotics were administered in varying doses and combinations. To be eligible for inclusion, the trials had to report on a measure of illness duration, such as the number of sick days or the number of days missed from school or work. The duration of probiotic treatment ranged from 3 weeks to 7 months. The researchers determined that the participants taking probiotics had significantly fewer days of illness and significantly fewer days of absence from school or work. The researchers commented that because their investigation included "a large number of high-quality studies that demonstrate a consistent trend . . ., the results are probably reliable."[8]

Probiotics May Help People Lose Weight

In a systematic review and meta-analysis published in 2015 in the *International Journal of Food Sciences and Nutrition*, researchers from China wanted to learn if probiotics would help people lose weight and improve their body mass index. Twenty studies with 25 trials and 1931 participants were included in the analyses. Nineteen studies were parallel randomized controlled trials, with 16 having a double-blind design. Twenty-one trials reported changes in body weight, and 19 trials reported changes in body mass index. The trials varied from 3 to 24 weeks in duration. Of the 21 trials with data on changes in body weight, 15 reported a reduction after using probiotics; of the 19 trials reporting data on body mass index, 16 noted reductions in those taking probiotics. Thus, the researchers concluded that "the consumption of probiotics significantly decreased body weight and BMI by a modest degree." This was most apparent when supplementation continued for more than 8 weeks in overweight and obese people. Multiple supplementation appeared more effective than single species probiotics.[9]

Probiotics May Be Helpful for High Blood Pressure (Hypertension)

In a systematic review and meta-analysis published in 2014 in the journal *Hypertension*, researchers from Australia wanted to learn if probiotics were useful for high blood pressure. Their analyses included nine trials with 543 participants. All of the studies were randomized controlled trials, with seven studies using a double-blind design. Seven trials used fermented dairy products for their probiotics. The researchers learned that consuming probiotics could significantly reduce both diastolic and systolic blood pressure. Studies that used more than one type of probiotics were more effective than those that used only one type of probiotic. While the reductions were "modest," even small reductions "may have important public health benefits." The researchers concluded that "the results of this study showed that consumption of probiotics may improve BP [blood pressure]."[10]

Probiotics May Support Psychological Health

In a systematic review and meta-analysis published in 2017 in *The Journal of Alternative and Complementary Medicine*, researchers from Australia evaluated the ability of probiotics to support psychological health. This is important because there is a prevailing hypothesis that there is an association between the gastrointestinal system and the functioning of the central nervous system. Seven randomized, placebo-controlled studies, with 394 participants, met the inclusion criteria. The studies measured preclinical psychological symptoms of depression, anxiety, and perceived stress in healthy volunteers both before and after supplementation with probiotics. The researchers determined that probiotic supplementation in healthy people significantly reduced the preclinical symptoms of anxiety, depression, and stress. The researchers noted that there is an "increasing need to understand the gut microbiome better and the role it plays in communication via the gut-brain axis."[11]

Probiotics May Reduce the Prevalence of Respiratory Tract Infection in Children Attending Preschool

In a double-blind, randomized, placebo-controlled pilot trial published in 2015 in the *European Journal of Clinical Nutrition*, researchers from Slovakia and the United Kingdom evaluated the use of probiotics and vitamin C supplementation to prevent respiratory tract infections in preschool children. The initial cohort consisted of 69 children between the ages of 3 and 6 years. For 6 months, 34 children took probiotic and vitamin C supplementation and 35 took placebos. Fifty-seven children were included in the final analyses. The researchers found that the children taking the supplementation had significant reductions in the incidence rates of upper respiratory infections, the number of days with infections, and the incidence rates of absence from preschool. The researchers commented that their results were "encouraging," but they need to be confirmed in larger studies. They concluded that "supplementation with a probiotic/vitamin C combination may be beneficial in the prevention and management of URTIs [upper respiratory tract infections]."[12]

Probiotics Do Not Appear to Be Useful for Atopic Dermatitis

In a randomized, double-blind, placebo-controlled trial published in 2014 in the journal *Allergy, Asthma & Immunology Research*, researchers from Korea tested the ability of probiotics to help children suffering with atopic dermatitis, also known as eczema. The initial cohort consisted of 100 children, between the ages of 2 and 10 years, with mild-to-moderate atopic dermatitis. The children were placed in a probiotics group or a placebo group. Measurements were taken at the beginning of the trial and when the trial ended at 6 weeks. Thirty-seven participants in the probiotics group and 34 in the placebo group completed the trial. While fecal cell counts for all probiotics strains were increased substantially, the researchers found significant improvements in both groups. The researchers commented that they were unable to find "an additional therapeutic or immunomodulatory effect on the treatment of AD [atopic dermatitis]."[13]

Probiotic Supplementation May Be Associated with Brain Fogginess, Gas, and Bloating

In a prospective, observational study published in 2018 in the journal *Clinical and Translational Gastroenterology*, researchers based in Augusta, Georgia (USA), examined the association between probiotics and brain fogginess, gas, and bloating. The researchers recruited 30 patients with brain fog and eight without brain fog. They found that abdominal bloating, pain, distension, and gas were the most severe symptoms that occurred at about the same rate in both groups. In the brain fog group, 28 of the 30 participants had fatigue and weakness after eating a meal (postprandial). Brain fog was so severe in the brain fog group that four participants had quit their jobs. All participants in the brain fog group were taking some form of probiotics. Many were also eating yogurt everyday. Only one participant in the no brain fog group took probiotics. When the researchers investigated further, they found that the brain fog group had large colonies of bacteria breeding in their small intestines and high levels of D-lactic acid being produced by the bacterial (*Lactobacillus*) fermentation of sugar. D-lactic acid has been shown to be temporarily toxic to brain cells, interfering with cognition. The researchers found that some of the brain fog participants had two to three times the normal amount of D-lactic acid in their blood. The participants with brain fog were given antibiotics that targeted their bacterial population and were told to discontinue taking probiotics. Those without small intestinal bacterial growth (SIBO) were told to stop probiotics and eliminate yogurt from the diet. Those with SIBO and D-lactic acidosis but no brain fog were also placed on antibiotics. After treatment, 70% of the participants reported significant improvement in symptoms and 85% said that their brain fogginess was gone. The researchers concluded that "clinicians should recognize and treat this condition."[14]

NOTES

1. Zhang, Yan, Lixiang Li, Chuanguo Guo, et al. "Effects of Probiotic Type, Dose and Treatment Duration on Irritable Bowel Syndrome Diagnosed by Rome III Criteria: A Meta-Analysis." *BMC Gastroenterology* 16 (2016): 62.

2. Moayyedi, P., A. C. Ford, N. J. Talley, et al. "The Efficacy of Probiotics in the Treatment of Irritable Bowel Syndrome: A Systematic Review." *Gut* 59, no. 3 (March 2010): 325–332.

3. Connell, M., A. Shin, T. James-Stevenson, et al. "Systematic Review and Meta-Analysis: Efficacy of Patented Probiotic, VSL #3, in Irritable Bowel Syndrome." *Neurogastroenterology & Mobility* 30, no. 12 (December 2018): e13227.

4. Hempel, S., S. J. Newberry, A. R. Maher, et al. "Probiotics for the Prevention and Treatment of Antibiotic-Associated Diarrhea: A Systematic Review and Meta-Analysis." *JAMA* 307, no. 18 (May 9, 2012): 1959–1969.

5. Hungin, A. P. S., C. Mulligan, B. Pot, et al. "Systematic Review: Probiotics in the Management of Lower Gastrointestinal Symptoms in Clinical Practice–An Evidence-Based International Guide." *Alimentary Pharmacology and Therapeutics* 38, no. 8 (October 2013): 864–886.

6. Shen, J., Z. X. Zuo, and A. P. Mao. "Effect of Probiotics on Inducing Remission and Maintaining Therapy in Ulcerative Colitis, Crohn's Disease, and Pouchitis: Meta-Analysis of Randomized Controlled Trials." *Inflammatory Bowel Diseases* 20, no. 1 (January 2014): 21–35.

7. Redman, M. G., E. J. Ward, and R. S. Phillips. "The Efficacy and Safety of Probiotics in People with Cancer: A Systematic Review." *Annals of Oncology* 25, no. 10 (October 2014): 1919–1929.

8. King, S., J. Glanville, M. E. Sanders, et al. "Effectiveness of Probiotics on the Duration of Illness in Healthy Children and Adults Who Develop Common Acute Respiratory Infection Conditions: A Systematic Review and Meta-Analysis." *British Journal of Nutrition* 112, no. 1 (July 14, 2014): 41–54.

9. Zhang, Qingqing, Yucheng Wu, and Xiaoqiang. "Effect of Probiotics on Body Weight and Body-Mass Index: A Systematic Review and Meta-Analysis of Randomized, Controlled Trials." *International Journal of Food Sciences & Nutrition* 66, no. 5 (August 2015): 571–580.

10. Khalesi, S., J. Sun, N. Buys, and R. Jayasinghe. "Effect of Probiotics on Blood Pressure: A Systematic Review and Meta-Analysis of Randomized, Controlled Trials." *Hypertension* 64, no. 4 (October 2014): 897–903.

11. McKean, J., H. Naug, E. Nikbakht, et al. "Probiotics and Subclinical Psychological Symptoms in Healthy Participants: A Systematic Review and Meta-Analysis." *The Journal of Alternative and Complementary Medicine* 23, no. 4 (2017): 249–258.

12. Garaiova, I., J. Muchova, Z. Nagyova, et al. "Probiotics and Vitamin C for the Prevention of Respiratory Tract Infections in Children Attending Preschool: A Randomised Controlled Pilot Study." *European Journal of Clinical Nutrition* 69 (2015): 373–379.

13. Yang, Hyeon-Jong, Taek Ki Min, Hae Won Lee, and Bok Yang Pyun. "Efficacy of Probiotic Therapy on Atopic Dermatitis in Children: A Randomized, Double-Blind, Placebo-Controlled Trial." *Allergy, Asthma & Immunology Research* 6, no. 3 (May 2014): 208–215.

14. Rao, Satish S. C., Abdul Rehman, Siegfried, and Nicole Martinez de Andino. "Brain Fogginess, Gas and Bloating: A Link between SIBO, Probiotics and Metabolic Acidosis." *Clinical and Translational Gastroenterology* 9 (2018): 162.

REFERENCE AND FURTHER READING

Connell, M., A. Shin, T. James-Stevenson, et al. "Systematic Review and Meta-Analysis: Efficacy of Patented Probiotic, VSL#3, in Irritable Bowel Syndrome." *Neurogastroenterology & Motility* 30, no. 12 (December 2018): e13427.

Garaiova, I., J. Muchova, Z. Nagyova, et al. "Probiotics and Vitamin C for the Prevention of Respiratory Tract Infections in Children Attending Preschool: A Randomised Controlled Pilot Study." *European Journal of Clinical Nutrition* 69 (2015): 373–379.

Hempel, S., S. J. Newberry, A. R. Maher, et al. "Probiotics for the Prevention and Treatment of Antibiotic-Associated Diarrhea: A Systematic Review and Meta-Analysis." *JAMA* 307, no. 18 (May 9, 2012): 1959–1969.

Hungin, A. P. S., C. Mulligan, B. Pot, et al. "Systematic Review: Probiotics in the Management of Lower Gastrointestinal Symptoms in Clinical Practice–An Evidence-Based International Guide." *Alimentary Pharmacology and Therapeutics* 38, no. 8 (October 2013): 864–886.

Khalesi, S., J. Sun, N. Buys, and R. Jayasinghe. "Effects of Probiotics on Blood Pressure: A Systematic Review and Meta-Analysis of Randomized, Controlled Trials." *Hypertension* 64, no. 4 (October 2014): 897–903.

King, S., J. Glanville, M. E. Sanders, et al. "Effectiveness of Probiotics on the Duration of Illness in Healthy Children and Adults who Develop Common Acute Respiratory Infections Conditions: A Systematic Review and Meta-Analysis." *British Journal of Nutrition* 112, no. 1 (July 14, 2014): 41–54.

McKean, J., H. Naug, E. Nikbakht, et al. "Probiotics and Subclinical Psychological Symptoms in Healthy Participants: A Systematic Review and Meta-Analysis." *The Journal of Alternative and Complementary Medicine* 23, no. 4 (April 2017): 249–258.

Moayyedi, P., A. C. Ford, N. J, Talley, et al. "The Efficacy of Probiotics in the Treatment of Irritable Bowel Syndrome: A Systematic Review." *Gut* 59, no. 3 (March 2010): 325–332.

Rao, Satish S. C., Abdul Rehman, Siegfried Yu, and Nicole Martinez de Andino. "Brain Fogginess, Gas, and Bloating: A Link between SIBO, Probiotics and Metabolic Acidosis." *Clinical and Translational Gastroenterology* 9 (2018): 162.

Redman, M. G., E. J. Ward, and R. S. Phillips. "The Efficacy and Safety of Probiotics in People with Cancer: A Systematic Review." *Annals of Oncology* 25, no. 10 (October 2014): 1919–1929.

Shen, J., Z. X. Zuo, and A. P. Mao. "Effect of Probiotics on Inducing Remission and Maintaining Therapy in Ulcerative Colitis, Crohn's Disease, and Pouchitis: Meta-Analysis of Randomized Controlled Trials." *Inflammatory Bowel Diseases* 20, no. 1 (January 2014): 21–35.

Yang, Hyeon-Jong, Taek Ki Min, Hae Won Lee, and Bok Yang Pyun. "Efficacy of Probiotic Therapy on Atopic Dermatitis in Children: A Randomized, Double-Blind, Placebo-Controlled Trial." *Allergy, Asthma & Immunology Research* 6, no. 3 (May 2014): 208–215.

Zhang, Qingqing, Yucheng Wu, Xiaoqiang Fei. "Effect of Probiotics on Body Weight and Body-Mass Index: A Systematic Review and Meta-Analysis of Randomized, Controlled Trials." *International Journal of Food Sciences and Nutrition* 66, no. 5 (August 2015): 571–580.

Zhang, Yan, Lixiang Li, Chuanguo Guo, et al. "Effect of Probiotic, Type, Dose and Treatment Duration on Irritable Bowel Syndrome Diagnosed by Rome III Criteria: A Meta-Analysis." *BMC Gastroenterology* 16 (2016): 62.

Red Yeast Rice

Red yeast rice is extracted from rice and fermented with a type of yeast known as *Monascus purpureus*. The powdery yeast–rice mixture is a dietary staple in Asian diet and has been used in traditional Chinese medicine for centuries. Today, many consider red yeast rice supplementation to be the most effective over-the-counter treatment for elevated levels of low-density lipoprotein (LDL) or bad cholesterol.

The exact composition of red yeast rice varies according to the yeast strains and culture conditions used in manufacturing. Because of this variability, it is important to obtain red yeast supplementation from a reliable source. Once a reliable source has been found, it is a good idea to keep buying the same brand.

HEALTH BENEFITS AND RISKS

In the United States, red yeast supplements are primarily sold as a means to support heart health and lower cholesterol levels. Red yeast rice products may contain monacolins, especially monacolin K, which are active compounds that inhibit the synthesis of cholesterol in the liver. Monacolin K is chemically identical to the active ingredient in the cholesterol-lowering drug lovastatin, the active ingredient in the prescription drug Mevacor. However, some products contain little or no monacolins, and consumers have no way of knowing the monacolin levels of the products they are buying as they are not listed on the label. Red yeast rice also contains sterols, isoflavones, and monounsaturated fats.

Some red yeast rice supplements have the same side effects as lovastatin and other cholesterol-lowering medications including myopathy (muscular pain and weakness), rhabdomyolysis (breakdown of muscle fibers and release of substances that may harm kidneys), and liver toxicity. Lovastatin should not be mixed with certain medications such as drugs used to treat fungal infections and certain antibiotics. Red yeast rice supplements that contain monacolin K could interact in the same way. On the other hand, people who are unable to tolerate statin medications appear to do well on red yeast rice supplementation.

People taking certain medications should not use red yeast rice supplementation. These include drugs that suppress the immune system, such as cyclosporine, antifungal drugs, such as fluconazole, and medications used to treat HIV. In addition, red yeast rice supplements may interact with medications for blood pressure, thyroid problems, and other supplements. People with liver or kidney disease or those who have received a transplant should not use red yeast rice. People who drink more than two alcoholic beverages per day or who have a serious infection or a physical problem should also avoid this supplement.

Some red yeast rice supplements may contain potentially harmful contaminants, such as citrinin, which may cause kidney failure. This is more likely to occur when the red yeast rice culturing process is not carefully controlled.

Other side effects associated with red yeast rice supplementation include headaches, heartburn, abdominal discomfort, gas, dizziness, and upset stomach. It is not known whether it is safe for pregnant or breastfeeding women to use red yeast rice supplements. Therefore, it is best for these women to avoid them. Unless under the care of a medical provider well versed in red yeast rice, children should not take red yeast rice supplementation. People already on prescription statin drugs should avoid this supplement.

HOW IT IS SOLD AND TAKEN

Red yeast rice supplementation is sold in tablets, capsules, powder, and extract. Though there are no dose recommendations for red yeast rice supplementation, some suggest 1200 mg once or twice a day with food.

RESEARCH FINDINGS

Red Yeast Rice Appears to Support Cardiovascular Health in People with Metabolic Syndrome

In a randomized, open-label, clinical trial published in 2018 in the journal *Biomedicine & Pharmacotherapy*, researchers from Italy and South Carolina (USA) examined the ability of red yeast rice to improve the high blood pressure and high levels of cholesterol in people suffering from metabolic syndrome. The cohort consisted of 104 patients suffering from metabolic syndrome, with a mean age of 57.4 years. Slightly over half were males. No one had a history of cardiovascular disease. For 2 months, 52 participants took daily supplementation containing red yeast rice and coenzyme Q10 and 52 followed a diet program. The researchers learned that the participants in the treatment group had significant improvements in lipid profile, blood pressure, and glucose levels. These changes were greater than the improvements in the other group. According to the researchers, the dietary supplementation of red yeast rice and coenzyme Q10 offers "promising strategies" for treating metabolic syndrome "with minimal side effects." They concluded that the treatment was "safe, well-tolerated, and effective."[1]

Monacolin K Improves Lipids and Metabolic Patterns of Hypertensive and Hypercholesterolemic Patients

In a single-site, randomized, open-label clinical trial published in 2018 in the journal *Food & Function*, researchers investigated the efficacy of using high doses of monacolin K (10 mg) to improve the lipid profile and glucose metabolism in participants with high blood pressure and high levels of cholesterol. The cohort consisted of 60 participants with high blood pressure and high levels of cholesterol. The treatment group of 30 participants took a daily supplementation containing monacolin K, policosanols, resveratrol, chromium picolinate, and black pepper. A control group of 30 participants only adhered to a diet program. Periodic assessments were conducted until the trial ended after 1 month. The researchers learned that the participants in the treatment group had significant reductions in total cholesterol, LDL, and glucose levels. The researchers noted that the supplement was effective, safe, and well-tolerated. They also commented that they paid particular attention to safety concerns, concluding that "the fact that no adverse event was detected, highlights the safety of the product."[2]

Monacolin K Reduces Concentrations of LDL

In a randomized, double-blind, placebo-controlled trial published in 2016 in the journal *Nutrition Research*, researchers from Germany tested the ability of a low dose (3 mg) of monacolin K from red yeast rice to lower serum concentrations of LDL. The cohort consisted of 142 adult participants who had elevated cholesterol levels but were not treated with statin medication. They were placed in the supplement group (n = 70) or the placebo group (n = 72). The intervention continued for 12 weeks. Blood samples were taken at baseline and after 6 and 12 weeks. The researchers found that even a lower dose of the supplement had a significant cholesterol-lowering effect. In fact, in the treatment group, levels of LDL cholesterol were reduced by about 15%. The researchers commented that their findings indicated "that borderline high LDL-C levels from nonstatin-treated participants can be effectively lowered despite the low dosage of 3 mg monacolin K."[3]

People Who Are Statin Intolerant May Wish to Try Red Yeast Rice

In a randomized, double-blind trial published in 2010 in the *American Journal of Cardiology*, researchers based in Pennsylvania (USA) wanted to learn if red yeast rice would be useful for people who develop statin-associated myalgia (statin-related muscle problems) and decide to discontinue their statin medications. Forty-three adults with dyslipidemia and a history of statin discontinuation because of myalgia were randomly assigned to red yeast rice 2,400 mg twice daily or 20 mg twice daily of pravastatin. There were 21 participants in the red yeast rice group and 22 in the pravastatin group. None of the participants had ever taken pravastatin. The trial continued for 12 weeks. The researchers found no difference in pain severity and muscle strength between the two groups. The LDL cholesterol levels decreased by 30% in the red yeast rice group and by 27% in the pravastatin group. Thus, red yeast rice and pravastatin were almost equally effective. While the researchers acknowledged that they are unable to offer any "definitive conclusions," their data "showed that the red yeast rice was as well tolerated as pravastatin and achieved similar and clinically significant levels of LDL cholesterol reduction in a population with previous statin intolerance."[4]

When Combined with a Mediterranean Diet, Red Yeast Rice Is Even More Effective for the Management of Hyperlipidemia in Statin-Intolerant People

In a trial published in 2013 in the journal *Evidence-Based Complementary and Alternative Medicine*, researchers from Italy compared the ability of red yeast rice supplementation combined with a Mediterranean diet or red yeast supplementation alone to manage elevated levels of cholesterol in statin-intolerant people with or without diabetes. The cohort consisted of 171 participants, of which 46 had type 2 diabetes and were treated only with a Mediterranean diet (group 1). Forty-four participants who had type 2 diabetes were treated with a Mediterranean diet and red yeast rice (group 2). Thirty-eight participants with elevated cholesterol levels were treated only with a Mediterranean diet (group 3), and 43 subjects with elevated cholesterol levels were treated with a Mediterranean diet and red yeast rice (group 4). The trial continued for 24 weeks, and there were follow-up visits after the trial ended. By the end of the trial, all participants had significant reductions in total cholesterol. While the Mediterranean diet alone was able to reduce LDL cholesterol level in statin-intolerant participants with moderately elevated levels of cholesterol. When the Mediterranean diet was combined with red yeast rice, there were even greater improvements. The reduction was "similar to the reduction obtained using statins."[5]

Red Yeast Rice Appears to Be an Effective and Safe Treatment for Dyslipidemia

In a meta-analysis published in 2014 in the online journal *PLoS ONE*, researchers from China examined the association between the intake of red yeast rice and dyslipidemia. Their cohort consisted of 13 randomized, placebo-controlled trials with a total of 804 participants; all trials were published in English and had treatments that continued for at least 4 weeks. Most trials were double-blind and had a low risk of bias. The researchers determined that red yeast rice demonstrated a significant lowering effect on total cholesterol, triglycerides, and LDL cholesterol, but it did not significantly increase HDL or good cholesterol levels. None of the trials reported any serious side effects. The researchers concluded that red yeast rice "is an effective and relatively safe approach for dyslipidemia." It may well be useful "for the primary and secondary prevention of coronary heart disease."[6]

In a double-blind, placebo-controlled, randomized trial published in 2013 in the journal *BMC Complementary and Alternative Medicine*, researchers from Belgium wanted to learn if red yeast rice would be useful for 52 physicians and physician spouses/partners who had elevated levels of cholesterol. They all had total cholesterol levels above 200 mg/dL. Participants already taking statin medications were excluded. For 8 weeks, the participants took red yeast rice supplementation or a placebo. The supplement contained 5025 mg of monacolin K per capsule, resulting in a daily dose of 10.05 mg, higher than most commercially available products. While the participants in the intervention group had significant reductions in total cholesterol and LDL, those in the placebo group experienced no reductions in total cholesterol and LDL. The magnitude of the effect in the intervention group ranged from −8.03% to 40.46%, with a mean difference of 22.17% and a median difference of 25.47%. While the difference was not statistically significant, there appeared to be slightly more muscle complaints in the intervention group. The researchers concluded that the possible indicators for using red yeast rice "are intolerance of statins or refusal to take synthetic drugs in people in whom lipid lowering therapy is indicated."[7]

Red Yeast Rice May or May Not Be as Effective as the Statin Medication Simvastatin in People with Elevated Cholesterol Levels

In a systematic review published in 2016 in the *Journal of Clinical Pharmacy and Therapeutics,* researchers from Malaysia compared the effectiveness and safety of red yeast rice and simvastatin for the management of elevated cholesterol levels. Their review included ten randomized controlled trials involving 905 Chinese participants who were treated for a minimum of 2 weeks. The total daily dose of red yeast rice used in the trials ranged from 1–2 to 3–6 g, while the daily dose of simvastatin was either 10 mg or 20 mg. Sample sizes ranged from 28 to 224 participants, and the duration of the trials varied from 4 to 12 weeks. The researchers determined that the trials found no significant differences in total cholesterol and LDL cholesterol between the participants treated with red yeast rice and simvastatin. However, the researchers cautioned that the trials had small sample sizes and lacked "methodological rigor." Hence, their findings do not support the use of red yeast rice instead of simvastatin, "except perhaps for those intolerant to the statins."[8]

Red Yeast Rice May Help Reduce the Negative Metabolic Impacts of Second-Generation Antipsychotic Medication

In a 30-day, open-label pilot trial published in 2018 in the journal *Complementary Therapies in Medicine,* researchers from Italy explained that second-generation antipsychotic medications place people at an increased risk for the development of metabolic syndrome. They wanted to learn if red yeast rice supplementation would reduce this effect of these drugs. This is important as metabolic syndrome increases the risk of cardiovascular disease and associated premature mortality. The cohort consisted of 30 psychiatric outpatients taking second-generation antipsychotic medications (clozapine, olanzapine, and quetiapine). There were 11 men and four women whose age ranged from 32 to 67 years. All participants were placed on 200 mg per day of red yeast rice supplementation. Assessments were made during three visits. Thirteen participants completed the trial. The researchers determined that the administration of red yeast rice resulted in a statistically significant reduction in LDL levels. The supplementation was well-tolerated, and no participants reported adverse effects. The researchers concluded that red yeast rice supplementation may prove to be useful to the growing number of people being treated with second-generation antipsychotic medications.

According to the researchers, "further adequately-powered and well-designed studies with long-term follow-up" are needed.[9]

There Appears to Be Strength Variability in Red Yeast Rice Supplements

In a study published in 2017 in the *European Journal of Preventive Cardiology*, researchers from the Boston area and Mississippi (USA) noted that in the United States, consumers spend about 20 million dollars a year on red yeast rice supplements. Therefore, they wanted to learn more about the usefulness of these supplements. Specifically, they hoped to determine the actual amount of monacolin K in 28 brands purchased at GNC, Walgreens, Walmart, and Whole Foods. The researchers found that two brands had no monacolin K. In the 26 brands that had monacolin K, the quantity ranged from 0.09 to 5.48 mg per 1200 mg of red yeast rice. None of the brands listed the quantity of monacolin K; only two products advised consumers not to take the supplement with prescription statins. The researchers concluded that the "strength and composition of red yeast supplements sold at mainstream retail stores in the United States remains unpredictable."[10]

Adverse Reactions to Red Yeast Rice May Occur

In a study published in 2017 in the *British Journal of Clinical Pharmacology*, researchers from Italy reviewed 52 reports with 55 red yeast rice adverse reactions collected by the Italian government from April 2002 to September 2015. The reports contained 37 women and 14 men aged 35–85 years—in one case gender was not reported. In all but four reports, the total daily dose of monacolin K was 3 mg. Nineteen people described muscle pain, including some who experienced an increase in creatine phosphokinase levels, an enzyme that is released when muscle tissue is damaged. Thirteen cases required hospitalization. Moreover, ten patients had liver damage, of which six were considered serious. These are the side effects associated with statin medications. Additionally, 12 patients reported gastrointestinal problems, such as upset stomach, nausea, vomiting, and diarrhea. Thirty-seven percent of the reactions occurred within 1 month of supplementation and 75% within 1 month. According to the researchers, it is important to note that statin medications are prescribed by medical providers; hence, during follow-up appointments, they should look out for side effects. On the other hand, people who decide to supplement their diets with red yeast rice may have side effects that go unnoticed. The researchers concluded that red yeast rice supplementation has a safety profile similar to statin medications. They commented that, "clinicians should be informed that monacolin K contained in RYR [red yeast rice] is identical to lovastatin, and consider early monitoring of liver function, and signs of muscle injury. In parallel, consumers should be discouraged from using RYR preparations as self-medication, particularly if they have experienced previous adverse reactions to statins."[11]

NOTES

1. Mazza, A., S. Lenti, L. Schiavon, et al. "Effect of Monacolin K and COQ10 Supplementation in Hypertensive and Hypercholesterolemic Subjects with Metabolic Syndrome." *Biomedicine & Pharmacotherapy* 105 (September 2018): 992–996.

2. Mazza, A., L. Schiavon, G. Rigatelli, et al. "The Short-term Supplementation of Monacolin K Improves the Lipid and Metabolic Patterns of Hypertensive and Hypercholesterolemic Subjects at Low Cardiovascular Risk." *Food & Function* 9, no. 7 (July 17, 2018): 3845–3852.

3. Heinz, T., J. P. Schuchardt, K. Möller, et al. "Low Daily Dose of 3 mg Moacolin K from RYR Reduces the Concentration of LDL-C in a Randomized, Placebo-Controlled Intervention." *Nutrition Research* 36, no. 10 (October 2016): 1162–1170.

4. Halbert, S. C., B. French, R. Y. Gordon, et al. "Tolerability of Red Yeast Rice (2,400 mg twice daily) versus Pravastatin (20 mg twice daily) in Patients with Previous Statin Intolerance." *American Journal of Cardiology* 105, no. 2 (January 15, 2010): 198–204.

5. Giovanni, Sartore, Burlina Silvia, Ragazzi Eugenio, et al. "Mediterranean Diet and Red Yeast Rice Supplementation for the Management of Hyperlipidemia in Statin-Intolerant Patients with or without Type 2 Diabetes." *Evidence-Based Complementary and Alternative Medicine* 2013 (2013): Article ID: 743473.

6. Li, Yinhua, Long Jiang, Zhangrong Jia, et al. "A Meta-Analysis of Red Yeast Rice: A Effective and Relatively Safe Alternative Approach for Dyslipidemia." *PLoS ONE* 9, no. 6 (2014): e98611.

7. Verhoeven, Veronique, Maja Lopez Hartmann, Roy Remmen, et al. "Red Yeast Rice Lowers Cholesterol in Physicians—A Double-Blind, Placebo-Controlled Randomized Trial." *BMC Complementary & Alternative Medicine* 13 (2013): 178.

8. Ong, Y. C. and Z. Aziz. "Systematic Review of Red Yeast Rice Compared with Simvastatin in Dyslipidaemia." *Journal of Clinical Pharmacy and Therapeutics* 41, no. 2 (April 2016): 170–179.

9. Bruno, Antonio, Gianluca Pandolfo, Manuela Crucitti, et al. "Red Yeast Rice (RYR) Supplementation in Patients Treated with Second-Generation Antipsychotics." *Complementary Therapies in Medicine* 37 (2018): 167–171.

10. Cohen, P. A., B. Avula, and I. A. Khan. "Variability in Strength of Red Yeast Rice Supplements Purchased from Mainstream Retailers." *European Journal of Preventive Cardiology* 24, no. 13 (September 2017): 1431–1434.

11. Mazzanti, Gabriela, Paola Angela Moro, Emanuel Raschi, et al. "Adverse Reactions to Dietary Supplements Containing Red Yeast Rice: Assessment of Cases from the Italian Surveillance System." *British Journal of Clinical Pharmacology* 83 (2017): 894–908.

REFERENCE AND FURTHER READING

Bruno, Antonio, Gianluca Pandolfo, Manuela Crucitti, et al. "Red Yeast Rice (RYR) Supplementation in Patients Treated with Second-Generation Antipsychotics." *Complementary Therapies in Medicine* 37 (2018): 167–171.

Cohen, P. A., B. Avula, and I. A. Khan. "Variability in Strength of Red Yeast Rice Supplements Purchased from Mainstream Retailers." *European Journal of Preventive Cardiology* 24, no. 13 (September 2017): 1431–1434.

Giovanni, Sartore, Burlina Silvia, Ragazzi Eugenio, et al. "Mediterranean Diet and Red Yeast Rice Supplements for the Management of Hyperlipidemia in Statin-

Intolerant Patients with or without Type 2 Diabetes." *Evidence-Based Complementary and Alternative Medicine* 2013 (2013): Article ID: 743473.

Halbert, S. C., B. French, R. Y. Gordon, et al. "Tolerability of Red Yeast Rice (2,400 mg twice daily) versus Pravastatin (20 mg twice daily) in Patients with Previous Statin Intolerance." *American Journal of Cardiology* 105, no. 2 (January 15, 2010): 198–204.

Heinz, T., J. P. Schuchardt, K. Möller, et al. "Low Daily Dose of 3 mg Monacolin K from RYR Reduces the Concentration of LDL-C in a Randomized, Placebo-Controlled Intervention." *Nutrition Research* 36, no. 10 (October 2016): 1162–1170.

Li, Yinhua, Long Jiang, Zhangrong Jia, et al. "A Meta-Analysis of Red Yeast Rice: An Effective and Relatively Safe Alternative Approach for Dyslipidemia." *PLoS ONE* 9, no. 6 (2014): e98611.

Mazza, A., S. Lenti, L. Schiavon, et al. "Effect of Monacolin K and COQ10 Supplementation in Hypertensive and Hypercholesterolmic Subjects with Metabolic Syndrome." *Biomedicine & Pharmacotherapy* 105 (September 2018): 992–996.

Mazza, A., L. Schiavon, G. Rigatelli, et al. "The Short-Term Supplementation of Monacolin K Improves the Lipid and Metabolic Patterns of Hypertensive and Hypercholesterolemic Subjects at Low Cardiovascular Risk." *Food & Function* 9, no. 7 (July 17, 2018): 3845–3852.

Mazzanti, Gabriela, Paola Angela Moro, Emanuel Raschi, et al. "Adverse Reactions to Dietary Supplements Containing Red Yeast Rice: Assessment of Cases from the Italian Surveillance System." *British Journal of Clinical Pharmacology* 83 (2017): 894–908.

Ong, Y. C., and Z. Aziz. "Systematic Review of Red Yeast Rice Compared with Simvastatin in Dyslipidaemia." *Journal of Clinical Pharmacy and Therapeutics* 41, no. 2 (April 2016): 170–179.

Verhoeven, Veronique, Maja Lopez Hartmann, Roy Remmen, et al. "Red Yeast Rice Lowers Cholesterol in Physicians—A Double Blind, Placebo Controlled Randomized Trial." *BMC Complementary and Alternative Medicine* 13 (2013): 178.

Resveratrol

Resveratrol is a member of a group of compounds called polyphenols that act like antioxidants and protect the body from free radicals that damage cells and increase the risk of heart disease and cancer.

Some contend that resveratrol may expand blood vessels and reduce blood clotting. Resveratrol may also reduce inflammation and heal acne, and may have mild estrogenic properties.

Though resveratrol is probably best known for being in red wine and the skin of red grapes, it is also found in other foods such as purple grape juice, peanuts, blueberries, raspberries, and cranberries. In the United States, most resveratrol sold contains extracts from an Asian plant called *Polygonum cuspidatrum.* However, they also may be manufactured from red wine or red grape extracts.

HEALTH BENEFITS AND RISKS

Resveratrol has received a good deal of attention for its many alleged health benefits. It is thought to improve cardiovascular health and reduce the risk of cancer. It is also believed to have antiaging and disease-fighting properties. Resveratrol may offer protection to nerve cells and fight the build-up of plaque associated with Alzheimer's disease. In addition, it appears to help prevent insulin resistance, a condition in which the body becomes less sensitive to insulin, the hormone that lowers blood sugar, which may lead to diabetes. Moreover, resveratrol is thought to activate the *SIRT1* gene, which protects the body against obesity.

It is possible that resveratrol may interact with blood-thinning medications, such as aspirin, or blood-thinning herbs or supplements, such as ginger and turmeric, which may increase the risk of bleeding. Resveratrol should be discontinued 2 weeks before any scheduled surgery. Because it has estrogen-like properties, resveratrol should not be used by anyone with an estrogen-sensitive condition, such as breast cancer, uterine cancer, ovarian cancer, endometriosis, and uterine fibroids. When a resveratrol supplement is taken with a high-fat meal, the amount of resveratrol actually absorbed into the body may be reduced.

It is best to avoid using resveratrol if one is already taking a medication that is altered or broken down by the liver. Resveratrol may decrease the rate at which this process occurs and increase the effects and side effects of such medications, for example, omeprazole (Prilosec), lansoprazole (Prevacid), diazepam (Valium), citalopram (Celexa), and amitriptyline (Elavil).

HOW IT IS SOLD AND TAKEN

Resveratrol is sold as tablets, capsules, softgels, powder, or liquid. There are no specific dosage recommendations. Recommendations may vary from supplement to supplement. However, the doses in supplements tend to be lower than the amounts used in research studies. Most supplements contain 250 to 500 mg, but there are supplements that have 2000 or 3000 mg.

RESEARCH FINDINGS

Resveratrol Supplementation Appears to Be Useful for People with Problematic Lipid Profiles

In a randomized, double-blind, placebo-controlled trial published in 2019 in the journal *Nutrition*, researchers from northern Mexico wanted to determine if resveratrol would be useful for apparently healthy people with problematic lipid levels. The cohort consisted of 71 people with newly diagnosed dyslipidemia. At baseline, there were no significant differences between the two groups in age, number of women, and total body fat percentage. For 2 months, thirty-five participants took 100 mg resveratrol per day and 36 took a placebo. The participants in both groups were advised to consume a diet with 50% carbohydrates, 30% lipids, and 20% protein. They were also told to perform physical activity for at least 30 min, three times per week. Sixty-two participants completed the study and follow-up. The researchers learned that resveratrol supplement significantly reduced the levels of total cholesterol and triacylglycerols. At the same time, it did not alter levels of high-density or low-density lipoprotein. The researchers commented that their findings "adds to the field that the beneficial effect of resveratrol on the TC [total cholesterol] levels also may be found in healthy individuals suggesting a potential role of this phenolic compound in prevention of CVDs [cardiovascular diseases]."[1]

Resveratrol Helps Lower High Blood Pressure

In a trial published in 2017 in the journal *Experimental and Therapeutic Medicine*, researchers from the Republic of Cyprus investigated the antihypertensive properties of resveratrol. The cohort consisted of 97 participants with high blood pressure. Based on the severity of high blood pressure, the participants were placed in group A (n = 46) or group b (n = 51). With a milder form of high blood pressure, group A had 25 males and 21 females. With more serious levels of high blood pressure, group B had 32 males and 19 females. The participants in these two groups were evenly divided in a random manner into two subgroups. Within each group, one subgroup received the standard treatment of Dapril and the other received Dapril plus Evelor, a resveratrol supplement. By the end of the trial, held from October 2010 to October 2012, the mean blood pressure of both groups was within the normal range. The researchers commented that their findings demonstrated that the addition of resveratrol to standard treatment for high blood pressure was "sufficient to reduce blood pressure to normal levels, without the need for additional antihypertensive drugs."[2]

Resveratrol May Play a Role in Treating Certain Aspects of Alzheimer's Disease

In a randomized, double-blind, placebo-controlled, 52-week trial published in 2015 in the journal *Neurology*, researchers from several locations in the United States but based in Washington, DC (USA), examined the use of resveratrol supplementation for people with mild-to-moderate Alzheimer's disease. The cohort consisted of 119 men and women; everyone was over the age of 49 years. The participants were initially placed on either 500 mg per day of resveratrol or a placebo. Over the course of the trial, the amount of resveratrol was periodically increased until it reached 1000 mg twice daily. During the trial, the researchers conducted periodic assessments. A total of 104 participants completed the trial, of which 57% were female and 91% were Caucasian. The researchers found that the high-dose oral resveratrol was safe and well-tolerated. The most common adverse effects of resveratrol were nausea, diarrhea, and weight loss. The researchers observed several important findings. First, resveratrol could penetrate the blood–brain barrier. Second, the participants treated with resveratrol showed little or no change in amyloid-beta 40 levels in the blood and cerebrospinal fluid, which was a good sign. A decrease in amyloid-beta 40 is associated with a worsening of Alzheimer's disease. In addition, the participants taking resveratrol lost weight, while those on placebo gained weight. Brain scans taken before and after the trial found that the participants on the supplement lost more brain volume than those on placebo. The researchers hypothesized that resveratrol reduced the brain swelling associated with Alzheimer's disease. The researchers concluded that a larger study is needed "to determine whether resveratrol may be beneficial."[3]

When Combined with Meloxicam, Resveratrol Appears to Be Useful for Knee Osteoarthritis

In a double-blind, placebo-controlled, randomized, multicenter trial published in 2018 in the journal *Clinical Interventions in Aging*, researchers from Iraq noted that resveratrol has demonstrated "remarkable" anti-inflammatory properties in experimental models. They wanted to learn if it would also be useful for people suffering from knee osteoarthritis. Their cohort consisted of 110 patients with knee osteoarthritis, of which 55 received 500 mg per day of resveratrol supplementation and 55 took a placebo. All patients were placed on 15 mg per day of meloxicam, a nonsteroidal anti-inflammatory drug. During the 90-day trial, the patients were assessed during four follow-up visits. Ninety-two patients completed the study and follow-up requirements. Compared to the placebo, the researchers determined that resveratrol supplementation significantly improved pain, function, and other symptoms associated with knee osteoarthritis. The researchers commented that their findings "suggest that resveratrol could be a potential analgesic that decreases pain and discomfort of knee OA [osteoarthritis] and improves the patient's general condition and quality of daily life."[4]

Short-Term Use of Resveratrol Supplementation Appears to Be Safe in Overweight Elders

In a double-blind, randomized, placebo-controlled trial published in 2014 in the journal *Experimental Gerontology*, researchers from Gainesville and Port Orange, Florida (USA), wanted to examine the safety and efficacy of resveratrol in older adults who were overweight. The cohort consisted of 32 adults with a mean age of 73 years. The participants were placed in one of the three groups—placebo (n = 10), 300 mg per day of resveratrol (n = 12), or 1000 mg per day of resveratrol (n = 10). The trial continued for 90 days; during that time, participants were periodically assessed. The researchers found that the participants on both doses of the supplement had significantly lower glucose levels than those taking the placebo. They also learned that both doses of resveratrol were well-tolerated, and that the supplement did not have an adverse effect on blood chemistries. They concluded that "these findings support the study of resveratrol for improving cardio-metabolic health in older adults in larger clinical trials."[5]

Resveratrol May Be Useful in the Treatment of Rheumatoid Arthritis

In a randomized controlled clinical trial published in 2018 in the journal *Clinical Rheumatology*, researchers from Saudi Arabia and Egypt investigated the role that resveratrol may play in the treatment of rheumatoid arthritis. The cohort consisted of 100 patients suffering from rheumatoid arthritis including 68 females and 32 males. During the trial, conducted between July 2016 and June 2017, 50 patients were assigned to take one softgel capsule containing 1 g of resveratrol each day for 3 months. Members of the control group continued with their regular treatment. The researchers learned that 41 participants in the treatment group had "moderate-to-good" responses to the supplement; nine participants (18%) in the treatment group had no response. However, some participants had good responses to their "standard antirheumatic" medications. Compared to the placebo group, the treatment group had a significant drop in the major clinical and biochemical markers of rheumatoid arthritis. According to the researchers, "the current study suggests the addition of RSV [resveratrol] as an adjuvant to the conventional anti-rheumatic drugs."[6]

Resveratrol Supplementation May Support Bone Health in People with Type 2 Diabetes

In a double-blind, randomized, placebo-controlled trial published in 2018 in the journal *Nutrition and Diabetes*, researchers from Italy noted that people with type 2 diabetes are at an increased risk for bone fractures. Therefore, the researchers wanted to learn if resveratrol supplementation would support their bone health. The cohort consisted of 192 participants with type 2 diabetes, with a median age of 66 years. For 6 months, they took either 40 mg per day of resveratrol (n = 65), 500 mg per day of resveratrol (n = 65), or a placebo (n = 62). Assessments were conducted at baseline and after 6 months. By the end of the trial, there were 62, 59, and

58 participants, respectively, in each group. The researchers found an association with "positive effects" on the intake of resveratrol and bone density in people with type 2 diabetes, "particularly in those with unfavorable conditions at baseline."[7]

Resveratrol Supplementation May Help Glucose Control and Insulin Sensitivity in People with Type 2 Diabetes

In a meta-analysis published in 2014 in the *American Journal of Clinical Nutrition*, researchers from China evaluated the effects of resveratrol on glucose control and insulin sensitivity. Their analysis included 11 randomized controlled trials with a total of 388 participants. All studies included at least 2 weeks of resveratrol supplementation and were parallel or crossover in design. Total number of participants ranged from 8 to 66, and doses of resveratrol ranged from 8 to 1500 mg per day. Five trials were deemed high quality. The researchers learned that resveratrol supplementation significantly improved glucose control and insulin sensitivity in people with type 2 diabetes; no significant effects were observed in people who did not have type 2 diabetes. The researchers commented that there is a need for more high quality randomly controlled trials "with durations longer than three months . . . to further confirm the effects of resveratrol on glucose control and insulin sensitivity."[8]

Resveratrol Supplementation May Be Useful for Polycystic Ovary Syndrome

In a double-blind, placebo-controlled trial published in 2016 in the *Journal of Clinical Endocrinology & Metabolism*, researchers from Poland and La Jolla, California (USA), wanted to learn if resveratrol would be useful for polycystic ovary syndrome, a common endocrine condition affecting women of reproductive age. Symptoms of this syndrome include irregular or absent menstrual periods, infertility, weight gain, acne, and excess hair on the face and body. It has been estimated that about five to six million women in the United States have this condition. The initial cohort consisted of 34 women, who were randomized to receive 3 months of 1500 mg resveratrol per day or a placebo. Blood samples were taken at the beginning and end of the trial. Thirty women completed the trial. The researchers learned that resveratrol helped moderate the hormone imbalance. In fact, total testosterone levels reduced by 23.1% in the women taking the supplement. Dehydroepiandrosterone sulfate, an adrenal androgen (a steroid hormone that controls the development and maintenance of masculine characteristics), reduced by 22.2% in the resveratrol group. Thus, resveratrol helped moderate the hormone imbalance that is the cornerstone of this medical problem. In addition, the women taking the supplement had improvements in risk factors for type 2 diabetes. For example, their fasting insulin levels reduced by 31.8%, and they become more responsive to the hormone insulin, which means they reduced their risk for developing type 2 diabetes. The researchers concluded that "resveratrol significantly reduced ovarian and adrenal androgens. This effect may be at least in part related to an improvement of insulin sensitivity and a decline of insulin level."[9]

Resveratrol Spray May Help Adults with Allergic Rhinitis

In a double-blind, placebo-controlled, randomized trial published in 2018 in the journal *International Archives of Allergy and Immunology*, researchers from China examined the ability of a nasal resveratrol spray to alleviate the symptoms of allergic rhinitis, such as nasal congestion and sneezing; allergic rhinitis is a very common disorder. The cohort consisted of 151 adults, aged between 18 and 60 years, who were diagnosed with allergic rhinitis. The participants were divided into a resveratrol nasal spray group (n = 51), a placebo group (n = 50), and a budesonide group (n = 50). (Budesonide is a corticosteroid used for allergic rhinitis.) Symptoms were assessed at baseline, at 2 weeks, at 4 weeks, and when the trial ended. The researchers determined that the participants in both treatment groups had significant reductions in allergic rhinitis symptoms. In contrast, the participants in the placebo group did not experience improvements. The researchers commented that their study demonstrated "that resveratrol alone is sufficient to reduce AR [allergic rhinitis] symptoms in adult patients."[10]

Resveratrol Does Not Appear to Be Useful for Nonalcoholic Fatty Liver Disease

In a prospective, placebo-controlled, randomized, and double-blind clinical trial published in 2016 in the *Scandinavian Journal of Gastroenterology*, researchers from various locations in Denmark investigated the use of resveratrol to treat nonalcoholic fatty liver disease. The initial cohort consisted of 28 overweight people with nonalcoholic fatty liver disease, who were recruited between October 2011 and February 2014. For 6 months, the participants were placed on either 500 mg resveratrol or a placebo; both were taken three times each day. Twenty-six participants completed the trial, and two left the trial early because of adverse effects. The researchers learned that resveratrol was not any better at improving plasma markers of liver injury than the placebo. They concluded that "in spite of resveratrol bioactivity, clinical NAFLD [non-alcoholic fatty liver disease] was not notably improved."[11]

A Gel Containing Resveratrol Appears Useful for Acne

In a single-blind trial published in 2011 in the *American Journal of Clinical Dermatology*, researchers from Italy wanted to learn if a gel containing resveratrol would be useful for acne. The cohort consisted of 20 participants, including 12 men and 8 women, who had acne vulgaris. At baseline, they ranged in age from 18 to 23 years. For 60 days, the participants applied the resveratrol-containing gel to the right side of their face and a hydrogel vehicle to the left side of their face. By the end of the trial, all participants had a visible clinical improvement in the resveratrol-treated side of the face, "including a remarkable decrease in inflammation and pustular lesions." Digital photographs documented the improvement. The resveratrol treatment was well-tolerated, and no adverse effects were reported. The researchers commented that their findings "should be considered a valid starting point for further research into the effectiveness of resveratrol at different concentrations, in innovative formulations, in larger groups of patients and for more widespread use on the body."[12]

NOTES

1. Simental-Mendía, Luis E., and Fernando Guerrero-Romero. "Effect of Resveratrol Supplementation on Lipid Profile in Subjects with Dyslipidemia: A Randomized Double-Blind, Placebo-Controlled Trial." *Nutrition* 58 (February 2019): 7–10.

2. Theodotou, Marios, Konstantinos Fokianos, Alexia Mouzouridou, et al. "The Effect of Resveratrol on Hypertension: A Clinical Trial." *Experimental and Therapeutic Medicine* 13 (2017): 295–301.

3. Turner, R. Scott, Ronald G. Thomas, Suzanne Craft, et al. "A Randomized, Double-Blind, Placebo-Controlled Trial of Resveratrol for Alzheimer Disease." *Neurology* 85 (2015): 1383–1391.

4. Hussain, S. A., B. H. Marouf, Z. S. Ali, and R. S. Ahmmad. "Efficacy and Safety of Co-Administration of Resveratrol with Meloxicam in Patients with Knee Osteoarthritis: A Pilot Interventional Study." *Clinical Interventions in Aging* 13 (September 5, 2018): 1621–1630.

5. Anton, Stephen D., Chelsea Embry, Michael Marsiske, et al. "Safety and Metabolic Outcomes of Resveratrol Supplementation in Older Adults: Results of a Twelve-Week, Placebo-Controlled Pilot Study." *Experimental Gerontology* 57 (September 2014): 181–187.

6. Khojah, H. M., S. Ahmed, M. S. Abedl-Rahman, and E. H. Elhakeim. "Resveratrol as an Effective Adjuvant Therapy in the Management of Rheumatoid Arthritis: A Clinical Study." *Clinical Rheumatology* 37, no. 8 (August 2018): 2035–2042.

7. Bo, S., R. Gambino, V. Ponzo, et al. "Effects of Resveratrol on Bone Health in Type 2 Diabetic Patients. A Double-Blind Randomized-Controlled Trial." *Nutrition and Diabetes* 8, no. 1 (September 20, 2018): 51.

8. Liu, K., R. Zhou, B. Wang, and M. T. Mi. "Effect of Resveratrol on Glucose Control and Insulin Sensitivity: A Meta-Analysis of 11 Randomized Controlled Trials." *American Journal of Clinical Nutrition* 99, no. 6 (June 2014): 1510–1519.

9. Banaszewska, B., J. Wrotyńska-Barczyńska, R. Z. Spaczynski, et al. "Effects of Resveratrol on Polycystic Ovary Syndrome: A Double-Blind, Randomized, Placebo-Controlled Trial." *Journal of Clinical Endocrinology & Metabolism* 101, no. 11 (November 2016): 4322–4328.

10. Lv, Chunjiang, Yongsheng Zhang, and Lili Shen. "Preliminary Clinical Evaluation of Resveratrol in Adults with Allergic Rhinitis." *International Archives of Allergy and Immunology* 175, no. 4 (2018): 231–236.

11. Heebóll, S., M. Kreuzfeldt, and S. Hamilton-Dutoit. "Placebo-Controlled, Randomised Clinical Trial: High-Dose Resveratrol Treatment for Non-Alcoholic Fatty Liver Disease." *Scandinavian Journal of Gastroenterology* 51, no.4 (2016): 456–464.

12. Fabbrocini, G., S. Staibano, G. De Rosa, et al. "Resveratrol-Containing Gel for the Treatment of Acne Vulgaris: A Single-Blind, Vehicle-Controlled, Pilot Study." *American Journal of Clinical Dermatology* 12, no. 2 (April 1, 2011): 133–141.

REFERENCES AND FURTHER READING

Anton, Stephen D., Chelsea Embry, Michael Marsiske, et al. "Safety and Metabolic Outcomes of Resveratrol Supplementation in Older Adults: Results of a Twelve-Week,

Placebo-Controlled Pilot Study." *Experimental Gerontology* 57 (September 2014): 181–187.

Banaszewska, B., J. Wrotyńska-Barczyńska, R. Z. Spaczynski, et al. "Effects of Resveratrol on Polycystic Ovary Syndrome: A Double-Blind, Randomized, Placebo-Controlled Trial." *Journal of Clinical Endocrinology & Metabolism* 101, no. 11 (November 2016): 4322–4328.

Bo, S., R. Gambino, V. Ponzo, et al. "Effects of Resveratrol on Bone Health in Type 2 Diabetic Patients. A Double-Blind Randomized-Controlled Trial." *Nutrition and Diabetes* 8, no. 1 (September 20, 2018): 51.

Fabbrocini, G., S. Staibano, G. De Rosa, et al. "Resveratrol-Containing Gel for the Treatment of Acne Vulgaris: A Single-Blind, Vehicle-Controlled, Pilot Study." *American Journal of Clinical Dermatology* 12, no. 2 (April 1, 2011): 133–141.

Heebøll, S., M. Kreuzfeldt, S. Hamilton-Dutoit, et al. "Placebo-Controlled, Randomised, Clinical Trial: High-Dose Resveratrol Treatment for Non-Alcoholic Fatty Liver Disease." *Scandinavian Journal of Gastroenterology* 51, no. 4 (2016): 456–464.

Hussain, S. A., B. H. Marouf, Z. S. Ali, and R. S. Ahmmad. "Efficacy and Safety of Co-Administration of Resveratrol with Meloxicam in Patients with Knee Osteoarthritis: A Pilot Interventional Study." *Clinical Interventions in Aging* 13 (September 5, 2018): 1621–1630.

Khojah, H. M., S. Ahmed, M. S. Abdel-Rahman, E. H. Elhakeim. "Resveratrol as an Effective Adjuvant Therapy in the Management of Rheumatoid Arthritis: A Clinical Study." *Clinical Rheumatology* 37, no. 8 (August 2018): 2035–2042.

Liu, K., R. Zhou, B. Wang, and M. T. Mi. "Effect of Resveratrol on Glucose Control and Insulin Sensitivity: A Meta-Analysis and 11 Randomized Controlled Trials." *American Journal of Clinical Nutrition* 99, no. 6 (June 2014): 1510–1519.

Lv, Chunjiang, Yongsheng Zhang, and Lili Shen. "Preliminary Clinical Effect Evaluation of Resveratrol Adults with Allergic Rhinitis." *International Archives of Allergy and Immunology* 175, no. 4 (2018): 231–236.

Simental-Mendía, Luis E., and Fernando Guerrero-Romero. "Effect of Resveratrol Supplementation on Lipid Profile in Subjects with Dyslipidemia: A Randomized Double-Blind, Placebo-Controlled Trial." *Nutrition* 58 (February 2019): 7–10.

Theodotou, Marios, Konstantinos Fokianos, Alexia Mouzouridou, et al. "The Effect of Resveratrol on Hypertension: A Clinical Trial." *Experimental and Therapeutic Medicine* 13 (2017): 295–301.

Turner, R. Scott, Ronald G. Thomas, Suzanne Craft, et al. "A Randomized, Double-Blind, Placebo-Controlled Trial of Resveratrol for Alzheimer Disease." *Neurology* 85 (2015): 1383–1391.

SAMe

SAMe, also known as S-adenosyl-L-methionine, S-adenosyl methionine, S-adenosylmethionine, or SAM-e, is a compound found naturally in human cells. It is made from methionine, an amino acid. SAMe helps produce and regulate hormones, and is used to maintain cell membranes and remove toxic substances from the body. In the United States, a synthetic version of SAMe is sold as a dietary supplement; in Europe, SAMe is a prescription medication.

People may experience improvements from SAMe in as little as 1 week, or it may require up to 1 month. It is possible that people may not observe any changes. SAMe works closely with vitamin B6, vitamin B12, and folate. Therefore, people taking SAMe may wish to increase their intake of foods containing these vitamins or add them in supplemental form.

SAMe was discovered in the early 1950s. Researchers found that people with liver diseases and depression had low levels of SAMe in their bodies, which led them to investigate whether SAMe might be useful for treating these conditions. When they evaluated people with depression who also had osteoarthritis, researchers found that SAMe improved the symptoms associated with osteoarthritis.

HEALTH BENEFITS AND RISKS

People take SAMe for various medical problems, especially depression, liver disease, and osteoarthritis. In addition, SAMe may be useful for fibromyalgia, bursitis, tendinitis, and chronic low back pain.

SAMe should not be taken by people on antidepressants or any medications or supplements that raise serotonin levels including antipsychotic medications, amphetamines, dextromethorphan, selective serotonin reuptake inhibitors, narcotics, and St. John's wort. The combination may cause excessive levels of the chemical serotonin to accumulate in the body.

Though believed to be rare, potential side effects from SAMe include upset stomach, nausea, mild insomnia, dizziness, irritability, anxiety, sweating, constipation, and diarrhea. Side effects are more likely to occur in people taking higher doses. People who have bipolar disorder or Parkinson's disease should avoid SAMe as it may increase anxiety and mania. Further, people with compromised immune systems should not take SAMe without the consent of a medical provider as it may increase their risk of an infection.

HOW IT IS SOLD AND TAKEN

Normally, SAMe is taken as an oral supplement. It is sold as tablets, capsules, caplets, and in a liquid. Dosing recommendations vary widely and tend to range from 200 to 1600 mg per day. It is best to take SAMe on an empty stomach with water. To prevent insomnia, SAMe should not be taken later in the day. Given a lack of safety evidence, breastfeeding women or children should not take SAMe. Pregnant women should only take this supplement under the close supervision of a medical provider.

In addition to oral supplementation, SAMe is available as an injection, which may be administered intravenously.

RESEARCH FINDINGS

SAMe Appears to Be Useful for Depression

In a single-center, randomized, double-blind trial published in 2010 in the *American Journal of Psychiatry*, researchers based in Boston, Massachusetts (USA), wanted to learn if SAMe supplementation would assist people with major depressive disorder who did not respond to serotonin reuptake inhibitor (SRI) medication. The cohort consisted of 73 men and women with major depressive disorder. All had received no symptom relief from their SRI medication. For 6 weeks, 39 participants were assigned to take SAMe and 34 took a placebo. Fifty-five participants (75.3%) completed the trial, of which 31 were in the SAMe group and 24 were in the placebo group. The researchers determined that significantly more participants treated with SAMe experienced clinical response and remission. The response rate for SAMe-treated versus placebo-treated participants was 36.1% versus 17.6%, respectively. The remission rates were 25.8% versus 11.7%, respectively. SAMe was well-tolerated, and no serious adverse effects were reported. The researchers concluded that "SAMe can be an effective relatively well-tolerated and self adjunctive treatment strategy for SRI nonresponders with major depressive disorder."[1]

In a trial published in 2013 in *The Scientific World Journal*, researchers from Italy, the Netherlands, and Miami, Florida (USA), investigated the ability of SAMe to help 25 outpatients (11 males and 14 females) with Stage II major depressive disorder who failed to respond to at least 8 weeks of traditional antidepressant treatment. In fact, for these participants, the mean duration of symptoms was 8 years. In addition to their antidepressant medication, all participants were treated with a fixed dose of 800 mg per day of SAMe for 8 weeks. During the trial, concurrent therapy, such as cognitive behavior therapy or psychoanalytic therapy, was not administered or allowed, and the participants could not add any new psychotropic medications or herbal supplements to their treatment plan. Assessments were conducted at baseline and during every week of the trial. Twenty-four participants completed the entire study. The researchers determined that a statistically significant clinical improvement appeared within the first week of treatment and continued until the end of the trial. SAMe supplementation was associated with "quite rapid improvement in depressive symptoms." Moreover, full remission was achieved by a remarkable 37.5% of the 24 participants. The researchers acknowledged several problems with their trial, specifically, a small sample size, the open-label design, the lack of a placebo or active control group, and the short treatment period. They concluded that "future randomized controlled trials are needed to confirm the efficacy and safety of such augmentation strategy."[2]

In a randomized, controlled, double-blind, 8-week trial published in 2018 in the journal *European Neuropsychopharmacology*, researchers from various locations in Australia assessed the ability of SAMe to treat people with major depressive disorder. The initial cohort consisted of 107 participants, who were placed on 800 mg per day of SAMe or a placebo. While the two groups were matched well, the placebo group had a higher mean years of education. Moreover, physical illness was significantly higher in the SAMe group than the placebo group. Seventy-two percent of the participants completed the entire trial; there were 40 participants in the SAMe group and 37 in the placebo group. During the course of the trial, 123 adverse events were noted—66 in the supplement group and 57 in the placebo group. The most commonly reported adverse events were diarrhea, sweating, irritability, hot and cold flashes, and cramping. The researchers learned that SAMe failed to outperform placebo in improving the symptoms of major depressive disorder. The researchers wondered if a longer duration study or a higher dose of SAMe may have produced different results. Moreover, they did not "rule out the possible therapeutic effect of SAMe."[3]

In a systematic review published in 2016 in the *Cochrane Database of Systematic Reviews*, researchers based in the United Kingdom compared the efficacy of SAMe to the antidepressants imipramine, desipramine, or escitalopram, and to placebos in adults suffering from depression. The researchers found eight relevant trials with a total of 934 men and women from inpatient and outpatient settings. The researchers included trials that used SAMe as a monotherapy or as an add-on therapy, with oral and parenteral administration of SAMe. The researchers learned that the results from the administration of SAMe were not different from the tested antidepressants and placebos. However, with imipramine, fewer participants experienced adverse effects when treated with parenteral SAMe. The researchers underscored the need for more high-quality randomized controlled studies on the ability of SAMe to mitigate the symptoms associated with depressive disorders. They noted that there was an "absence of high quality evidence."[4]

When Combined with Vitamin B Complex, SAMe May Be Useful for Mild-to-Moderate Depression

In a randomized, placebo-controlled trial published in 2017 in the journal *Hippokratia*, researchers from Serbia examined the use of SAMe and vitamin B complex for mild-to-moderate symptoms of depression. The cohort consisted of 60 outpatients diagnosed with mild-or-moderate depressive symptoms, but who refused to take antidepressant medications. For 3 months, members of the supplement group took SAMe and vitamin B complex, and members of the control group took a placebo. The mean age of the study group was almost 50 years, and the mean age of the control group was slightly over 51 years. While the members of the treatment group experienced significant improvements in their depressive symptoms, the members of the control group had "no change or minimally worsening." The researchers concluded that "three months supplementation with SAMe-vitamin B complex is effective in the treatment of mild and moderate depressive symptoms, with significant differences compared to the placebo."[5]

SAMe May Help with Cognitive Impairment Associated with Depression

In a 6-week, double-blind, randomized trial published in 2012 in the journal *European Psychiatry*, researchers from Israel and Boston, Massachusetts (USA), explained that major depressive disorder is often accompanied by significant cognitive impairment. They wanted to learn if SAMe supplementation would support cognition and prevent some degree of that deterioration. The cohort consisted of 46 participants with major depressive disorder who had not responded to SRI medication. During the course of the trial, the participants took SAMe supplementation or a placebo. Assessments were conducted at baseline and when the trial ended. The researchers learned that SAMe was effective for improving memory-related cognitive functioning in participants with depression. The researchers commented that SAMe "may represent a potential treatment option for MDD [major depressive disorder] patients who also present with significant memory impairment from comorbid disorders such as Alzheimer's disease."[6]

SAMe Supplementation May Have Limited Value for People with Chronic Liver Disease

In a meta-analysis and systematic review published in 2015 in the online journal *PLoS ONE*, researchers from China wanted to learn if SAMe would help people with chronic liver disease. Their cohort consisted of 12 randomized controlled trials from 11 studies, which included 705 participants with seven types of chronic liver disease. The researchers learned that SAMe supplementation could improve liver function in people with chronic liver diseases. Further, it improved some liver function test results. However, results varied, and there was a lack of evidence regarding the type of data used. On the other hand, SAMe appeared to be safe, and there was no significant difference in the adverse effects experienced from SAMe and placebos. The researchers concluded that, although SAMe may be used as a "basis of medication program," it "does not improve outcome or reduce the occurrence of adverse events for chronic liver disease."[7]

SAMe May Be Useful for Liver Toxicity from Chemotherapy

In a trial published in 2012 in the journal *Supportive Care in Cancer*, researchers from Italy evaluated the ability of SAMe to help people with liver toxicity caused by chemotherapy treatments, a rather common occurrence. The cohort consisted of 78 patients with metastatic colorectal cancer. The patients either treated with their chemotherapy medication alone or combined with twice daily 400 mg of SAMe supplementation. Assessments were made at baseline and at every therapy cycle. Chemotherapy course delays, discontinuations, and dose reductions due to liver toxicity were recorded. The researchers found that SAMe supplementation reduced the levels of liver toxicity. For example, the increase in liver enzymes from chemotherapy was significantly lower in the patients on supplementation. Because they had lower rates of toxicity, the patients taking SAMe had less need for chemotherapy delays and dose reductions. They were able to have "greater regularity of chemotherapy administration." Still, the researchers cautioned that "the reliability of the results obtained is limited by retrospective nature of the present study and the small sample size of the patients included."[8]

SAMe May Help People with Osteoarthritis

In a somewhat dated but important prospective, randomized, double-blind, crossover trial published in 2004 in the journal *BMC Musculoskeletal Disorders*, researchers from Orange, California (USA), compared the use of SAMe and the prescription medication celecoxib (Celebrex) for the pain and functional impairment associated with osteoarthritis. The initial cohort consisted of 61 adults suffering from knee osteoarthritis. The trial was divided into two 8-week testing periods, with a 1-week wash-out period in between phases. During the first phase, the participants were treated with 600 mg twice daily of SAMe or 100 mg twice daily of Celebrex; during the second phase, they were treated with the alternate treatment. Fifty-six participants completed the trials. The participants were assessed during five monthly visits. Forty-six participants reported adverse effects during the Celebrex period and 36 reported adverse effects during the SAMe period. The most common adverse effects were gastrointestinal disorders, anxiety, and dyspepsia. The researchers found that SAMe was equivalent "in almost all measures" to Celebrex in relieving pain and improving function in participants with knee osteoarthritis. However, SAMe required more time—up to 1 month—to achieve the level of improvement obtained far more rapidly from Celebrex. The researchers concluded that their findings "confirm results from prior studies indicating a possible role for SAMe in the management of osteoarthritis."[9]

In an 8-week, multicenter, randomized, double-blind trial published in 2009 in the journal *Clinical Therapeutics*, researchers from Korea compared the ability of SAMe and nabumetone, a nonsteroidal anti-inflammatory drug, to treat the symptoms of knee osteoarthritis. The initial cohort consisted of 134 Asian patients with knee osteoarthritis, who were placed in one of the two treatment groups—1200 mg per day of SAMe (n = 67) or 1000 mg per day of nabumetone (n = 67). Assessments were conducted at baseline, at 4 weeks, and at the end of the trial. Ninety-seven participants completed the trial. Twenty-three in the SAMe group and 14 in the nabumetone group failed to complete the trial. On analyzing changes in pain intensity from 0 to 8 weeks, the researchers learned that both SAMe and nabumetone effectively reduced pain. Interestingly, the degree of pain relief was not significantly different between the two groups, and there were no significant differences between the treatments in the proportion of participants with adverse events. The researchers concluded that SAMe "was not significantly different from nabumetone in terms of pain relief and tolerability over 8 weeks in these Korean patients with knee OA [osteoarthritis]."[10]

SAMe May Improve the Quality of Life and Reduce Aggression in People Suffering from Schizophrenia

In a small pilot trial published in 2009 in the journal *European Neuropsychopharmacology*, researchers from Israel and Bronx, New York (USA), wanted to learn if SAMe supplementation would help people suffering from schizophrenia, a profound and debilitating psychiatric disorder. For 8 weeks, 18 participants (12 males and 6 females aged 27–65 years) with chronic schizophrenia were randomly assigned to take either 800 mg of SAMe or a placebo. During the trial, they continued to take their regular medication. Participants were assessed at baseline and every 2 weeks. Thirteen participants completed the entire trial, which is a dropout rate of 28% from a sample that was already small. Although the sample numbers were low, the researchers found that the administration of SAMe lowered aggression levels and improved the quality of life among participants. There was no evidence of worsening of any cognitive measures in the participants treated with SAMe, with no significant difference between the groups. The researchers commented that their findings "may have identified, albeit in a very cautious fashion, an agent capable of augmenting antipsychotic medication and assisting in the management of aggressive behavior and improvement of quality of life in this patient subpopulation."[11]

NOTES

1. Papakostas, George I., David Mischoulon, Irene Shyu, et al. "S-Adenosyl Methionine (SAMe) Augmentation of Serotonin Reuptake Inhibitors for Antidepressant Nonresponders with Major Depressive Disorder: A Double-Blind, Randomized Clinical Trial." *American Journal of Psychiatry* 167 (2010): 942–948.

2. De Berardis, Domenico, Stefano Marini, Nicola Serroni, et al. "S-Adenosyl-L-Methionine Augmentation in Patients with Stage II Treatment-Resistant Major Depressive Disorder: An Open Label, Fixed Dose, Single-Blind Study." *The Scientific World Journal* 2013 (2013): Article ID: 204649.

3. Sarris, Jerome, Gerard J. Byrne, Chad Bousman, et al. "Adjunctive S-Adenosylmethionine (SAMe) in Treating Non-Remittent Major Depressive Disorder: An 8-Week Double-Blind, Randomized, Controlled Trial." *European Neuropsychopharmacology* 28, no. 10 (October 2018): 1126–1136.

4. Galizia, I., L. Oldani, K. Macritchie, et al. "S-Adenosyl Methionine (SAMe) for Depression in Adults." *Cochrane Database of Systematic Reviews* 10 (October 2016): CD011286.

5. Djokic, G., D. Korcok, V. Djordjevic, et al. "The Effects of S-Adenosyl-L-Methionine-Vitamin B Complex on Mild and Moderate Depressive Symptoms." *Hippokratia* 21, no. 3 (July–September 2017): 140–143.

6. Levkovitz, Y., J. E. Alpert, C. E. Brintz, et al. "Effects of S-Adenosylmethionine Augmentation of Serotonin-Reuptake Inhibitor Antidepressants on Cognitive Symptoms of Major Depressive Disorder." *European Psychiatry* 27, no. 7 (October 2012): 518–521.

7. Guo, Tao, Lei Chang, Yusha Xiao, and Quanyan Liu. "S-Adenosyl-L-Methionine for the Treatment of Chronic Liver Disease: A Systematic Review and Meta-Analysis." *PLoS ONE* 10, no. 3 (2015): e0122124.

8. Vincenzi, Bruno, Santini Daniele, Anna Maria Frezza, et al. "The Role of S-Adenosylmethionine in Preventing Oxaliplatin-Induced Liver Toxicity: A Retrospective Analysis in Metastatic Colorectal Cancer Patients Treated with Bevacizumab Plus Oxaliplatin-Based Regimen." *Supportive Care in Cancer* 20, no. 1 (January 2012): 135–139.

9. Najm, Wadie I., Sibylle Reinsch, Fred Hoehler, et al. "S-Adenosyl Methionine (SAMe) versus Celecoxib for the Treatment of Osteoarthritis Symptoms: A Double-Blind Cross-over Trial." *BMC Musculoskeletal Disorders* 5, no. 1 (March 2004): 6.

10. Kim, J., E. Y. Lee, E. M. Koh, et al. "Comparative Clinical Trial of S-Adenosylmethionine versus Nabumetone for the Treatment of Knee Osteoarthritis: A 8-Week, Multicenter, Randomized, Double-Blind, Double-Dummy, Phase IV Study in Korean Patients." *Clinical Therapeutics* 31, no. 12 (December 2009): 2860–2872.

11. Strous, R. D., M. S. Ritsner, S. Adler, et al. "Improvement of Aggressive Behavior and Quality of Life Impairment Following S-Adenosyl-Methionine (SAM-e) Augmentation in Schizophrenia." *European Neuropsychopharmacology* 19, no. 1 (January 2009): 14–22.

REFERENCES AND FURTHER READING

De Berardis, Domenico, Stefano Marini, Nicola Serroni, et al. "S-Adenosyl-L-Methionine Augmentation in Patients with Stage II Treatment-Resistant Major Depressive Disorder: An Open Label, Fixed Dose, Single-Blind Study." *The Scientific World Journal* 2013 (2013): Article ID: 204649.

Djokic, G., D. Korcok, V. Djordjevic, et al. "The Effects of S-Adenosyl-L-Methionine-Vitamin B Complex on Mild and Moderate Depressive Symptoms." *Hippokratia* 21, no. 3 (July–September 2017): 140–143.

Galizia, I., L. Oldano, K. Macritchie, et al. "S-Adenosyl Methionine (SAMe) for Depression in Adults." *Cochrane Database of Systematic Reviews* 10 (October 2016): CD011286.

Guo, Tao, Lei Chang, Yusha Xiao, Quanyan Liu. "S-Adenosyl-L-Methionine for the Treatment of Chronic Liver Disease: A Systematic Review and Meta-Analysis." *PLoS ONE* 10, no. 3 (2015): e0122124.

Kim, J., E. Y. Lee, E. M. Koh, et al. "Comparative Clinical Trial of S-Adenosylmethionine versus Nabumetone for the Treatment of Knee Osteoarthritis: A 8-Week, Multicenter, Randomized, Double-Blind, Double-Dummy, Phase IV Study in Korean Patients." *Clinical Therapeutics* 31, no. 12 (December 2009): 2860–2872.

Levkovitz, Y., J. E. Alpert, C. E. Brintz, et al. "Effects of S-Adenosylmethionine Augmentation of Serotonin-Reuptake Inhibitor Antidepressants on Cognitive Symptoms of Major Depressive Disorder." *European Psychiatry* 27, no. 7 (October 2012): 518–521.

Najm, Wadie I., Sibylle Reinsch, Fred Hoehler, et al. "S-Adenylyl Methionine (SAMe) versus Celecoxib for the Treatment of Osteoarthritis Symptoms: A Double-Blind Cross-over Trial." *BMC Musculoskeletal Disorders* 5, no. 1 (March 2004): 6.

Papakostas, George I., David Mischoulon, Irene Shyu, et al. "S-Adenosyl Methionine (SAMe) Augmentation of Serotonin Reuptake Inhibitors for Antidepressant Nonresponders with Major Depressive Disorder: A Double-Blind, Randomized Clinical Trial." *American Journal of Psychiatry* 167 (2010): 942–948.

Sarris, Jerome, Gerard J. Byrne, Chad Bousman, et al. "Adjunctive S-Adenosylmethionine (SAMe) in Treating Non-Remittent Major Depressive Disorder: An 8-Week Double Blind, Randomized, Controlled Trial." *European Neuropsychopharmacology* 28, no. 10 (October 2018): 1126–1136.

Strous, R. D., M. S. Ritsner, S. Adler, et al. "Improvement of Aggressive Behavior and Quality of Life Impairment Following S-Adenosyl-Methionine (SAM-e) Augmentation in Schizophrenia." *European Neuropsychopharmacology* 19, no. 1 (January 2009): 14–22.

Vincenzi, Bruno, Santini Daniele, Anna Maria Frezza, et al. "The Role of S-Adenosylmethionine in Preventing Oxaliplatin-Induced Liver Toxicity: A Retrospective Analysis in Metastatic Colorectal Cancer Patients Treated with Bevacizumab Plus Oxaliplatin-Based Regimen." *Supportive Care in Cancer* 20, no. 1 (January 2012): 135–139.

Saw Palmetto

Saw palmetto, also known as *Serenoa repens*, is a small, low-growing palm tree native to southeastern United States, especially Florida. The leaves have a sharp, spiny edge. The saw palmetto plant produces egg-shaped berries, which when ripe, are almost black in color. Though edible, they have an unpleasant taste.

Historically, the fruit was considered a medicine and used by Native Americans in Florida to treat prostate gland swelling and inflammation, testicular atrophy, and erectile dysfunction. Moreover, saw palmetto was also thought to be useful for a wide variety of medical concerns, especially male urinary problems.

Even the early American settlers found saw palmetto useful. They drank the juice from saw palmetto berries to gain weight, improve general disposition, support sleep, and promote reproductive health.

The saw palmetto berry contains over 100 known compounds. The active ingredients appear to be contained in the purified lipid-soluble extract of the saw palmetto berry. This has been found to contain 85% to 95% fatty acids, long-chain alcohols, and sterols.

HEALTH BENEFITS AND RISKS

Today, saw palmetto is a dietary supplement primarily used for urinary symptoms associated with an enlarged prostate gland, also known as benign prostatic hyperplasia or BPH. This is a very common disorder in men over the age of 40, and it has been estimated that at least half of all men develop this problem. Symptoms of BPH include excessive urination, sense of incomplete emptying of the bladder, an urge to urinate, and a weak urinary stream.

One of the main components of saw palmetto is beta-sitosterol, a substance that inhibits the activity of 5-alpha-reductase enzyme. This enzyme promotes the growth of prostate cells, thereby contributing to an enlarged prostate. Saw palmetto also appears to reduce dihydrotestosterone levels, a hormone which, at elevated levels, causes the prostate to become enlarged. In addition, saw palmetto may be used for chronic pelvic pain, sex drive, migraines, and hair loss.

Saw palmetto is generally well-tolerated. In some people, it may cause digestive symptoms, such as diarrhea and nausea, or headaches. In very rare instances, it has been associated with allergic reactions including difficulty in breathing, constriction of the throat, hives, and swelling of the lips, tongue, or face.

Saw palmetto does not appear to affect prostate-specific antigen (PSA) levels, even when taken in larger amounts. (A protein produced by the prostate gland,

PSA levels are often used to screen for prostate cancer and monitor patients who have been diagnosed with prostate cancer.) The vast majority of studies including saw palmetto have been conducted among men. Little is known about the use of this supplement by women or children.

Because saw palmetto may decrease the effects of estrogen in the body, it may reduce the effectiveness of birth control pills that contain estrogen. Women taking birth control pills with estrogen who also take saw palmetto must be extra vigilant about birth control. Further, as saw palmetto may slow blood clotting, people who take medications or supplements that slow clotting may have increased risk for bruising or bleeding

HOW IT IS SOLD AND TAKEN

Extracts of the saw palmetto fruit are sold in tablets and capsules. It may also be used as ground, dried, or whole berries and as a liquid extract or tea. In pill form, the usual dose recommendation is 320 mg of saw palmetto extract once or twice a day. It may take up to 4 weeks to notice any benefits.

RESEARCH FINDINGS

Saw Palmetto Supplementation Appears to Be Effective and Safe for the Treatment of Lower Urinary Tract Symptoms Associated with BPH

In a meta-analysis and systematic review published in 2018 in the journal *BJU International*, researchers from various locations in Spain investigated the use of saw palmetto supplementation for the lower urinary tract symptoms associated with an enlarged prostate. They included data from 15 randomized controlled trials and 12 observational studies. In total, there were 5800 participants, who took Permixon® (saw palmetto) at a daily dose of 320 mg. The researchers determined that saw palmetto supplementation had a positive effect "over and above placebo" in several of the measures used to assess lower urinary tract symptoms in men with enlarged prostate glands. Moreover, saw palmetto worked about as well as tamsulosin and 5-alpha reductase inhibitor, medications used to treat an enlarged prostate. The researchers concluded that Permixon "appears to be an efficacious and well-tolerated therapeutic option."[1]

Long-Term Use of Saw Palmetto May Be Useful for Mild and Moderate Symptoms of BPH

In a trial published in 2011 in the journal *Urologia Internationalis*, researchers based in Romania evaluated the ability of the long-term use of saw palmetto to assist men with mild and moderate lower urinary symptoms caused by BPH. The vast majority of the men had moderate symptoms, and only 7% had mild symptoms. The initial cohort consisted of 120 men who had experienced symptoms for at least 6 months. They were all treated with one daily capsule of 320 mg saw palmetto (Prostamol Uno). Assessments were conducted at baseline, at 6 months, at 12 months, at 18 months, and at 24 months. By the end of the trial, 45% of the men had mild symptoms—a significant improvement over 7%. In fact, the assessments demonstrated several areas of significant improvement. Moreover, none of the men experienced a treatment-related adverse event. The researchers underscored the need for "more randomized, place-controlled, long-term trials . . . in order to eliminate all skepticism."[2]

The Combination of Saw Palmetto Supplement and Tamsulosin Is "Slightly" More Effective Than Monotherapy with Tamsulosin for Treating BPH

In a 12-month, single-center, open-label trial published in 2015 in *Urologia Internationalis*, researchers from Korea compared using tamsulosin alone or in combination with Permixon to treat BPH. The cohort consisted of 120 men who had symptoms associated with their enlarged prostate. Sixty men were randomly assigned to take 0.2 mg per day of tamsulosin, and another 60 were randomly assigned to take 0.2 mg per day of tamsulosin and 320 mg per day of Permixon. At baseline, there were no meaningful differences between the men in the two treatment groups; the study participants had a mean age of 62.5. During the study year, the men attended follow-up assessments, and 103 completed the trial. The researchers learned that the combination therapy was "slightly more beneficial" than tamsulosin alone. They concluded that "the combination of tamsulosin plus Permixon showed symptomatic improvements in men with concomitant voiding and storage symptoms compared with tamsulosin monotherapy."[3]

Adding Saw Palmetto to Silodosin, a BPH Medication, May Increase the Effectiveness of Silodosin

In a retrospective trial published in 2017 in the journal *Scientific Reports*, researchers from Milan, Italy wanted to learn if adding saw palmetto supplementation to the enlarged prostate medication, silodosin, would improve its effectiveness. The cohort consisted of 186 men with enlarged prostate glands. Ninety-three men were placed on silodosin alone, and 93 were placed on silodosin and saw palmetto. The two groups were demographically similar. At a mean follow-up of 13.5 months, the men in the combination group had significantly better overall improvements, and had "greater clinically meaningful improvements." Treatment-related adverse effects were experienced by 27 men in the silodosin group and 29 men in the combination group, with no significant differences between the two groups. None of the men discontinued the trial because of the side effects. The researchers concluded that "finding a therapeutic option which leads to greater clinically meaningful improvements in symptomatic terms along with a comparable rate of drug-related adverse events as compared with the most widely first-line drugs clearly emerges as a major clinical need."[4]

Saw Palmetto May Be Useful for Painful Urination in Men with an Enlarged Prostate Gland

In a retrospective study published in 2012 in the journal *Archivio Italiano di Uropogia e Andrologia*, researchers based in Italy investigated the association between saw palmetto supplementation and several symptoms associated with BPH. Their study was conducted at eight different centers throughout Italy from September 2010 to November 2011. Data were obtained from 298 men, with an average age of 63 years. The men were either taking a daily dose of saw palmetto or a daily dose of saw palmetto and an alpha-blocker to treat their enlarged prostate. All but two of the participants used Permixon as their source of saw palmetto. The researchers observed "a substantial decreasing" in the numbers of men with severe prostatic symptoms, and saw palmetto "demonstrated its efficacy reducing dysuria," or painful urination.[5]

Saw Palmetto Supplementation Appears to Be Useful for Men with Prostatic Inflammation

In a randomized, double-blind clinical trial published in 2019 in the *World Journal of Urology*, researchers from Greece wanted to learn more about the ability of saw palmetto supplementation to reduce prostatic inflammation. The cohort consisted of 97 men with biopsy-diagnosed prostatic inflammation. The biopsies were performed because the men had elevated PSA levels and/or positive digital rectal exams. For 6 months, the men were randomly assigned to take 320 mg per day of saw palmetto supplementation or no treatment. After 6 months, all men underwent a second biopsy, and the degree of inflammation was assessed a second time. The researchers found that the men taking saw palmetto supplementation had significantly less inflammation than those taking no treatment. All the various measures studied were significantly lower in the men taking the supplement. The researchers concluded that saw palmetto supplementation "seems to reduce prostatic inflammation in terms of histological and immunohistochemical parameters in patients who underwent two biopsies due to elevated PSA and/or suspicious DRE [digital rectal exams]."[6]

Combining Saw Palmetto with Lycopene, Selenium, and Tamsulosin Works Better Than Monotherapy for Treating the Symptoms Associated with an Enlarged Prostate Gland

In a 1-year, randomized, double-blind, 11-center trial published in 2014 in the journal *The Prostate*, researchers from various locations in Italy examined the efficacy and tolerability of saw palmetto, lycopene, selenium, and the drug tamsulosin verses single therapies. The initial cohort consisted of 225 men, with a median age of 65 years, who were enrolled from March 2011 to March 2012. All the men had enlarged prostate glands. The men in group A took saw palmetto, lycopene, selenium, and a placebo. The men in group B took 0.4 mg tamsulosin and a placebo. The men in group C took the three supplements and 0.4 mg tamsulosin. Identical tablets were used in all groups. Two hundred and nineteen men completed the trial. The researchers learned that the combination of the three supplements and tamsulosin resulted in significant improvement in symptoms associated with an enlarged prostate. The researchers concluded that the addition of saw palmetto, lycopene, and selenium to tamsulosin "may give rise to significant improvements of both LUTS [lower urinary tract symptoms] and the urinary flow."[7]

Saw Palmetto May Not Be as Useful as Some Think. In Fact, Increasing Doses of Saw Palmetto Did Not Help Lower Urinary Tract Symptoms Associated with an Enlarged Prostate Gland

In a multicenter, randomized, placebo-controlled, clinical trial published in 2011 in *JAMA*, researchers from many locations in the United States but based in Boston, Massachusetts (USA), tested the ability of increasing doses of saw palmetto to reduce lower urinary tract symptoms experienced by men with an enlarged prostate gland. The initial cohort consisted of 369 men who were at least 45 years old. All the men met specific enlarged prostate criteria. For 72 weeks, the men received one, two, and then three 320 mg per day doses of saw palmetto extract or a placebo, with dose increases at 24 and 48 weeks. The men were seen at baseline and at 12, 24, 36, 48, 60, and 72 weeks for outcome assessments. During these visits, various tests were administered. Though saw palmetto appeared to be safe and without negative side effects, it did not improve enlarged prostate symptoms. It was about as useful as the placebo. Even three times the normal dose had no effect. The researchers concluded that "increasing doses of a saw palmetto fruit extract did not reduce lower urinary tract symptoms more than placebo."[8]

In a meta-analysis and systematic review published in 2012 in the *Cochrane Database of Systematic Reviews*, researchers based in Minneapolis, Minnesota (USA), assessed the effects of saw palmetto in treating men with symptoms of an enlarged prostate gland. The researchers included 32 randomized controlled trials, with 5666 men; trial duration ranged from 4 to 72 weeks. Twenty-seven of the trials were double-blinded. The primary outcome measure was to compare the effectiveness of saw palmetto with active or inert controls. However, the researchers also looked for changes in nocturia and urodynamic measures. The researchers found that saw palmetto, even at double and triples doses, did not improve urinary flow measures or prostate sizes. Therefore, the researchers concluded that saw palmetto is not useful for the symptoms associated with an enlarged prostate gland.[9]

Topical Saw Palmetto May Be of Some Limited Help to Men with Male Androgenetic Alopecia or Male Pattern Baldness

In a pilot, prospective, open trial published in 2016 in the *Australasian Journal of Dermatology*, researchers from Thailand assessed the ability of topical saw palmetto to help men dealing with male androgenetic alopecia or male pattern baldness. Symptoms of this common disorder include thinning and baldness. The cohort consisted of 50 men between the ages of 20 and 50 years who had mild-to-moderate hair loss. All men used concentrated topical saw palmetto for 24 weeks with a follow-up period of 4 weeks. Hair counts were conducted at baseline and at 12 and 24 weeks. During those times, the men also reviewed their hair changes. Forty-nine men completed the trial. Minor side effects were common including feeling of coldness, mild burning, an unpleasant smell, an itchy scalp, and acne on the forehead. The researchers learned that topical saw palmetto significantly increased the amount of total hair. Improvements appeared by week 12, but the positive gains declined at week 24. The researchers concluded that the topical application of saw palmetto "could be an alternative treatment in male pattern baldness in male patients who do not want or cannot tolerate the side-effects of standard medications."[10]

In an open-label trial published in 2012 in the *International Journal of Immunopathology and Pharmacology*, researchers from Rome, Italy compared the treatment of male pattern hair loss with oral saw palmetto or finasteride, a medication used for male pattern hair loss and an enlarged prostate. The cohort consisted of 100 male participants, who had been clinically diagnosed with mild-to-moderate male pattern hair loss. They were randomly assigned to take 320 mg per day of saw palmetto or 1 mg per day of finasteride. Both groups were followed for 24 months. The researchers learned that both therapies had good results and were well-tolerated by the men. But, those taking saw palmetto had more improvement in the vertex or crown of the scalp and finasteride improved hair growth in the front area and the vertex. The most common side effect of saw palmetto was mild stomach upset, which was relieved if the supplement/medication was taken after eating. The researchers concluded that saw palmetto "could be considered as a valid approach in treating low or moderate AGA [male androgenetic alopecia]."[11]

NOTES

1. Vela-Navarrete, R., A. Alcaraz, A. Rodriquez-Antolin, et al. "Efficacy and Safety of a Hexanic Extract of Serenoa Repens (Permixon®) for the Treatment of Lower Urinary Tract Symptoms Associated with Benign Prostatic Hyperplasia (LUTS/BPH): Systematic Review and Meta-Analysis of Randomised Controlled Trials and Observational Studies." *BJU International* 122, no. 6 (December 2018): 1049–1065.

2. Sinescu, I., P. Geaviete, R. Multescu, et al. "Long-Term Efficacy of *Serenoa Repens* Treatment in Patients with Mild and Moderate Symptomatic Benign Prostatic Hyperplasia." *Urologia Internationalis* 86, no. 3 (2011): 284–289.

3. Ryu, Y. W., S. W. Lim, J. H. Kim, et al. "Comparison of Tamsulosin Plus Serenoa Repens with Tamsulosin in the Treatment of Benign Prostatic Hyperplasia in Korean Men: 1-Year Randomized Open Label Study." *Urologia Internationalis* 94, no. 2 (2015): 187–193.

4. Boeri, Luca, Paolo Capogrosso, Eugenio Ventimiglia, et al. "Clinically Meaningful Improvements in LUTS/BPH Severity in Men Treated with Silodosin Plus Hexanic Extract of Serenoa Repens or Silodosin Alone." *Scientific Reports* 7 (2017): Article Number 15179.

5. Bertaccini, Alessandro, Marco Giampaoli, Riccardo Cividini, et al. "Observational Database Serenoa Repens (DOSSER): Overview, Analysis and Results. A Multicentric SIUrO (Italian Society of Oncological Urology) Project." *Archivio Italiano di Urologia e Andrologia* 84, no. 3 (September 2012): 117–122.

6. Gravas, S., M. Samarinas, K. Zacharouli, et al. "The Effect of Hexanic Extract of *Serenoa repens* on Prostatic Inflammation: Results from a Randomized Biopsy Study." *World Journal of Urology* 37, no. 3 (March 2019): 539–544.

7. Morgia, G., G. I. Russo, S. Voce, et al. "Serenoa Repens, Lycopene and Selenium versus Tamsulosin for the Treatment of LUTS/BPH. An Italian Multicenter Double-Blinded

Randomized Study between Single or Combination Therapy (PROCOMB Trial)." *The Prostate* 74, no. 15 (November 2014): 1471–1480.

8. Barry, Michael J., Sreelatha Meleth, Jeannette Y. Lee, et al. "Effect of Increasing Doses of Saw Palmetto on Lower Urinary Tract Symptoms: A Randomized Trial." *JAMA* 306, no. 12 (September 28, 2011): 1344–1351.

9. Tacklind, J., R. Macdonald, I. Rutks, et al. "Serenoa Repens for Benign Prostatic Hyperplasia." *Cochrane Database of Systematic Reviews* 12 (December 12, 2012): CD001423.

10. Wessagowit, V., C. Tangjaturonrusamee, T. Kootiratrakarn, et al. "Treatment of Male Androgenetic Alopecia with Topical Products Containing Serenoa Repens Extract." *Australasian Journal of Dermatology* 57, no. 3 (August 2016): e76–e82.

11. Rossi, A., E. Mari, M. Scarno, et al. "Comparative Effectiveness of Finasteride vs. Serenoa Repens in Male Androgenetic Alopecia: A Two-Year Study." *International Journal of Immunopathology and Pharmacology* 25, no. 4 (October–December 2012): 1167–1173.

REFERENCES AND FURTHER READING

Barry, Michael J., Sreelatha Meleth, Jeannette Y. Lee, et al. "Effect of Increasing Doses of Saw Palmetto on Lower Urinary Tract Symptoms: A Randomized Trial." *JAMA* 306, no. 12 (September 28, 2011): 1344–1351.

Bertaccini, A., M. Giampaoli, R. Cividini, et al. "Observational Database Serenoa Repens (DOSSER): Overview, Analysis and Results. A Multicentric SIUrO (Italian Society of Oncological Urology) Project." *Archivio Italiano di Urologia e Andrologia* 84, no. 3 (September 2012): 117–122.

Boeri, Luca, Paolo Capogrosso, Eugenio Ventimiglia, et al. "Clinically Meaningful Improvements in LUTS/BPH Severity in Men Treated with Silodosin Plus Hexanic Extract of Serenoa Repens or Silodosin Alone." *Scientific Reports* 7 (2017): Article Number 15179.

Gravas, S., M. Samarinas, K. Zacharouli, et al. "The Effect of Hexanic Extract of *Serenoa Repens* on Prostatic Inflammation: Results from a Randomized Biopsy Study." *World Journal of Urology* 37, no. 3 (March 2019): 539–544.

Morgia, G., G. I. Russo, S. Voce, et al. "Serenoa Repens, Lycopene, and Selenium versus Tamsulosin for the Treatment of LUTS/BPH. An Italian Multicenter Double-Blinded Randomized Study between Single or Combination Therapy (PROCOMB Trial)." *The Prostate* 74, no. 15 (November 2014): 1471–1480.

Rossi, A., E. Mari, M. Scarnò, et al. "Comparative Effectiveness of Finasteride vs. Serenoa Repens in Male Androgenetic Alopecia: A Two-Year Study." *International Journal of Immunopathology and Pharmacology* 25, no. 4 (October–December 2012): 1167–1173.

Ryu, Y. W., S. W. Lim, J. H. Kim, et al. "Comparison of Tamulosin Plus Serenoa Repens with Tamulosin in the Treatment of Benign Prostatic Hyperplasia in Korean Men: 1-Year Randomized Open Label Study." *Urologia Internationalis* 94, no. 2 (2015): 187–93.

Sinescu, I., P. Geavlete, R. Multescu, et al. "Long-Term Efficacy of *Serenoa repens* Treatment in Patients with Mild and Moderate Symptomatic Benign Prostatic Hyperplasia." *Urologia Internationalis* 86, no. 3 (2011): 284–289.

Tacklind, J., R. Macdonald, I. Rutks, et al. "Serenoa Repens for Benign Prostatic Hyperplasia." *Cochrane Database of Systematic Reviews* 12 (December 12, 2012): CD001423.

Vela-Navarrete, R., A. Alcaraz, A. Rodriguez-Antolin, et al. "Efficacy and Safety of a Hexanic Extract of *Serenoa Repens* (Permixon®) for the Treatment of Lower Urinary Tract Symptoms Associated with Benign Prostatic Hyperplasia (LUTS/ BPH): Systematic Review and Meta-Analysis of Randomized Controlled Trials and Observational Studies." *BJU International* 122, no. 6 (December 2018): 1049–1065.

Wessagowit, V., C. Tangjaturonrusamee, T. Kootiratrakarn, et al. "Treating of Male Androgenetic Alopecia with Topical Products Containing Serenoa Repens Extract." *Australasian Journal of Dermatology* 57, no. 3 (August 2016): e76–e82.

Spirulina

Spirulina, also known as *Arthrospira platensis*, is one of the world's most popular supplements. Able to grow in fresh and salt water, spirulina is rich in vitamins, nutrients, and antioxidants including protein, carbohydrate, fat, calcium, magnesium, phosphorous, vitamin A, vitamin B1, vitamin B2, vitamin B3, vitamin C, vitamin K, copper, iron, and omega-3 and omega-6 fatty acids.

Spirulina is a type of cyanobacteria, which is a family of single-celled microbes often referred to as blue-green algae. Its main active component is phycocyanin, from which it derives its blue-green color. Phycocyanin fights free radicals and has anti-inflammatory properties.

It is known that spirulina was consumed by the ancient Aztecs. But, it grew in popularity several decades ago when NASA proposed that it could be grown in space.

HEALTH BENEFITS AND RISKS

Spirulina is believed to have a number of health benefits. It is thought to lower low-density lipoprotein (LDL) or "bad" cholesterol, total cholesterol, and triglycerides while raising "good" or high-density lipoprotein (HDL) cholesterol. Spirulina may lower blood pressure, and it appears to have anticancer properties. Some researchers contend that spirulina helps people who have allergic rhinitis or inflammation of nasal passages, and it may be useful for anemia. Some have suggested that spirulina improves physical endurance and significantly increases the time before people becomes fatigued. It may even help control blood sugar levels in people with diabetes.

Although spirulina is believed to have few adverse side effects, it has the potential to cause headaches, allergic reactions, muscle pain, sweating, diarrhea, nausea, vomiting, anxiety, and insomnia. People who are allergic to seafood, seaweed, and other sea vegetables should avoid spirulina. It is possible that spirulina grown in the wild may absorb toxins, pollutants, and heavy metals from the water. Contaminated spirulina may cause liver damage, nausea, vomiting, thirst, weakness, rapid heartbeat, shock, and even death. It is important to purchase spirulina only from the most reputable sources. In addition, spirulina may interact with certain medications, such as immune-suppressing drugs, and may harm people dealing with an autoimmune disease, such as lupus or rheumatoid arthritis.

HOW IT IS SOLD AND TAKEN

Spirulina is generally sold in tablets or a powder. A standard dose tends to be between 1 and 3 g, but it is not uncommon for people to take higher doses.

RESEARCH FINDINGS

Spirulina Appears to Have Properties That Support Cardiovascular and Overall Health

In a meta-analysis published in 2018 in the journal *Diabetes, Metabolic Syndrome and Obesity: Targets and Therapy*, researchers from China examined the effects of spirulina on serum lipid profile, glucose management, blood pressure, and body weight. The analysis included 12 clinical trials with 14 arms. Only trials on humans were included, and all the trials were published in English. The amount of spirulina ranged from 1 to 19 g per day, and the duration of the trials ranged from 2 to 48 weeks. The researchers found that the participants taking spirulina supplementation had significantly lower levels of total cholesterol, LDL cholesterol, very low-density LDL, triglycerides, fasting blood sugar, and diastolic blood pressure than the control participants. However, spirulina supplementation did not substantially alter other cardiovascular parameters such as HDL cholesterol, body weight, systolic blood pressure, hemoglobin A1C (test for diabetes), and body mass index (BMI). The researchers concluded that "spirulina consumption may be considered as an adjunct to the prevention and treatment of CVD [cardiovascular disease] in humans."[1]

In a meta-analysis and systematic review published in 2016 in the journal *Clinical Nutrition*, researchers from Romania, Australia, and Poland investigated the impact of spirulina supplementation on plasma lipid concentrations. The researchers found seven randomized controlled trials with either a case-control or case-crossover design that met their criteria. In total, 522 participants were randomized. Three hundred and twelve took spirulina supplementation and 210 were in control groups. The number of participants in the trials ranged from 23 to 169. Four studies were conducted in India, two in Korea, and one in Cameroon. Spirulina doses ranged from 1 to 10 g per day, and duration of supplementation ranged between 2 and 12 months. The researchers learned that spirulina supplementation significantly reduced levels of total cholesterol, LDL cholesterol, and triglycerides, while it increased levels of HDL cholesterol. The impact of spirulina on total cholesterol and triglycerides was independent of the dose administered. The researchers underscored the need for more well-designed trials "to clarify the clinical value of spirulina supplementation as add-on to conventional and novel lipid-lowering therapies in dyslipidemic patients."[2]

In a prospective, open label, 3-month study published in 2014 in the *Journal of the Science of Food and Agriculture*, researchers from Greece evaluated the ability of spirulina to lower lipid levels in patients with elevated lipid levels. The cohort consisted of 52 adult participants; there were 32 men and 20 women aged between 37 and 61 years who were overweight or obese, with a mean age of

47 years. All the participants were placed on 1 g of spirulina per day. Blood samples were taken at baseline and when the trial ended. The researchers learned that the participants experienced significant reductions in several lipid markers such as total cholesterol, LDL cholesterol, and triglycerides. While HDL levels were higher, the difference was not significant. The researchers emphasized that the role of spirulina in improving lipid health "should not be overlooked."[3]

People with Nonalcoholic Fatty Liver Disease May Benefit from Spirulina Supplementation

In an open label, nonrandomized pilot trial published in 2014 in the journal *Annals of Gastroenterology*, some of the same researchers from the previous trial as well as additional Greek researchers examined the ability of spirulina supplementation to help people dealing with nonalcoholic fatty liver disease, a rather common medical disorder characterized by lipid accumulation in the liver. The cohort consisted of 13 men and two women aged between 29 and 63 years, with a median age of 48 years. All participants had metabolic syndrome, central obesity, nonalcoholic fatty liver disease, and normal blood pressure. While 80% were obese, only 20% had diabetes. The participants were placed on 6 g per day of spirulina for six months. Blood samples were taken at baseline and at the end of the trial. The researchers determined that the supplements helped several problems. These included a significant reduction in serum liver enzymes and lipids and an improvement in scores on health-related quality of life. The researchers suggested that spirulina be used as a dietary supplement for people with this disorder. They concluded that "the role of spirulina supplementation as a natural food supplement in NAFLD [non-alcoholic fatty liver disease] patients should not be overlooked."[4]

Spirulina Appears to Be Useful for Allergic Rhinitis

In a randomized, double-blind, placebo-controlled trial published in 2008 in the journal *European Archives of Oto-Rhino-Laryngology*, researchers from Turkey examined the ability of spirulina to help people who suffer from allergic rhinitis, a very common medical problem. The cohort consisted of 150 participants between the ages of 19 and 49 years, all of whom had a history of allergic rhinitis. For 6 months, the participants took 2000 mg per day of spirulina supplementation or a placebo. The supplements and placebos were identical in appearance. During the trial, the participants, who kept diaries listing their symptoms, were not allowed to take any allergy or rhinitis medication. The final analyses were conducted on 129 participants; of these, 85 participants took spirulina and 44 took placebos. The researchers determined that spirulina consumption significantly improved the symptoms associated with allergic rhinitis, such as nasal discharge, sneezing, nasal congestion, and itching. The researchers concluded that "spirulina is clinically effective on allergic rhinitis when compared to placebo."[5]

When Added to Sunscreen, Spirulina Appears to Help Prevent Sun-Induced Skin Damage

In a 3-month, single-blind trial published in 2017 in the *European Journal of Pharmaceutical Sciences*, researchers from Brazil investigated the ability of spirulina and the antioxidant dimethylmethoxy chromanol to improve the sunprotective properties of sunscreen. The researchers wanted to determine if the addition of these antioxidants to a broad-spectrum sunscreen would increase its photoprotective effect in "real-use conditions." According to the researchers, little is known about the benefits of the topical application of spirulina. The cohort consisted of 44 healthy participants between the ages of 30 and 50 years; twice each day, they applied one of three formulations of sunscreens that were prepared with or without these antioxidants. Different skin parameters were analyzed, such as pigmentation and skin elasticity, at baseline, and after 28, 56, and 84 days. The researchers found that sunscreen with or without these antioxidants protected the skin against sun-induced damages. However, the addition of these antioxidants to the sunscreen significantly improved skin pigmentation and elasticity. The researchers concluded that their findings "contribute to elucidate the in vivo effect of sunscreens containing antioxidants and gives new insights to encourage additional studies to develop more effective and safer sunscreens."[6]

Undernourished Children May Benefit from Spirulina Supplementation

In a prospective trial published in 2016 in the *International Journal of Pediatrics*, researchers from the Democratic Republic of the Congo evaluated the ability of spirulina to assist undernourished children, a very common problem in the country and throughout the developing world. The cohort consisted of 50 undernourished children between the age of 6 and 60 months, with a median age of 41.2 months. Eighty-eight percent of the children were more than 24 months, and all of them had anemia. Seventy-eight percent of the children demonstrated a failure to thrive and 84% had "growth retardation." The intervention group consisted of 16 children who received 10 g of spirulina daily, as well as a local diet administered by a nutritional center; the children in the control group ate the local diet. The children were assessed at baseline, after 15 days, and on the thirtieth day. The researchers found that the spirulina "significantly and quickly improved the nutritional status of undernourished children in the intervention group when compared to the control group." For example, the rate of global malnutrition decreased from 30% before the spirulina supplements to 20% on day 30.[7]

Spirulina May Improve Anemia and Immune Function in Seniors

In an open-label trial published in 2011 in the journal *Cellular & Molecular Immunology*, researchers from Italy, California, and Hawaii (USA) tested their hypothesis that spirulina would benefit older men and women with anemia and lower levels of immune function, common challenging conditions among this population. The cohort consisted of 40 participants who were over 50 years old. While none of the participants had a history of chronic illness, they had all been diagnosed with anemia during the previous year. Enrolled participants completed an online dietary questionnaire and were told to take six tablets of 500 mg spirulina per day for 12 weeks. Blood samples were collected at baseline, at week 6, and at week 12. Thirty participants, with a mean age of 63 years, completed the trial. Of these, 14 were between the ages of 50 and 60, ten were between 61 and 70, and six were over 70 years. The researchers found that spirulina improved both anemia and immune function. The researchers noted that older people tend to eat "enormous" amounts of fast food and often make "poor health nutrition decisions." The researchers "encourage the design of larger clinical studies with solid endpoints and sufficiently long follow-up with appropriate randomization."[8]

Spirulina May Be Useful for Athletes, Especially Rowers

In a double-blind trial published in 2018 in the *Journal of the International Society of Sports Nutrition*, researchers from Poland wanted to learn if spirulina supplementation would benefit 19 male members of the Polish Rowing Team. For 6 weeks, while the rowers attended a training camp, ten participants were randomly assigned to take 1500 mg of spirulina per day, and nine participants were randomly assigned to the placebo group. At baseline, the rowers in the two groups did not differ significantly in age, height, body weight, and years of training. After a number of different assessments, the researchers found that the supplementation protected against "a deficit in immune function" or lowered immune functioning related to strenuous exercise. In addition, spirulina "may cause a beneficial shift in 'overtraining threshold' preventing a radical deterioration of immunity." Additionally, they commented that supplementation with spirulina "may modulate some components of the immune system in athletes exposed to repeated strenuous exercise."[9]

Spirulina May Improve Mental and Physical Fatigue

In a randomized, double-blind, placebo-controlled trial published in 2016 in the *International Journal of Food Sciences and Nutrition*, researchers from Columbus, Ohio (USA), evaluated the ability of spirulina supplementation to improve mental and physical fatigue in men. The cohort consisted of 18 healthy males between the ages of 20 and 43, who were graduate students and staff at Ohio State University. The selected males had to be able to maintain aerobic exercise for 30 min, but they could not be people who were highly trained for aerobic exercise. The males in the treatment group took six 500 mg spirulina tablets per day, and the males in the placebo group took six gelatin capsules per day. At baseline, the participants participated in tests that evaluated aerobic exercise and mental and physical fatigue. At least 1 week later, the participants took the first spirulina supplement or placebo. The baseline tests were then repeated, and repeated once more 1 week later. The participants took the supplement or placebo for about 8 weeks. At the end of the trial, the baseline tests were again administered. The researchers found that spirulina improved mental and physical fatigue in the men. They concluded that "future work can examine larger subject numbers, other testing methods, and females."[10]

Spirulina May Benefit People Who Exercise

In a double-blind, placebo-controlled, crossover trial published in 2010 in the journal *Medicine & Science in Sports & Exercise*, researchers from Greece and the United Kingdom investigated the association between exercise and spirulina supplementation. The cohort consisted of nine males with an average age of 23.3 years. The participants were recreational runners who had trained for a minimum of 1 year; their training took place at least two times per week for at least 45 min. They were deemed "moderately trained." During the first 4 weeks of the trial, half of the participants took 6 g per day of spirulina supplementation and the other half took a placebo. After a 2-week washout period, the supplementation was reversed. The participants who had taken spirulina were placed on 4 weeks of the placebo, and the participants who had taken the placebo were placed on 4 weeks of 6 g per day of spirulina. At baseline, all participants underwent a V02 max test, which is a treadmill test used to determine the maximum amount of oxygen the body can transport and use during exercise. The V02 max test was readministered after the first 4 weeks and after the end of the trial. Though the average intensity of exercise during the V02 max test was similar for all participants, the time to fatigue was significantly higher in those on spirulina supplementation. Spirulina supplementation also increased the fat oxidation rate. According to the researchers, "the reasons behind the enhanced performance and increased fat oxidation after spirulina supplementation are poorly understood, and more research is needed to elucidate this."[11]

Obese Elderly Do Not Appear to Experience the Same Spirulina Benefits as Normal Weight Elderly

In a double-blind, placebo-controlled trial published in 2016 in the journal *Nutrition Research and Practice*, researchers from Korea compared how obese and normal weight elders respond to spirulina supplementation. The cohort consisted of 43 men and 35 women between the ages of 60 and 87. For 16 consecutive weeks, they were randomly assigned to take either 8 g per day of spirulina or a placebo that was 100% starch. Blood samples were taken at baseline and at the end of the trial, and the participants were interviewed individually. In addition, the participants were divided into obese and nonobese based on Asian standards of obesity. While the nonobese group experienced a significant lowering of total cholesterol and LDL cholesterol, these changes did not occur in the obese group. Similarly, while the nonobese group had improvement in immune function and antioxidant status, the members of the obese group did not obtain these benefits. The researchers concluded "that obesity may influence the effect of spirulina supplementation." It is possible, the researchers noted, that "obesity itself may impair immunity and can also induce oxidative stress."[12]

Overweight and Obese People May Benefit from Spirulina Supplementation

In a randomized, double-blind, placebo-controlled clinical trial published in 2018 in the journal *Complementary Therapies in Medicine*, researchers from Iran investigated the ability of spirulina to alter anthropometric measures, appetite, and metabolic parameters in overweight and obese healthy people. The initial cohort consisted of 52 men and women between the ages of 20 and 60 years, who were all overweight or obese. For 12 weeks, the participants were placed on four daily 500 mg spirulina supplements and a restricted calorie diet or a placebo with a restricted calorie diet. Body weight and body fat were measured; BMI levels were calculated; waist and hip circumferences were measured; and blood samples were collected. Thirty-eight participants completed the trial. The researchers learned that the participants taking the supplementation had significant reductions in body weight, waist circumference, body fat, and BMI. In addition, the participants taking the supplement had significant reduction in triglycerides and highly sensitive C-reactive protein. They even had significant reductions in their appetite scores. Still, the researchers commented that the participants were metabolically healthy, and the results may or may not apply to an unhealthy overweight and obese population. Nevertheless, according to the researchers, spirulina may "have favorable effects on weight management."[13]

In a randomized, double-blind, placebo-controlled clinical trial published in 2017 in the journal *BMC Complementary and Alternative Medicine*, researchers from Iran examined the same effects in obese men and women. Their cohort consisted of 64 obese participants between the ages of 20 and 50 years. They were placed in one of the two groups. For 12 weeks, 32 participants took 500 mg of spirulina twice each day and 32 took placebos. The participants were followed by phone every 7 days. Medical assessments were conducted at baseline and at the end of the trial. Dietary intakes were evaluated by a 24-h recall method, and appetite was measured using a standard visual analog scale. Fifty-six participants completed the trial; there were 29 participants in the spirulina group and 27 in the placebo group. The researchers determined that the body weight and BMI in both groups were decreased, though the decrease was significantly greater in the spirulina group. Serum total cholesterol was significantly reduced in the spirulina group, and spirulina significantly reduced the appetites of the participants. Serum levels of HDL cholesterol increased in both groups. The researchers noted that spirulina supplementation at a dose of 1 g per day "was effective in weight reduction, serum total cholesterol and appetite reduction." And, they added that "further studies with higher dose, sample sized and study duration are warranted."[14]

NOTES

1. Huang, Haohai, Dan Liao, Rong Pu, and Yejia Cui. "Quantifying the Effects of Spirulina Supplementation on Plasma Lipid and Glucose Concentrations, Body Weight, and Blood Pressure." *Diabetes, Metabolic Syndrome and Obesity: Targets and Therapy* 11 (2018): 729–742.

2. Serban, M. C., A. Sahebkar, S. Dragan, et al. "A Systematic Review and Meta-Analysis of the Impact of Spirulina Supplementation on Plasma Lipid Concentrations." *Clinical Nutrition* 35, no. 4 (August 2016): 842–851.

3. Mazokopakis, E. E., I. K. Starakis, M. G. Papadomanolaki, et al. "The Hypolipidaemic Effect of Spirulina (*Arthrospira platensis*) Supplementation in a Cretan Population: A Prospective Study." *Journal of the Science of Food and Agriculture* 94, no. 3 (February 2014): 432–437.

4. Mazokppakis, Elias E., Maria G. Papadomanolaki, Andreas A. Fousteris, et al. "The Hepatoprotective and Hypolipidemic Effects of Spirulina (*Arthrospira platensis*) Supplementation in a Cretan Population with Non-Alcoholic Fatty Liver Disease: A Prospective Pilot Study." *Annals of Gastroenterology* 27 (2014): 387–397.

5. Cingi, Cemal, Meltem Conk-Dalay, Hamdi Cakli, and Cengiz Bal. "The Effects of Spirulina on Allergic Rhinitis." *European Archives of Oto-Rhino-Laryngology* 265 (2008): 1219–1223.

6. Souza, C. and P. M. B. G. M. Campos. "Development and Photoprotective Effect of a Sunscreen Containing the Antioxidants Spirulina and Dimethylmethoxy Chromanol on Sun-Induced Skin Damage." *European Journal of Pharmaceutical Sciences* 104 (June 15, 2017): 52–64.

7. Matondo, F. K., K. Takaisi, A. B. Nkuadiolandu, et al. "Spirulina Supplements Improved the Nutritional Status of Undernourished Children Quickly and Significantly: Experience fro, Kisantu, the Democratic Republic of the Congo." *International Journal of Pediatrics* 2016 (2016): Article ID: 1296414.

8. Selmi, Carlo, Patrick S. C. Leung, Laura Fischer, et al. "The Effects of Spirulina on Anemia and Immune Function in Senior Citizens." *Cellular & Molecular Immunology* 8 (2011): 248–254.

9. Juszkiewicz, A., P. Basta, E. Petriczko, et al. "An Attempt to Induce an Immunomodulatory Effect in Rowers with Spirulina Extract." *Journal of the International Society of Sports Nutrition* 15 (2018): 9.

10. Johnson, M., L. Hassinger, J. Davis, et al. "A Randomized, Double Blind, Placebo Controlled Study of Spirulina Supplementation on Indices of Mental and Physical Fatigue in Men." *International Journal of Food Sciences and Nutrition* 67, no. 2 (2016): 203–206.

11. Kalafati, M., A. Z. Jamurtas, M. G. Nikiolaidis, et al. "Ergogenic and Antioxidant Effects of Spirulina Supplementation in Humans." *Medicine & Science in Sports & Exercise* 42, no. 1 (January 2010): 142–151.

12. Park, Hee-Jung and Hyun-Sook Lee. "The Influence of Obesity on the Effects of Spirulina Supplementation in the Human Metabolic Response of Korean Elderly." *Nutrition Research and Practice* 10, no. 4 (2016): 418–423.

13. Yousefi, R., A. Mottaghi, and A. Saidpour. "*Spirulina Platensis* Effectively Ameliorates Anthropometric Measurements and Obesity-Related Metabolic Disorders in Obese or Overweight Healthy Individuals: A Randomized Controlled Trial." *Complementary Therapies in Medicine* 40 (October 2018): 106–112.

14. Zeinalian, Reihaneh, Mahdieh Abbasalizad Farhangi, Atefeh Shariat, and Maryam Saghafi-Asl. "The Effects of Spirulina Platensis on Anthropometric Indices, Appetite, Lipid Profile and Serum Vascular Endothelial Growth Factor (VEGF) in Obese Individuals: A Randomized Double Blinded Placebo Controlled Trial." *BMC Complementary and Alternative Medicine* 17 (2017): 225.

REFERENCES AND FURTHER READING

Cingi, Cemal, Meltem Conk-Dalay, Hamdi Cakli, and Cengiz Bal. "The Effects of Spirulina on Allergic Rhinitis." *European Archives of Oto-Rhino-Laryngology* 265 (2008): 1219–1223.

Huang, Haohai, Dan Liao, Rong Pu, and Yejia Cui. "Quantifying the Effects of Spirulina Supplementation on Plasma Lipid and Glucose Concentrations, Body Weight, and Blood Pressure." *Diabetes, Metabolic Syndrome and Obesity: Targets and Therapy* 11 (2018): 729–742.

Johnson, M., L. Hassinger, J. Davis, et al. "A Randomized, Double Blind, Placebo Controlled Study of Spirulina Supplementation on Indices of Mental and Physical Fatigue in Men." *International Journal of Food Sciences and Nutrition* 67, no. 2 (2016): 203–206.

Juszkiewicz, A., P. Basta, E. Petriczzko, et al. "An Attempt to Induce an Immunomodulatory Effect in Rowers with Spirulina Extract." *Journal of the International Society of Sports Nutrition* 15 (2018): 9.

Kalafati, M., A. Z. Jamurtas, M. G. Nikolaidis, et al. "Ergogenic and Antioxidant Effects of Spirulina Supplementation in Humans." *Medicine & Science in Sports & Exercise* 42, no. 1 (January 2010): 142–151.

Matondo, F. K., K. Takaisi, A. B. Nkuadiolandu, et al. "Spirulina Supplements Improved the Nutritional Status of Undernourished Children Quickly and Significantly: Experience from Kisantu, the Democratic Republic of the Congo." *International Journal of Pediatrics* 2016 (2016): Article ID: 1296414.

Mazokopakis, E. E., I. K. Starakis, M. G. Papadomanolaki, et al. "The Hypolipidaemic Effects of Spirulina (*Arthrospira platensis*) Supplementation in a Cretan Population: A Prospective Study." *Journal of the Science of Food and Agriculture* 94, no. 3 (February 2014): 432–437.

Mazokopakis, Elias E., Maria G. Papadomanolaki, Andreas A. Fousteris, et al. "The Hepatoprotective and Hypolipidemic Effects of Spirulina (*Arthrospira platensis*) Supplementation in a Cretan Population with Non-Alcoholic Fatty Liver Disease: A Prospective Pilot Study." *Annals of Gastroenterology* 27 (2014): 387–394.

Park, Hee-Jung and Hyun-Sook Lee. "The Influence of Obesity on the Effects of Spirulina Supplementation in the Human Metabolic Response of Korean Elderly." *Nutrition Research and Practice* 10, no. 4 (2016): 418–423.

Selmi, Carlo, Patrick S. C. Leung, Laura Fischer, et al. "The Effects of Spirulina on Anemia and Immune Function in Senior Citizens." *Cellular & Molecular Immunology* 8 (2011): 248–254.

Serban, M. C., A. Sahebkar, S. Dragan, et al. "A Systematic Review and Meta-Analysis of the Impact of Spirulina Supplementation on Plasma Lipid Concentrations." *Clinical Nutrition* 35, no. 4 (August 2016): 842–851.

Souza, C. and P. M. B. G. M. Campos. "Development and Photoprotective Effect of a Sunscreen Containing the Antioxidants Spirulina and Dimethylmethoxy Chromanol on Sun-Induced Skin Damage." *European Journal of Pharmaceutical Sciences* 104 (June 15, 2017): 52–64.

Yousefi, R., A. Mottaghi, and A. Saidpour. "*Spirulina Platensis* Effectively Ameliorates Anthropometric Measurements and Obesity-Related Disorders in Obese or Overweight Healthy Individuals: A Randomized Controlled Trial." *Complementary Therapies in Medicine* 40 (October 2018): 106–112.

Zinalian, Reihaneh, Mahdieh Abbasalizad Farhangi, Atefeh Shariat, and Maryam Saghafi-Asl. "The Effects of Spirulina Platensis on Anthropometric Indices, Appetite, Lipid Profile and Serum Vascular Endothelial Growth Factor (VEGF) in Obese Individuals: A Randomized Double Blinded Placebo Controlled Trial." *BMC Complementary and Alternative Medicine* 17 (2017): 225.

St. John's Wort

St. John's wort, also known as *Hypericum perforatum*, is a plant with yellow flowers that has been used in traditional European medicine since the ancient Greeks. It is believed that the name St. John's refers to John the Baptist; the plant is in full bloom around June 24—the time of the feast of St. John the Baptist. Red spots appear on the plant's leaves on August 29 in the northern hemisphere, the anniversary of the death of St. John. The spots supposedly represent the blood spilled when St. John was beheaded

St. John's wort plant contains the active chemical hypericin, which is believed to give the herb most of its useful properties. Other ingredients, such as hyperforin and flavonoids, appear to play an additional role.

HEALTH BENEFITS AND RISKS

Historically, St. John's wort was used for various medical problems such as depression, kidney and lung illnesses, insomnia, and wound healing. Today, it is most often used for depression. But, it is also considered as a supplement to treat menopausal symptoms, attention deficit hyperactivity disorder, and obsessive-compulsive disorder. Because of its antiviral and antibacterial activity, it has been used as a topical treatment for wounds.

St. John's wort may interact with a number of different medications, including antidepressants, birth control pills, cyclosporine, digoxin, some cancer and HIV medications, and warfarin. Taking St. John's wort with medications that affect serotonin levels may lead to very high serotonin levels, a condition known as serotonin syndrome, which is characterized by confusion, fever, agitation, rapid heart rate, shivering, perspiration, diarrhea, and muscle spasms. St. John's wort may weaken the effects of some medications such as Xanax, an antianxiety medication. Side effects associated with St. John's wort include increased sensitivity to sunlight, anxiety, panic attacks, aggression, amnesia, dry mouth, dizziness, gastrointestinal upset, vomiting, fatigue, headache, and sexual dysfunction. Pregnant or breastfeeding women should avoid St. John's wort.

HOW IT IS SOLD AND TAKEN

St. John's wort is sold in tablets, capsules, liquid extracts, tinctures, topical preparations, and teas. Dosing recommendations tend to vary widely. A normal dose may range from 300 to 1200 mg per day. However, it is usually taken in divided doses of 300 or 600 mg. In most countries, St. John's wort is sold as an over-the-counter product. However, in some countries, a prescription is required.

RESEARCH FINDINGS

St. John's Wort May or May Not Have Antidepressive Properties

In a systematic review published in 2016 in the journal *Systematic Reviews*, researchers from Santa Monica, California (USA), evaluated the ability of St. John's wort to relieve the symptoms of major depressive disorder. Their review included 35 studies with a total of 6993 participants. All the studies addressed the efficacy of St. John's wort, reported on the rate of treatment responders, provided mean scores on depression scales, or the number of participants in remission. All but one of the studies reported on the safety issues and the number of participants with adverse effects. Very few studies dealt with quality of life issues and relapses. The researchers learned that St. John's wort was an effective treatment for participants with mild-to-moderate major depressive disorder. St. John's wort appeared to have fewer adverse effects than antidepressants. However, there was a lack of research on the use of St. John's wort in severe depression. Still, the researchers concluded that St. John's wort "is a herbal alternative to antidepressant medication with fewer adverse events without compromising effectiveness in symptom improvement in mild and moderate depression."[1]

In a meta-analysis and systematic review published in 2017 in the *Journal of Affective Disorders*, researchers from Singapore and the United Kingdom investigated the ability of St. John's wort to ease the symptoms of depression. Their cohort consisted of 27 clinical trials with a total of 3808 patients; the duration of the studies ranged from 4 to 12 weeks. All the studies compared the use of St. John's wort to selective serotonin reuptake inhibitor medications or SSRIs. The researchers determined that the studies supported the clinical use of St. John's wort for the management of depression. For people suffering from depression, St. John's wort worked as well as SSRIs, with about the same rates of remission and significantly lower discontinuation rates than SSRIs. Though generally well-tolerated, the most frequent reported side effects of St. John's wort were nausea, rash, fatigue, restlessness, and photosensitivity. A more serious concern is the many interactions St. Johns interaction has with other drugs. The researchers concluded that future studies "should be done to ascertain that the clinical improvement with St. John's wort use is stable in the long term."[2]

In a 12-week, three-arm, clinical trial published in 2011 in the *Journal of Psychiatric Research*, researchers from Los Angeles, California, Boston, Massachusetts, and Pittsburgh, Pennsylvania (USA), assessed the ability of St. John's wort to treat mild forms of depression. The cohort consisted of 73 participants who had symptoms of minor depression. They were placed on 810 mg per day of St. John's wort or 20 mg per day of citalopram (Celexa, an SSRI), or a placebo. The participants in all three groups responded well to the treatments. Neither St. John's wort or citalopram provided benefit over the placebo. At the same time, 84.6% of the St. John's wort-treated group, 100% of the citalopram-treated group, and 91.3% of the placebo group reported the development of a new adverse event or exacerbation of one present at baseline. The percentage of participants reporting any emerging or worsening depression-related symptoms was 69% for St. John's wort. The figure for the placebo group was 65% and 92% for the citalopram group. The participants taking St. John's wort or citalopram had substantially more gastrointestinal and sleep problems than those taking the placebo. The researchers concluded that minor depression "was not responsive to either a conventional antidepressant or a nutraceutical, and both compounds were associated with a notable side effects burden."[3]

St. John's Wort Appears to Improve Mood in Healthy Volunteers

In a trial published in 2019 in the *Journal of Psychopharmacology*, researchers from the United Kingdom wondered if St. John's wort supplementation would improve the mood of healthy volunteers. For 7 days, 48 healthy participants were given 300 mg tablets of St. John's wort or a placebo containing lactose. They took three pills per day for 6 days. On the seventh day, they took one pill 2 h before the testing session, where they underwent tests that measured emotional processing and elements of cognition. The participants also completed daily visual analog scales and side-effect questionnaires. One participant was excluded from the final analyses. The researchers found that the short-term treatment of St. John's wort produced changes in emotional processing similar to those seen with antidepressants. According to the researchers, St. John's wort supplementation "decreased the perception of disgusted facial expressions, increased memory recall for positive stimuli, and reduced attentional vigilance to unmasked fearful faces."[4]

Low Doses of St. John's Wort May Improve Short-Term Memory in Healthy Adults

In a single-dose, randomized, double-blind, placebo-controlled trial published in 2019 in the journal *Psychopharmacology*, researchers from Israel wanted to learn more about the ability of St. John's wort to improve short-term memory in healthy adults. The cohort consisted of 82 adult Technion (technical university) students, with 49 men and 33 women, with a mean age of 24.9 years. The trial was conducted during two sessions separated by at least 2 weeks. In one session, each participant received a placebo; during the other session, each participant took a 250 mg or 500 mg doses of St. John's wort (Remotiv 250 or Remotiv 500). During both approximately 3-h sessions, the participants completed an identical battery of tests that assessed short-term memory capacity and sustained attention. The researchers found that the lower dose of St. John's wort had a positive effect on short-term memory, whereas the larger dose had a negative effect on memory. However, the researcher noted that their findings "should be interpreted with caution." Still, the researcher concluded that a low dosage of St. John's wort "seems to have not only a positive effect on mood, but also a positive effect on short-term verbal memory."[5]

St. John's Wort May Help People with Migraines Who Take the Medication Sodium Valproate

In a clinical trial published in 2012 in the *Journal of Medicinal Plants Research*, researchers from Iran and the United Kingdom evaluated the use of St. John's wort to help people suffering from migraine headaches. The initial cohort consisted of 100 participants between the ages of 15 and 45 years, who had at least three migraine attacks per month. The trial was conducted in four phases of 45 days. In the first phase, the participants were drug-free. During the first treatment phase, all the participants took 200 mg per day of sodium valproate, twice each day. (Sodium valproate is a medication used to treat migraines and other medical problems. It has been shown to reduce the frequency and intensity of migraine headaches.) In the second treatment phase, participants were divided into two groups. In one group, the participants continued to take sodium valproate; the participants in the other group took sodium valproate and St. John's wort supplementation. During the trial, the participants rated the frequency and intensity of their headaches. Seventy-six participants completed the trial. The researchers learned that the administration of both sodium valproate and St. John's wort reduced the intensity and frequency of migraine attacks. The researchers concluded that people who suffer from migraines may well benefit from this combination treatment.[6]

Topical St. John's Wort Has Wound Healing Properties

In a retrospective review published in 2014 in the journal *Forschende Komplementärmedizin* (*Research in Contemporary Medicine*), researchers from Switzerland examined the efficacy and cost-effectiveness of a wound healing dressing that contained a mixture of St. John's wort oil and neem oil. The cohort consisted of 15 patients, with a mean age of 76.87 years, who had scalp wounds with exposed bones following the removal of skin tumors. All the wounds had failed treatment with split-thickness skin grafts, the usual first therapy. As a second option, the researchers tried daily treatment with the combination oil, and the treatment continued until the wounds healed. A wound care specialist saw the patients at least every 2 weeks. The researchers determined that the mean treatment period for complete wound healing was 8.1 weeks. No patient reported severe wound discomfort, and the dressing changes were not painful. The researchers concluded that "controlled studies, with a larger population, are still required to further assess the effectiveness and economy of this wound spray."[7]

In a case study published in 2017 in the *Journal of Ethnopharmacology*, researchers from Turkey examined the ability of St. John's wort oily extract to treat a pressure sore on an 82-year-old critically ill male patient in the intensive care unit. During his hospital stay, the patient developed a stage-2 pressure ulcer wound. For 40 successive days, the wound was cleaned twice daily and treated with an oily extract of St. John's wort. Photographs of the treated area were taken every 5 days. The researchers determined that the St. John's wort oily extract "provided significant efficacy" for the treatment of the pressure sore. They concluded that "St. John's wort oily extract may be suggested as a cost-effective option for the prevention or treatment of pressure sores in ICU patients."[8]

St. John's Wort Does Not Appear to Be Useful for Attention Deficit Hyperactivity Disorder in Children and Adolescents

In a randomized, double-blind, placebo-controlled trial published in 2008 in *JAMA*, researchers from Washington and Massachusetts (United States) evaluated the ability of St. John's wort to help children and adolescents with attention deficit hyperactivity disorder. The researchers explained that between 3% and 12% of the children in the United States have this disorder. Could St. John's wort reduce the severity of the symptoms? The cohort consisted of 54 participants between the ages of 6 and 17 years; all participants met the criteria for attention deficit hyperactivity disorder. For 8 weeks, the participants took either 300 mg of St. John's wort three times a day or a matching placebo. The researchers determined that there was no significant difference between the two groups in symptoms; the group taking St. John's wort did not have any significant relief from symptoms. The participants in the St. John's wort group "experienced neither more nor fewer adverse events than the placebo group."[9]

People Tend to Use St. John's Wort for Depression or Anxiety Because It Is "Less Like a Drug Than a Drug"

In a study published in 2014 in the journal *Complementary Therapies in Medicine*, researchers from Australia noted that people frequently begin taking St. John's wort with or without the advice of a health professional. They wanted to learn more about the consumer perspectives on the use of St. John's wort. Specifically, they wanted to determine how and why people use St. John's wort for "self-identified depression, stress, or worries." The researchers interviewed 41 participants for 1 to 3 h; the cohort included both men and women and people of varying ages. Most participants used St. John's wort tablets, often preferring a specific brand that was thought to be of a better quality or cheaper. They were generally aware of potential drug interactions from reading the label, information that is required in Australia. Most women had used antidepressant medications; only three men had used antidepressant medication. The participants liked the fact that they could take St. John's wort without visiting a doctor and had positive perceptions of the supplement. The participants tended to prefer a more "natural" product over antidepressant medications; St. John's wort "was perceived as being outside of conventional medicine."[10]

St. John's Wort Does Not Appear to Be Useful for Smoking Cessation

In a randomized, blinded, placebo-controlled clinical trial published in 2010 in the *Journal of Alternative and Complementary Medicine*, researchers based in Rochester, Minnesota (USA), wanted to learn if St. John's wort would be useful for people who want to stop smoking cigarettes. For 12 weeks, 118 participants, with a mean age of 37.6 years, were allocated to receive 300 mg of St. John's wort three times per day, 600 mg of St. John's wort three times per day, or a matching placebo three times a day; these supplements were combined with behavioral interventions. The dropout rate was 43%, which was considered high. At week 12 of the trial and 12 weeks after the trial ended, the researchers found no significant differences between the two St. John's wort groups and the placebo group. According to the researchers, St. John's wort failed to attenuate withdrawal symptoms among the abstinent participants. The researchers concluded that, because a number of studies have found that St. John's wort is not useful for smoking cessation, "further testing for SJW [St. John's wort] for tobacco cessation may not be warranted."[11]

Until Further Research Yields More Definitive Data, It Is Best to Avoid St. John's Wort during Pregnancy

In a study published in 2015 in the journal *Reproductive Toxicology*, researchers from Denmark and Australia evaluated the potential side effects of using St. John's wort during pregnancy. Using data from the Danish National Birth Cohort, they investigated the outcomes of 38 out of 90,128 women who were exposed to Sr. John's wort during pregnancy. The researchers examined associations between intake of St. John's wort and gestational age, preterm birth, birth weight, malformations, and Apgar scores (medical assessments made immediately after birth). The researchers found that the pregnancy outcomes in the women who did and did not use St. Johns wort were similar. There were 37 live births in the St. John's wort group and 86,745 in the unexposed group, with the live birth rate at 97.4% and 98.5%, respectively. Malformations were identified in three of the 37 babies (8.1%) exposed to St. John's wort, which is in contrast to 289 (3.3%) of the 86,745 unexposed babies. Still, the researchers commented that "the increased prevalence was based on only three exposed cases and could be a chance finding." Though they had a large cohort, no definitive results could be obtained. Too few babies were exposed to St. John's wort. The researchers emphasized the need for more research on the safety of St. John's wort during pregnancy.[12]

The Content of St. John's Wort Supplements May Vary Widely

In a study published in 2018 in the journal *Phytomedicine*, researchers from the United Kingdom and Switzerland evaluated the quality of 47 commercially sold St. John's wort products; they tested powders and extracts. The researchers noted that their previous research has found that herbal food supplements "are often of poor quality or adulterated." The researchers purchased St. John's wort supplements from various locations and countries, and the samples were analyzed. The researchers found significant differences in the products. More than one-third of the products were adulterated with *Hypericum* species from China, "which were not acceptable," and almost one-fifth of the samples had been adulterated with food dyes.[13]

NOTES

1. Apaydin, Eric A., Alicia R. Maher, Roberta Shanman, et al. "A Systematic Review of St. John's Wort for Major Depressive Disorder." *Systematic Reviews* 5, no. 1 (2016): 148.

2. Ng, Qin Xiang, Nandini Venkatanarayanan, and Collin Yih Xian Ho. "Clinical Use of *Hypericum perforatum* (St. John's Wort) in Depression: A Meta-Analysis." *Journal of Affective Disorders* 210 (2017): 211–221.

3. Rapaport, Mark Hyman, Andrew A. Nierenberg, Robert Howland, et al. "The Treatment of Minor Depression with St. John's Wort or Citalopram: Failure to Show Benefit Over Placebo." *Journal of Psychiatry Research* 45, no. 7 (July 2011): 931–941.

4. Warren, Matthew B., Philip J. Cowen, and Catherine J. Harmer. "Subchronic Treatment with St. John's Wort Produces a Positive Shift in Emotional Processing in Healthy Volunteers." *Journal of Psychopharmacology* 33, no. 2 (2019): 194–201.

5. Yechiam, E., D. Ben Eliezer, N. J. S. Ashby, and M. Bar-Shaked. "The Acute Effect of *Hypericum perforatum* on Short-Term Memory in Healthy Adults." *Psychopharmacology* 236, no. 2 (February 2019): 613–623.

6. Mirzaei, Mahmoud Gh., Robert D. E. Sewell, Soleiman Kheiri, and Mahmoud Rafieian-Kopaei. "A Clinical Trial of the Effect of St. John's Wort on Migraine Headaches in Patients Receiving Sodium Valproate." *Journal of Medicinal Plant Research* 6, no. 9 (March 9, 2012): 1519–1523.

7. Läuchli, Severin, Stefanie Vannotti, Jürg Hafner, et al. "A Plant-Derived Wound Therapeutic for Cost-Effective Treatment of Post-Surgical Scalp Wounds with Exposed Bone." *Forschende Komplementärmedizin* (*Research in Contemporary Medicine*) 21 (2014): 88–93.

8. Yücel, Ali, Yüksel Kan, Erdem Yesilada, and Onat Akin. "Effect of St. John's Wort (*Hypericum perforatum*) Oily Extract for the Care and Treatment of Pressure Sores: A Case Report." *Journal of Ethnopharmacology* 196 (2017): 236–241.

9. Weber, Wendy, Ann Vander Stoep, Rachelle L. McCarty, et al. "A Randomized Placebo Controlled Trial of *Hypericum perforatum* for Attention Deficit Hyperactivity Disorder in Children and Adolescents." *JAMA* 299, no. 22 (June 11, 2008): 2633–2641.

10. Pirotta, M., K. Willis, M. Carter, et al. "'Less Like a Drug Than a Drug': The Use of St. John's Wort among People Who Self-Identify as Having Depression and/or Anxiety Symptoms." *Complementary Therapies in Medicine* 22, no. 5 (October 2014): 870–876.

11. Sood, Amit, Jon O. Ebbert, Kavita Prasad, et al. "A Randomized Clinical Trial of St. John's Wort for Smoking Cessation." *Journal of Alternative and Complementary Medicine* 16, no. 7 (2010): 761–767.

12. Kolding, Line, Lars Henning Pedersen, Tine Brink Henriksen, et al. "Hypericum perforatum Use during Pregnancy and Pregnancy Outcome." *Reproductive Toxicology* 58 (2015): 234–237.

13. Booker, A., A. Agapouda, D. A. Frommenwiler, et al. "St. John's Wort (Hypericum perforatum) Products—An Assessment of Their Authenticity and Quality." *Phytomedicine* 40 (February 1, 2018): 158–164.

REFERENCES AND FURTHER READING

Apaydin, Eric A., Alicia R. Maher, Roberta Shanman, et al. "A Systematic Review of St. John's Wort for Major Depressive Disorder." *Systematic Reviews* 5, no. 1 (2016): 148.

Booker, A., A. Agapouda, D. A. Frommenwiler, et al. "St. John's Wort (Hypericum perforatum) Products—An Assessment of their Authenticity and Quality." *Phytomedicine* 40 (February 1, 2018): 158–164.

Kolding, Line, Lars Henning Pedersen, Tine Brink Henriksen, et al. "Hypericum perforatum Use during Pregnancy and Pregnancy Outcome." *Reproductive Toxicology* 58 (2015): 234–237.

Läuchli, Severin, Stefanie Vannotti, Jürg Hafner, et al. "A Plant-Derived Wound Therapeutic for Cost-Effective Treatment of Post-Surgical Scalp Wounds with Exposed Bone." *Forschende Komplementärmedizin* (*Research in Contemporary Medicine*) 21 (2014): 88–93.

Mirzaei, Mahmoud Gh., Robert D. E. Sewell, Soleiman Kheiri, and Mahmoud Rafieian-Kopaei. "A Clinical Trial of the Effect of St. John's Wort on Migraine Headaches in Patients Receiving Sodium Valproate." *Journal of Medicinal Plants Research* 6, no. 9 (March 9, 2012): 1519–1523.

Ng, Qin Xiang, Nandini Venkatanarayanan, and Collin Yih Xian Ho. "Clinical Use of *Hypericum perforatum* (St. John's Wort) in Depression: A Meta-Analysis." *Journal of Affective Disorders* 210 (2017): 211–221.

Pirotta, M., K. Willis, M. Carter, et al. "'Less Like a Drug Than a Drug': The Use of St. Johns Wort among People Who Self-Identify as Having Depression and/or Anxiety Symptoms." *Complementary Therapies in Medicine* 22, no. 5 (October 2014): 870–876.

Rapaport, Mark Hyman, Andrew A. Nirenberg, Robert Howland, et al. "The Treatment of Minor Depression with St. John's Wort or Citalopram: Failure to Show Benefit over Placebo." *Journal of Psychiatric Research* 45, no. 7 (July 2011): 931–941.

Sood, Amit, Jon O. Ebbert, Kavita Prasad, et al. "A Randomized Clinical Trial of St. John's Wort for Smoking Cessation." *Journal of Alternative and Complementary Medicine* 16, no. 7 (2010): 761–767.

Warren, Matthew E., Philip J. Cowen, and Catherine J. Harmer. "Subchronic Treatment with St. John's Wort Produces a Positive Shift in Emotional Processing in Healthy Volunteers." *Journal of Psychopharmacology* 33, no. 2 (2019): 194–201.

Weber, Wendy, Ann Vander Stoep, Rachelle L. McCarty, et al. "A Randomized Placebo Controlled Trial of *Hypericum perforatum* for Attention Deficit Hyperactivity Disorder in Children and Adolescents." *JAMA* 299, no. 22 (June 11, 2008): 2633–2641.

Yechiam, E, D. Ben-Eliezer, N. J. S. Ashby, and M. Bar-Shaked. "The Acute Effect of Hypericum perforatum on Short-Term Memory in Healthy Adults." *Psychopharmacology* 236, no. 2 (February 2019): 613–623.

Yücel, Ali, Kan Yüksel, Erdem Yesilada, and Onat Akin. "Effect of St. John's Wort (*Hypericum perforatum*) Oily Extract for the Care and Treatment of Pressure Sores: A Case Report." *Journal of Ethnopharmacology* 196 (2017): 236–241.

Turmeric (Curcumin)

Turmeric, grown in Asia and Central America, is a tall plant containing bioactive compounds, known as curcuminoids, with powerful medicinal properties. The most important curcumoinoid is curcumin, the main active ingredient in turmeric. Curcumin, which is yellow in color, has strong anti-inflammatory and antioxidant properties.

However, the curcumin content of turmeric is only about 3% by weight. So, to obtain a sufficient amount of curcumin, people need to select supplements that have larger amounts of curcumin. People also need to be aware that curcumin is poorly absorbed by the body. To improve absorption, curcumin should be combined with black pepper, which contains piperine, a natural substance that enhances the absorption of curcumin.

HEALTH BENEFITS AND RISKS

Turmeric is probably best known for its antipain and anti-inflammatory properties. Therefore, it is frequently recommended for people dealing with the pain associated with arthritis. It is also thought to be useful for a host of other medical concerns, such as supporting liver function and digestion, reducing the risk of cancer, especially cancers of the digestive tract, reducing the risk of Alzheimer's disease, and helping those dealing with depression, skin problems, and premenstrual syndrome. It is believed that curcumin, which crosses the blood–brain barrier, may increase levels of brain-derived neurotropic factor (BDNF), a type of growth hormone that functions in the brain. Certain brain disorders, such as Alzheimer's disease and depression, have been linked to lower levels of BDNF. In addition, curcumin improves the functioning of the endothelium or the lining of blood vessels, and may lower triglyceride levels.

Pregnant women may use turmeric spice, but they should not take the supplement. People on medications that slow blood clotting, such as aspirin, may increase their risk of bruising and bleeding if turmeric supplementation is taken. High doses of turmeric may also cause digestive problems in some people.

HOW IT IS SOLD AND TAKEN

The underground stems of turmeric, known as rhizomes, are dried and made into capsules, tablets, teas, and extracts. Turmeric powder may be made into a paste for skin conditions. There are no official dosage recommendations for either turmeric or curcumin, although they tend to begin at either 400 or 500 mg a few times each day. But, higher doses may be advised. It is best to use a product from a highly reputable company and follow the directions on the label. Curcumin supplements should also include black pepper extract, as it improves absorption.

RESEARCH FINDINGS

Turmeric Appears to Have Some Useful Properties for People with Arthritis

In a randomized, single-blind, 2-month pilot trial published in 2012 in the journal *Phytotherapy Research*, researchers from India and Dallas, Texas (USA), assessed the usefulness of curcumin supplementation for people with active rheumatoid arthritis. Forty-five participants (38 females and seven males, with a mean age of 47.88 years) with rheumatoid arthritis were placed into one of three groups; each group had 15 participants. The participants were given 500 mg per day of curcumin or 50 mg per day of diclofenac sodium, a pain medication, or both 500 mg per day of curcumin and 50 mg per day of diclofenac sodium. The participants in all three groups had significant improvement in the levels of disease activity. However, those in the curcumin group had the highest percentage of improvement. Interestingly, the combination of curcumin and diclofenac sodium was "slightly less efficacious than curcumin alone." While curcumin was safe, the participants in the diclofenac sodium group "experienced several adverse events." The researchers concluded that "curcumin can provide significant improvement in treatment efficacy in active RA [rheumatoid arthritis]."[1]

In a randomized, double-blind, placebo-controlled, three-arm, parallel-group trial published in 2017 in the *Journal of Medicinal Food*, researchers from India and Omaha, Nebraska (USA), also examined the usefulness of curcumin for people with rheumatoid arthritis. The cohort consisted of 36 participants between the ages of 22 and 55 years who had rheumatoid arthritis. For 90 days, the participants took either 250 mg of curcumin twice daily or 500 mg of curcumin extract twice daily, or 500 mg of a food-grade starch twice daily, a placebo. To determine the efficacy of curcumin, the researchers conducted a number of rheumatoid arthritis assessments, and significant improvements were seen in the participants taking both doses of curcumin. For example, compared to the participants taking the placebo, those on curcumin had significant improvements in the following tests—C-reactive protein, erythrocyte sedimentation rate, rheumatoid factor, and visual analog scale. Any changes in the placebo group were minimal and not statistically significant. The researchers commented that "both doses of the study product were well tolerated and without side effects."[2]

In a randomized, double-blind, placebo-controlled, prospective clinical trial published in 2014 in the *Journal of Orthopaedic Science*, researchers from Japan investigated the use of curcumin (Theracurmin) for treating knee osteoarthritis. The initial cohort consisted of 50 patients with knee osteoarthritis, which was confirmed by radiographic analysis; all participants were over the age of 40.

For 8 weeks, the participants took a daily supplement containing 180 mg of curcumin or a placebo. Blood biochemistry tests were administered at baseline and at the end of the trial. The participants' knee symptoms were evaluated at baseline, at 2 weeks, at 4 weeks, at 6 weeks, and when the trial ended. Forty-one participants completed the trial. Almost 80% of the participants were female. The researchers learned that the curcumin supplement was very effective. The participants taking the supplement had significantly lower levels of knee pain, which was true for all the participants except for those who initially had virtually no pain. The curcumin supplement "lowered the celecoxib [pain and inflammation medication] dependence significantly more than placebo," and the supplement had no major side effects.[3]

Knee osteoarthritis was also the subject of a trial published in 2009 in the *Journal of Alternative and Complementary Medicine*. In this trial, after discontinuing their osteoarthritis pain medication, researchers from Thailand randomly placed 107 participants with knee osteoarthritis and pain levels of at least five out of ten on 2 g per day of turmeric extract (n = 52) or 800 mg per day of ibuprofen (n = 55). During this 6-week trial, the participants were assessed every 2 weeks by the same assessor. The researchers were primarily interested in the degree of pain that the participants experienced during level walking and walking on stairs. Forty-five participants in the turmeric group and 46 in the ibuprofen group completed the trial. The prevalence of adverse effects was the same between the two groups. The researchers learned that turmeric "might be as effective as ibuprofen in alleviating knee pain and improving knee function." However, they were "unable to claim that the efficacy of both treatments was equivalent."[4]

Turmeric Appears to Support Skin Health

In a systematic review published in 2016 in the journal *Phytotherapy Research*, researchers from Pennsylvania and California (USA) examined studies that evaluated the association between turmeric supplementation and skin health. Their cohort consisted of nine studies that addressed the effects of the oral intake of turmeric and eight studies investigated the effects of the topical use of turmeric. In an additional study, the participants took oral turmeric and used turmeric topically. The studies included various skin conditions, such as acne, alopecia, atopic dermatitis, facial photoaging, oral lichen planus, pruritus, psoriasis, radiodermatitis, and vitiligo. The researchers found that ten studies noted statistically significant improvement in the severity of skin conditions in the supplement groups. The researchers concluded that "more thorough and large-scale clinical studies are needed to assess how turmeric could be used orally and topically to treat skin diseases."[5]

Curcumin Supplementation May Help People with Depressive Disorder and Anxiety

In a randomized, double-blind, placebo-controlled trial published in 2017 in the *Journal of Affective Disorders*, researchers from Australia investigated the association between curcumin and curcumin/saffron supplementation and major depressive disorder. The cohort consisted of 123 participants with major depressive disorder. For 12 weeks, they were assigned to receive one of four different treatments—low-dose curcumin extract (250 mg twice per day), high-dose curcumin extract (500 mg twice per day), low-dose curcumin extract and 15 mg saffron supplementation twice per day, or a placebo. Assessments were conducted every 4 weeks. The researchers learned that the participants taking the supplement had significant improvement in their depressive symptoms. There were no significant differences in the efficacy of the low and high doses of curcumin. On the other hand, in people taking placebos, depressive symptoms improved only during the first 4 weeks. The researchers emphasized the need for more studies on the association between curcumin and depressive disorder.[6]

In a meta-analysis published in 2017 in the *Journal of the American Directors Association*, researchers from Singapore and Australia reviewed studies on the use of curcumin supplementation for depression. The cohort consisted of six clinical trials with a total of 377 participants. The researchers found that the data supported the antidepressant effects of curcumin supplementation in depressed participants. None of the trials reported any adverse events from the supplements. In addition, in three trials, curcumin demonstrated antianxiety effects. Most trials had a generally low risk of bias. The researchers concluded that there is a need for "more robust randomized controlled trials [on curcumin] with larger sample sizes and follow-up studies carried out over a longer duration."[7]

In a double-blind, crossover trial published in 2015 in the *Chinese Journal of Integrative Medicine*, researchers from Iran examined the use of curcumin supplementation in obese people with anxiety. The cohort consisted of 30 obese participants; 83% were female. They were randomized to receive either 1 g per day of curcumin or a placebo. After 30 days, there was a washout period of 2 weeks, which was followed by the participants using the alternate regimen for 30 days. The researchers conducted assessments of anxiety and depression at baseline, at 4 weeks, at 6 weeks, and at 10 weeks. The researchers found that after 4 weeks the curcumin supplementation had a significant antianxiety effect in their participants, but there were no observed improvements in depressive symptoms. The researchers concluded that "curcumin has a potential anti-anxiety effect in individuals with obesity."[8]

Curcumin Supplementation May Be Useful for People with Ulcerative Colitis

In an analysis published in 2017 in the journal *Acta Medica Indonesiana*, researchers from Indonesia reviewed three randomized controlled trials on the use of curcumin supplementation as an adjuvant therapy for ulcerative colitis. Two trials examined the use of curcumin to induce remission and one examined the use of curcumin to help maintain remission. The sample sizes were 50, 45, and 89. The researchers learned that in all three trials, curcumin supplementation was significantly more effective than the placebo in inducing or maintaining ulcerative colitis remission. According to the researchers, curcumin has the potential to "be used in clinical settings." Still, they added that "further studies with larger sample sizes are needed to recommend it as adjuvant therapy of ulcerative colitis."[9]

Curcumin Supplementation Improves Metabolic Parameters in Overweight People

In a randomized, double-blind, placebo-controlled trial published in 2019 in the *European Journal of Nutrition*, researchers from Italy and Iran evaluated the ability of curcumin supplementation to improve metabolic parameters in overweight people. The cohort consisted of 80 overweight participants with "suboptimal fasting plasma glucose." For 8 weeks, the participants took 800 mg phytosomal curcumin, a highly absorbable form of curcumin supplement, or an identical looking placebo. Clinical and laboratory data were obtained at baseline, after 4 weeks, and at the end of the trial. All participants completed the trial, and none experienced any ill effects. Both groups had a 92% rate of compliance. The researchers learned that curcumin supplementation significantly improved glycemic and hepatic function indices and serum cortisol concentrations. They added that "future studies are warranted to verify the present results."[10]

Turmeric and Curcumin May Help People at Increased Risk for Cardiovascular Disease to Lower Their Lipid Levels

In a meta-analysis published in 2017 in *Nutrition Journal*, researchers from China assessed the efficacy and safety of turmeric and curcumin in lowering lipid levels in people at an increased risk for cardiovascular problems. Their analysis included seven studies with a total of 649 patients. Two studies were performed in Iran, and two were conducted in India. The remaining studies were from Pakistan, Taiwan, and Thailand. The duration of the studies ranged from 4 weeks to 6 months. Four studies were classified as high quality, and the three additional studies were thought to be of moderate quality. The researchers found that turmeric and curcumin had "beneficial effects" on the levels of triglycerides and LDL cholesterol ("bad" cholesterol). No significant effects were observed on HDL cholesterol ("good" cholesterol) or total cholesterol. The researchers concluded that "turmeric and curcumin may protect patients at risk of CVD [cardiovascular disease] through improving serum lipid levels."[11]

Curcumin Supplementation May Play a Role in Weight Loss

In a 2-month randomized, controlled clinical trial published in 2015 in the journal *European Review for Medical and Pharmacological Sciences*, researchers from different locations in Italy wanted to determine if curcumin supplementation could play a role in weight loss. The initial cohort consisted of 127 adults who were overweight and diagnosed with metabolic syndrome; they were placed on a standard weight loss regime for 30 days. Forty-four participants, who lost less than 2% of their body weight during the previous month, were then placed on 30 days of either curcumin supplementation with phosphatidylserine or pure phosphatidylserine. The results were notable. The people on curcumin supplementation increased their weight loss and reduced body fat, and experienced more waistline and hip reduction. There were even improvements in the BMI levels. The participants taking only the pure phosphatidylserine did not experience health benefits. The researchers concluded that their findings demonstrated that "a bioavailable form of curcumin is tolerated and can affect weight management protocols and approaches."[12]

Curcumin Appears to Be Useful for the Symptoms Associated with Premenstrual Syndrome

In a randomized, double-blind, placebo-controlled clinical trial published in 2015 in the journal *Complementary Therapies in Medicine*, researchers from Iran wanted to learn if curcumin supplementation would be useful for symptoms associated with premenstrual syndrome. The cohort consisted of 70 female students at the Tehran University of Medical Sciences. Data were collected over a period of 8 months. The participants recorded symptoms in a daily questionnaire, which included mood symptoms, physical symptoms, and behavioral characteristics. At baseline, the two groups had similar premenstrual symptoms. Thirty-five participants were placed in the curcumin supplement group and 35 were placed in the placebo group. Each participant received two capsules daily for 7 days before their periods and for 3 days after their periods for three successive cycles. Doses of curcumin and placebo were 100 mg per 12 hours. Three participants in the curcumin group and four in the placebo group did not complete the trial. The researchers learned that the participants in the curcumin group experienced significant reductions in the mean scores of the evaluated symptoms and characteristics. The researchers concluded that their findings "showed a potential advantageous effect of curcumin in attenuating severity of PMS symptoms, which were probably mediated by modulation of neurotransmitters and anti-inflammatory effects of curcumin."[13]

Curcumin Supplementation May Play a Role in the Prevention of Type 2 Diabetes

In a randomized, double-blind, placebo-controlled trial published in 2012 in the journal *Diabetes Care*, researchers from Thailand and Boston, Massachusetts (USA), investigated the ability of curcumin supplementation to prevent the development of type 2 diabetes in people diagnosed with prediabetes. The initial cohort consisted of 240 participants (at least 35 years old) with prediabetes. For 9 months, the participants took either six capsules per day of curcumin or a placebo. Each of the curcumin capsules had curcuminoid content of 250 mg. Assessments were conducted at baseline, and after 3, 6, and 9 months. During the trial, while none of the participants in the curcumin group developed type 2 diabetes, 16.4% in the placebo group developed the illness. The participants in the curcumin group also had significant improvement in glucose tolerance, hemoglobin A1C, insulin sensitivity, fasting blood sugar levels, and beta cell function. Moreover, no adverse effects were reported in the supplement group. The researchers concluded "that curcumin extract may be used for an intervention therapy for the prediabetic population."[14]

Oral Curcumin Does Not Appear to Be Useful for Breast Cancer Patients with Radiation Dermatitis

In a randomized, double-blinded, placebo-controlled, multisite trial published in 2018 in the journal *Supportive Care in Cancer*, researchers from several locations in the United States but based in Rochester, New York (USA), noted that there is no standard and effective way to prevent or control radiation-induced dermatitis, a very frequent occurrence in breast cancer patients treated with radiation. Therefore, they evaluated the usefulness of curcumin supplementation for this problem. The initial cohort consisted of 686 breast cancer patients. During the course of their radiation treatment and during the week after the treatment ended, the participants took four 500 mg capsules of curcumin or placebo three times each day. Five hundred and seventy-eight patients completed the trial. The vast majority of the patients were white females with a mean age of 58 years. All participants had a high compliance rate and experienced minimal adverse symptoms. Yet, the researchers failed to find a significant difference between the participants taking curcumin and those taking the placebo. According to the researchers, curcumin supplementation "did not reduce radiation dermatitis severity compared to placebo."[15]

NOTES

1. Chandran, B. and A. Goel. "A Randomized, Pilot Study to Assess the Efficacy and Safety of Curcumin in Patients with Active Rheumatoid Arthritis." *Phytotherapy Research* 26, no. 11 (November 2012): 1719–1725.

2. Amalraj, A., K. Varma, J. Jacob, et al. "A Novel Highly Bioavailable Curcumin Formulation Improves Symptoms and Diagnostic Indictors in Rheumatoid Arthritis Patients: A Randomized, Double-Blind, Placebo-Controlled, Two-Dose, Three-Arm, and Parallel-Group Study." *Journal of Medicinal Food* 20, no. 10 (October 2017): 1022–1030.

3. Nakagawa, Yasuaki, Shogo Mukai, Shigeru Yamada, et al. "Short-Term Effects of Highly-Bioavailable Curcumin for Treating Knee Osteoarthritis: A Randomized, Double-Blind, Placebo-Controlled Prospective Study." *Journal of Orthopaedic Science* 19 (2014): 933–939.

4. Kuptniratsaikul, V., S. Thanakhumtorn, P. Chinswangwatanakul, et al. "Efficacy and Safety of *Curcuma domestica* Extracts in Patients with Knee Osteoarthritis." *Journal of Alternative and Complementary Medicine* 15, no. 8 (August 2009): 891–897.

5. Vaughn, A. R., A. Branum, and R. K. Sivamani. "Effects of Turmeric (*Curcuma longa*) on Skin Health: A Systematic Review of the Clinical Evidence." *Phytotherapy Research* 30, no. 8 (August 2016): 1243–1264.

6. Lopresti, A. L., and P. D. Drummond. "Efficacy of Curcumin, and a Saffron/Curcumin Combination for the Treatment of Major Depression: A Randomised, Double-Blind, Placebo-Controlled Study." *Journal of Affective Disorders* 207 (January 2017): 188–196.

7. Ng, Q. X., S. S. H. Koh, H. W. Chan, and C. Y. X. Ho. "Clinical Use of Curcumin in Depression: A Meta-Analysis." *Journal of the American Directors Association* 18, no. 6 (June 1, 2017): 503–508.

8. Esmaily, H., A. Sahebkar, M. Iranshahi, et al. "An Investigation of the Effects of Curcumin on Anxiety and Depression in Obese Individuals: A Randomized Controlled Trial." *Chinese Journal Fin Integrative Medicine* 21, no. 5 (May 2015): 332–338.

9. Simadibrata, M., C. C. Halimkesuma, and B. M. Suwita. "Efficacy of Curcumin as Adjuvant Therapy to Induce or Maintain Remission in Ulcerative Colitis Patients: An Evidence-Based Clinical Review." *Acta Medica Indonesiana* 49, no. 4 (October 2017): 363–368.

10. Cicero, A. F. G., A. Sahebkar, F. Fogacci, et al. "Effects of Phytosomal Curcumin on Anthropometric Parameters, Insulin Resistance, Cortisolemia and Non-Alcoholic Fatty Liver Disease Indices: A Double-Blind, Placebo-Controlled Clinical Trial." *European Journal of Nutrition* (2019). Published Online.

11. Qin, Si, Lifan Huang, Jiaojiao Gong, et al. "Efficacy and Safety of Turmeric and Curcumin in Lowering Blood Lipid Levels in Patients with Cardiovascular Risk Factors: A Meta-Analysis of Randomized Controlled Trials." *Nutrition Journal* 16, no. 1 (2017): 68.

12. Di Pierro, F., A. Bressan, D. Ranaldi, et al. "Potential Role of Bioavailable Curcumin in Weight Loss and Omental Adipose Tissue Decrease: Preliminary Data of a Randomized, Controlled Trial in Overweight People with Metabolic Syndrome. Preliminary Study." *European Review for Medical and Pharmacological Sciences* 19 (2015): 4195–4202.

13. Khayat, S., H. Fanaei, M. Kheirkhah, et al. "Curcumin Attenuates Severity of Premenstrual Syndrome Symptoms: A Randomized, Double-Blind, Placebo-Controlled Trial." *Complementary Therapies in Medicine* 23, no. 3 (June 2015): 318–324.

14. Chuengsamarn, Somlak, Suthee Rattanamongkolgul, Rataya Luechapudiporn, et al. "Curcumin Extract for Prevention of Type 2 Diabetes." *Diabetes Care* 35 (2012): 2121–2127.

15. Ryan Wolf, J., C. E. Heckler, J. J. Guido, et al. "Oral Curcumin for Radiation Dermatitis: A URCC NCORP Study of 686 Breast Cancer Patients." *Supportive Care in Cancer* 26, no. 5 (May 2018): 1543–1552.

REFERENCES AND FURTHER READING

Amalraj, A., K. Varma, J. Jacob, et al. "A Novel Highly Bioavailable Curcumin Formulation Improves Symptoms and Diagnostic Indicators in Rheumatoid Arthritis Patients: A Randomized, Double-Blind, Placebo-Controlled, Two-Dose, Three-Arm, and Parallel-Group Study." *Journal of Medicinal Food* 20, no. 10 (October 2017): 1022–1030.

Chandran, B., and A. Goel. "A Randomized, Pilot Study to Assess the Efficacy and Safety of Curcumin in Patients with Active Rheumatoid Arthritis." *Phytotherapy Research* 26, no. 11 (November 2012): 1719–1725.

Chuengsamarn, Somlak, Suthee Rattanamongkolgul, Rataya Luechapudiporn, et al. "Curcumin Extract for Prevention of Type 2 Diabetes." *Diabetes Care* 35 (2012): 2121–2127.

Cicero, A. F. G., A. Sahebkar, F. Fogacci, et al. "Effects of Phytosomal Curcumin on Anthropometric Parameters, Insulin Resistance, Cortisolemia, and Non-Alcoholic Fatty Liver Disease Indices: A Double-Blind, Placebo-Controlled Clinical Trial." *European Journal of Nutrition* (2019). Published Online.

Di Pierro, F., A. Bressan, D. Ranaldi, et al. "Potential Role of Bioavailable Curcumin in Weight Loss and Omental Adipose Tissue Decrease: Preliminary Data of a Randomized, Controlled Trial in Overweight People with Metabolic Syndrome.

Preliminary Study." *European Review for Medical and Pharmacological Sciences* 19 (2015): 4195–4202.

Esmaily, H., A. Sahebkar, M. Iranshahi, et al. "An Investigation of the Effects of Curcumin on Anxiety and Depression in Obese Individuals: A Randomized Controlled Trial." *Chinese Journal of Integrative Medicine* 21, no. 5 (May 2015): 332–338.

Khayat, S., H. Fanaei, M. Kheirkhah, et al. "Curcumin Attenuates Severity of Premenstrual Syndrome Symptoms: A Randomized, Double-Blind, Placebo-Controlled Trial." *Complementary Therapies in Medicine* 23, no. 3 (June 2015): 318–324.

Kuptniratsaikul, K., S. Thanakhumtorn, P. Chinswangwatanakul, et al. "Efficacy and Safety of *Curcuma domestica* Extracts in Patients with Knee Osteoarthritis." *Journal of Alternative and Complementary Medicine* 15, no. 8 (August 2009): 891–897.

Lopresti, A. L., and P. D. Drummond. "Efficacy of Curcumin, and a Saffron/Curcumin Combination for the Treatment of Major Depression: A Randomised, Double-Blind, Placebo-Controlled Study." *Journal of Effective Disorders* 207 (January 1, 2017): 188–196.

Nakagawa, Yasuaki, Shogo Mukai, Shigeru Yamada, et al. "Short-Term Effects of Highly-Bioavailable Curcumin for Treating Knee Osteoarthritis: A Randomized, Double-Blind, Placebo-Controlled Prospective Study." *Journal of Orthopaedic Science* 19 (2014): 933–939.

Ng, Q. X., S. S. H. Koh, H. W. Chan, and C. Y. X. Ho. "Clinical Use of Curcumin in Depression: A Meta-Analysis." *Journal of the American Directors Association* 18, no. 6 (June 1, 2017): 503–508.

Qin, Si, Lifan Huang, Jiaojiao Gong, et al. "Efficacy and Safety of Turmeric and Curcumin in Lowering Blood Lipid Levels in Patients with Cardiovascular Risk Factors: A Meta-Analysis of Randomized Controlled Trials." *Nutrition Journal* 16, no. 1 (2017): 68.

Ryan Wolf, J., C. E. Heckler, J. J. Guido, et al. "Oral Curcumin for Radiation Dermatitis: A URCC NCORP Study of 686 Breast Cancer Patients." *Supportive Care in Cancer* 26, no. 5 (May 2018): 1543–1552.

Simadibrata, M., C. C. Halimkesume, and B. M. Suwita. "Efficacy of Curcumin as Adjunct Therapy to Induce or Maintain Remission in Ulcerative Colitis Patients: An Evidence-Based Clinical Review." *Acta Medica Indonesiana* 49, no. 4 (October 2017): 363–368.

Vaughn, A. R., A. Branum, and R. K. Sivamani. "Effect of Turmeric (*Curcuma longa*) on Skin Health: A Systematic Review of the Clinical Evidence." *Phytotherapy Research* 30, no. 8 (August 2016): 1243–1264.

Appendix: Supplements That May Be Useful for Specific Health Concerns

Acid Reflux
Hyaluronic Acid

Acne
Aloe Vera
Evening Primrose Oil

Age-Related Macular Degeneration
Fish Oil
Lutein and Zeaxanthin

Alzheimer's Disease
Acai
Alpha Lipoic Acid
Melatonin
Resveratrol
Turmeric (Curcumin)

Antibiotic-Associated Diarrhea
Probiotics

Anxiety
Ashwagandha
5-HTP
Ginkgo Biloba
L-Theanine

Athletic Performance and Muscle Building
Ashwagandha
Branched-Chain Amino Acids

Creatine
Ginseng
Spirulina

Attention Deficit Hyperactivity Disorder (ADHD)
Fish Oil
5-HTP
Ginseng
L-Theanine

Bacterial and Fungal Infections
Cinnamon
Cranberry
Echinacea
Ginseng

Benign Prostatic Hyperplasia
Saw Palmetto

Blood Flow Improvement
Acai
Ginkgo Biloba
L-Theanine

Bone Health
Chia
Cod Liver Oil
Collagen
Flaxseed Oil
Krill Oil

Cancer Prevention
Acai
Ashwagandha
Cranberry
Ginseng
Green Tea
Krill Oil
Spirulina
Turmeric (Curcumin)

Cataracts
Lutein and Zeaxanthin

Cognitive Improvement
Ginkgo Biloba
Green Tea
Krill Oil
L-Theanine

Common Cold and Other Respiratory Infections
Echinacea
Ginseng
Spirulina

Constipation
Aloe Vera
Flaxseed Oil

Depression
Ashwagandha
Fish Oil
5-HTP
L-Theanine
SAMe
St. John's Wort
Turmeric (Curcumin)

Diabetes and Blood Sugar Management
Alpha Lipoic Acid
Ashwagandha
Chia
Cinnamon
Coenzyme Q10
Flaxseed Oil
Ginseng

Green Tea
Milk Thistle
Resveratrol
Spirulina

Diabetic Neuropathy
Alpha Lipoic Acid
Evening Primrose Oil

Dry Eye
Fish Oil
Hyaluronic Acid

Fatigue
Evening Primrose Oil
Ginseng

Fibromyalgia
Melatonin
SAMe

Gastrointestinal Health
Collagen
Probiotics
Turmeric (Curcumin)

High Blood Pressure
Chia
Coenzyme Q10
Fish Oil
Ginseng
Resveratrol
Spirulina

High Cholesterol
Acai
Aloe Vera
Alpha Lipoic Acid
Ashwagandha
Chia
Coenzyme Q10
Cranberry
Fish Oil
Flaxseed Oil
Milk Thistle
Red Yeast Rice
Resveratrol
Spirulina

Indigestion
Ginger
Milk Thistle
Turmeric (Curcumin)

Inflammation
Acai
Alpha Lipoic Acid
Ashwagandha
Cinnamon
Fish Oil
Ginger
Ginseng
Green Tea
Milk Thistle
Turmeric (Curcumin)

Insomnia and Other Sleep Disorders
5-HTP
Melatonin

Joint Health
Cod Liver Oil
Collagen
Glucosamine and Chondroitin
Hyaluronic Acid
Krill Oil

Liver Disease
Branched-Chain Amino Acids
Milk Thistle
SAMe

Male Pattern Baldness
Saw Palmetto

Memory Problems
Acai
Alpha Lipoic Acid
Ginkgo Biloba
Ginseng

Metabolic Syndrome
Acai
Alpha Lipoic Acid
Chia
Green Tea

Migraines and Headaches
Coenzyme Q10
Fish Oil
5-HTP
Melatonin

Mood Improvement
5-HTP
Ginseng
L-Theanine
St. John's Wort

Nausea
Ginger

Negative Effects of Statin Medications
Coenzyme Q10

Osteoarthritis
Acai
Aloe Vera
Cod Liver Oil
Fish Oil
Flaxseed Oil
Ginger
Glucosamine and Chrondroitin
Hyaluronic Acid
SAMe
Turmeric (Curcumin)

Pain
5-HTP
Ginseng
SAMe
Turmeric (Curcumin)

Premenstrual Syndrome and Menstrual Pain
Black Cohosh
5-HTP
Ginger

Problems Associated with Menopause
Black Cohosh
Evening Primrose Oil
Flaxseed Oil

Ginseng
Melatonin

Psoriasis
Aloe Vera
Evening Primrose Oil

Rheumatoid Arthritis
Cod Liver Oil
Evening Primrose Oil
Fish Oil
Ginger
Ginseng
Milk Thistle

Skin Health
Aloe Vera
Alpha Lipoic Acid
Collagen
Hyaluronic Acid
Krill Oil

Stress
Ashwagandha
Ginseng
L-Theanine

Urinary Tract Infections
Cranberry

Weight Management
Acai
Aloe Vera
Alpha Lipoic Acid
Ashwagandha
Chia
Cinnamon
Green Tea
Krill Oil
Probiotics

Wound Healing
Aloe Vera
Hyaluronic Acid
St. John's Wort

Glossary

Adrenal androgen: A steroid hormone synthesized in the adrenal glands that controls the development and maintenance of masculine characteristics

Age-related macular degeneration: An age-related medical problem in which people lose central vision

Alopecia: Loss of hair anywhere in the body

Alzheimer's disease: The most common form of dementia

Anaerobic: Without oxygen

Angina pectoris: Short-lasting squeezing pain in the chest that radiates beyond

Arterial stiffness: Thickening and stiffening of arterial walls

Ascites: Accumulation of fluid in the peritoneal cavity causing abdominal swelling

Asthenopia: Also known as eyestrain, symptoms include pain in and around the eyes, blurred vision, headache, and occasional double vision

Atherogenic diet: A diet that promotes the development of atheromas or inflamed plaques on the inside of arteries

Atherosclerosis: Build-up of plaque in the arteries of the body

Atopic dermatitis: A condition that makes skin inflamed red and itchy

Augmentation index: A measure of arterial stiffness

Benign prostatic hyperplasia: An enlarged prostate gland

Body Mass Index (BMI): Body weight in pounds divided by the square of the body height in inches times 703

Cardiometabolic risk: Risk of cardiovascular disease, diabetes, or stroke

Cartilage: Connective tissue found in many parts of the body

Cholecystectomy: Surgical removal of the gallbladder

Cinnamon contact stomatitis: A rare reaction caused by the use of products containing artificial cinnamon flavored ingredients

Claudication distance: The distance walked before the onset of claudication pain

Dry eye disease: A medical problem characterized by symptoms of ocular (eye) discomfort, visual disturbance, and tear film instability

Dyslipidemia: Abnormal amounts of lipids in the blood

Dysmenorrhea: Pain and pelvic cramps associated with menstruation

Dyspepsia: Pain or uncomfortable feeling in the upper-middle part of the abdomen

Dyspnea: Shortness of breath

Dysuria: Painful urination

Eczema: A chronic inflammatory skin condition that usually begins in early childhood

Ergogenic agent: A substance that enhances physical performance

Erythema: Redness of the skin or mucous membranes caused by increased blood flow

Ethanol: Alcohol for human consumption

Euglycemia: Normal levels of sugar in the blood

Fibromyalgia: A chronic syndrome characterized by generalized pain, muscle dysfunction, disability, fatigue, psychological distress, cognitive dysfunction, and sleep and mood disturbances

Glycemia: Related to glucose in the blood

Heart failure: Failure of the heart to function properly

Helicobacter pylori: The gram-negative bacterium that is the primary cause of gastritis and peptic ulcer disease

Hepatotoxicity: Chemical-driven liver damage

Hyperlipidemia: Elevated lipid levels such as elevated levels of total cholesterol

Hyperplasia: The enlargement of an organ or tissue caused by increases in the reproduction rate of its cells

Hypertension: High blood pressure

Hyponatremia: A condition in which blood has low levels of sodium. Symptoms may include confusion, seizures, and coma

Insulin resistance: A condition in which the body becomes less sensitive to insulin, the hormone that lowers blood sugar levels, which may lead to diabetes

Insulin sensitivity: The body's sensitivity to insulin. A person who is insulin sensitive needs only a small amount of insulin to maintain blood glucose levels in the normal range

Intermittent claudication: Pain in the legs caused by too little blood flow

Knee osteoarthritis: An illness associated with pain and stiffness in the knee joints

Male androgenetic alopecia: Male pattern baldness

Melasma: Increased pigmentation of the skin characterized by symmetrical and confluent gray-brown patches, usually on the areas of the face exposed to the sun

Metabolic syndrome: A condition characterized by central obesity, hypertension, and disturbed glucose and insulin metabolism. The syndrome has been linked to an increased risk of type 2 diabetes and cardiovascular disease

Metabolite: Product of metabolism

Molluscum contagiosum: A skin infection caused by a virus that produces benign raised lesions or bumps in the outer layers of the skin

Mucositis: Painful inflammation and ulceration of mucous membranes lining the digestive tract

Myalgia: Muscle pain

Mydriatic: Dilated pupil(s)

Myocardial infarction: Heart attack

Oral dryness: Dry mouth

Oral lichen planus: Chronic inflammatory disease that affects the mucous membranes of the oral cavity

Osteoarthritis: The most common form of inflammatory joint disease associated with severe pain, stiffness, limitation of joint movement, and disability

Otitis media: Middle ear infection

Peritonitis: Inflammation of the peritoneum, the tissue that lines the inner wall of the abdomen and covers and supports the abdominal organs

Polycystic ovary syndrome: Women suffering from this disorder have slightly higher amounts of testosterone and other androgen hormones than average. These elevated hormones levels may contribute to irregular or absent menstrual periods, infertility, weight gain, acne, and excess hair on the face and the body

Postprandial glycemia: Glucose levels in the blood after eating a meal

Prostate-specific antigen (PSA): A protein produced by the prostate gland. PSA levels may be used to screen for prostate cancer and monitor patients who have been diagnosed with prostate cancer

Pyuria: White cells in urine

Radical prostatectomy: The surgical removal of the prostate gland and the surrounding tissues, such as seminal vesicles and nearby lymph nodes

Reactive aggression: Aggression in response to provocation

Rheumatoid arthritis: A chronic autoimmune disease that may lead to joint destruction and disability

Sarcopenia: Loss of skeletal muscle mass and function

Selective serotonin reuptake inhibitors (SSRIs): A class of drugs that are typically used in the treatment of major depressive disorder and anxiety disorders

Serotonin syndrome: A potentially life-threatening drug reaction that may occur when an excessive amount of serotonin-raising medications are taken. Signs and symptoms include agitation, restlessness, confusion, rapid heart rate, high blood pressure, dilated pupils, loss of muscle coordination, twitching muscles, muscle rigidity, heaving sweating, diarrhea, headache, shivering, and goose bumps. Sign and symptoms of a severe case include high fever, seizures, irregular heartbeat, and unconsciousness.

Sleep latency: Length of time it takes to transition from full wakefulness to sleep

Somnolence: Sleepiness

Superoxide dismutase: Enzyme that speeds up certain chemical reactions in the body

Tamsulosin: An alpha-blocker drug used for an enlarged prostate. It helps relax muscles in the prostate and in the opening of the bladder

Tinnitus: A perception of ringing, buzzing, and other sounds in the ear in the absence of actual noise

Vitiligo: A long-term skin condition in which patches of skin lose pigment

V02 max: Also known as maximal oxygen, it is the maximum rate of oxygen consumption measured during incremental exercise or exercise of increasing intensity

Index

Page numbers in **bold** indicate main entries in this volume.

About the Authors

Myrna Chandler Goldstein, MA, has been a freelance writer and independent scholar for 30 years. She is the author of Greenwood's *Vitamins and Minerals: Fact versus Fiction, The 50 Healthiest Habits and Lifestyle Changes*, and other Greenwood books.

Mark A. Goldstein, MD, is the founding chief of the Division of Adolescent and Young Adult Medicine at Massachusetts General Hospital and associate professor of pediatrics at Harvard Medical School. He is the author of numerous professional and lay publications and editor in chief of *Current Pediatrics Reports*. His research interests include studying the effects of eating disorders and malnutrition on bone mineralization in adolescents and young adults.